# Telephone Numbers & Information

Emergency Medical Service (EMS): _____

Fire: _____ Police: _____

Poison Control Center: 1-800-POISON1 (764-7661) Suicide Prevention: _____

## Health Care Providers

| Name | Specialty | Telephone Number(s) |
|------|-----------|---------------------|
| _____ | _____ | _____ |
| _____ | _____ | _____ |
| _____ | _____ | _____ |

Hospital: _____ Pharmacy: _____

Employee Assistance Program (EAP): _____

## Health Insurance Information (See also "Health Insurance Checklist" on page 48.)

Company Number 1: _____ Phone Number: _____

Policyholder's Name: _____ Policy Number: _____

Company Number 2: _____ Phone Number: _____

Policyholder's Name: _____ Policy Number: _____

# What to Tell Your Doctor

Use this summary when you call or visit a provider. See pages 27–28 for more information. (Make copies as needed.)

## Symptoms

❏ Pain
❏ Skin problems
❏ Bowel/bladder problems

❏ Fever/chills
❏ Stomach problems
❏ Muscle or joint problems

❏ Breathing problems
❏ Eye, ear, nose, throat problems

Other problems/specific questions I have now: _____

What I need to do: _____

## Medications

(See "Medicine Log" on page 46 for a list of all medicines you take.)

Medications I'm allergic to: _____ _____

1

**Note:** This book is not meant to substitute for expert medical advice or treatment. The information is given to help you make informed choices about your health. Follow your doctor's or health care provider's advice if it differs from what is given in this book.

Please know that many of the designations used by manufacturers and sellers to distinguish their products are claimed as trademarks. Where those designations appear in this book and the American Institute for Preventive Medicine was aware of a trademark claim, the designations have been printed in initial capital letters (e.g., Tums).

{**Note:** "LifeArt image copyright, 1998, Williams & Wilkens. All rights reserved" applies to illustrations in this book noted with a single *.}

This guide is one of a series of publications and programs offered by the American Institute for Preventive Medicine designed to help individuals reduce health care costs and improve the quality of their lives. Other booklets in the series include:

**HealthyLife® Self-Care Guides** – Each booklet discusses the most common health problems and teaches when to see the doctor or use self-care. Each booklet addresses specific needs. The titles are: *Self-Care Guide; Women's Self-Care Guide; Children's Self-Care Guide; Seniors' Self-Care Guide; Prenatal Self-Care Guide; Alternative Medicine Self-Care Guide;* and *Mental Fitness Guide*. Some guides are also available in a low literacy format and Spanish. The books *Health at Home* and *HealthySelf* are also available.

**For more information, call or write:**
American Institute for Preventive Medicine
30445 Northwestern Hwy., Suite 350
Farmington Hills, MI 48334-3102
(248) 539-1800 / FAX (248) 539-1808

e-mail: aipm@healthy.net

**365 Health Topics**
To access 365 additional health topics, go to the American Institiute for Preventive Medicine's web site: www.HealthyLife.com, and double-click on "365 Health Topics."

ISBN 0-9635612-9-4

# Seniors' Health at Home®

## Your Complete Guide to Symptoms, Solutions, and Self-Care

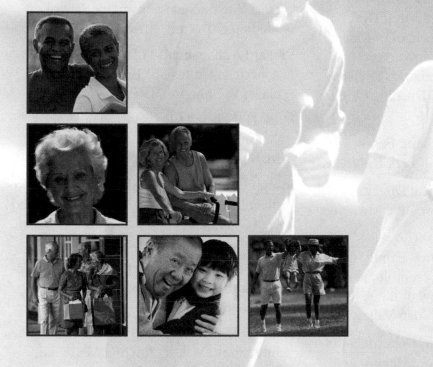

*Written by*

**Don R. Powell, Ph.D.**

*and the*

**American Institute for Preventive Medicine**

*Published by*

**American Institute for Preventive Medicine Press**
**Farmington Hills, Michigan**

# Acknowledgements

The material in this book has undergone an extensive process in order to ensure medical accuracy and present the latest medical research. We are indebted to the physicians and other health professionals who served on our clinical review team.

June Chang, M.D., Associate Medical Director of Geriatrics, Independent Health Plan, Buffalo, NY

Cathryn Devons, M.D., M.P.H., Assistant Professor of Geriatrics and Adult Development at the Mount Sinai School of Medicine, New York, NY and Director of Geriatric Services and Geriatrics Division Chief at Phelps Memorial Hospital Center Sleep Hollow, NY

Nichelle Harvey, M.D., Geriatric Fellow, Lutheran General Hospital, Park Ridge, IL

Thomas J. Hazy, M.D., Medical Director, American Institute for Preventive Medicine, Farmington Hills, MI

Marcie Parker, Ph.D., Certified Family Life Educator, Fellow of the Gerontological Society of America, Fellow of the American Institute on Stress, Golden Valley, MN

Susan Schooley, M.D., Chair, Department of Family Practice, Henry Ford Health System, Detroit, MI

Joel Shoolin, D.O., AAFP, Medical Director, Advocate Lutheran General Health Partners, Mt. Prospect, IL

Richard S. Lang, M.D., M.P.H., Head, Section of Preventive Medicine, Department of Internal Medicine, Cleveland Clinic Foundation, Cleveland, OH

Edward Adler, M.D., S.A.C.P., Attending Physician, Division of Geriatric Medicine, William Beaumont Hospital, Royal Oak, MI; Clinical Assistant Professor of Medicine, Wayne State University School of Medicine, Detroit, MI

Richard Aghababian, M.D., Past President, American College of Emergency Physicians, Washington, DC

Mark H. Beers, M.D., Senior Director of Geriatrics and Associate Editor, Merck Manual, West Point, PA

Joseph Berenholz, M.D., F.A.C.O.G., Diplomate, American College of Obstetrics and Gynecology, Faculty and Staff Physician, Detroit Medical Center, Detroit, MI

Dwight L. Blackburn, M.D., Medical Director, Anthem Blue Cross/Blue Shield, Louisville, KY

Douglas D. Blevins, M.D., Departments of Infectious Disease, Internal Medicine, Lewis-Gale Clinic, Salem, VA

Peter Fass, M.D., Medical Director, KeyCorp, Albany, NY

Gerald Freidman, M.D., Medical Director, Physicians Health Plan, Kalamazoo, MI

Abe Gershonowicz, D.D.S., Family Dentistry, Sterling Heights, MI

Gary P. Gross, M.D., Dermatologist, Lewis-Gale Clinic, Salem, VA

J. Bruce Hagadorn, M.D., Otolaryngologist, Lewis-Gale Clinic, Salem, VA

William Hettler, M.D., Director, University Health Service, University of Wisconsin, Stevens Point, WI

Jeanette Karwan, R.D., Director, Product Development, American Institute for Preventive Medicine, Farmington Hills, MI

James Kohlenberg, M.D., Internal Medicine, John R. Medical Clinic, Madison Heights, MI

Herb Martin, Ph.D., CEAP, Director, Employee Assistance Program, Vista Health Plans, San Diego, CA

Dan Mayer, M.D., Associate Professor, Emergency Medicine, Albany Medical College, Emergency Department, Albany Medical Center, Albany, NY

Myron Miller, M.D., Vice Chairman and Professor, Department of Geriatrics and Adult Development, The Mount Sinai School of Medicine, New York, NY

Alonzo H. Myers, Jr., M.D., Orthopaedic Surgeon, Lewis-Gale Clinic, Salem, VA

Joseph L. Nelson, III, M.D., Gastroenterologist, Lewis-Gale Clinic, Salem, VA

E. Blackford Noland, M.D., Department of Internal Medicine, Lewis-Gale Clinic, Salem, VA

William A. Pankey, M.D., Senior Vice President, Corporate Medical Director, D.C. Chartered Health Plan, Inc., Washington, D.C.

Anthony Pelonero, M.D., Associate Professor of Psychiatry, Medical College of Virginia-Virginia Commonwealth University and Medical Director, Mental Health Care, Trigon Blue Cross/Blue Shield, Richmond, VA

J. Courtland Robinson, M.D., M.P.H., Associate Professor, Dept. Gynecology and Obstetrics, Johns Hopkins School of Medicine, Baltimore, MD; joint appointment in the Department of Population Dynamics at the Johns Hopkins School of Hygiene and Public Health, Baltimore, MD

Mark A. Schmidt, M.D., Urologist, Lewis-Gale Clinic, Salem, VA

Ian Shaffer, M.D., Executive Vice President and Chief Medical Officer, Value Behavioral Health, Falls Church, VA

E.A. Shaptini, M.D., Vice President and Medical Director, American Natural Resources Company, Detroit, MI

Bruce Stewart, M.D., Department of Internal Medicine, Lewis-Gale Clinic, Salem, VA

J. Steven Strosnider, M.D., Director of Psychological Counseling, Lewis-Gale Clinic, Salem, VA

David J. Thaler, D.O., Internal Medicine, Lewis-Gale Clinic, Salem, VA

Neill D. Varner, D.O., M.P.H., Medical Director, Saginaw Steering Division, General Motors Corporation, Member of the UAW-GM Health Promotion Task Force, and Medical Director, Saginaw County Department of Public Health, Saginaw, MI

Mark Werner, M.D., Obstetrics and Gynecology, Staff Physician, William Beaumont Hospital, Royal Oak, MI

Yael Zoldan, Manager, Graphic Design, American Institute for Preventive Medicine, Farmington Hills, MI

# Table of Contents

## Chapter 11. Abdominal & Urinary Problems

## Chapter 12. Heart & Circulation Problems

## Chapter 13. Brain & Nervous System Conditions

# SECTION I

## You & Your Health

## Introduction

You are the most important person in caring for your health. What you do from this day on affects your health and how you feel.

This section helps you know what to do to take care of your own health and well-being.

Ways to stay well and prevent disease are presented in Chapter 1.

Chapters 2 through 5 give many tips and guidelines to help be a wise medical consumer.

Chapter 6 gives tips on making plans for healthy living.

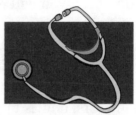

**Staying Well**

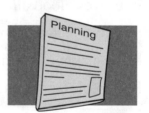

**You & Your Doctor**

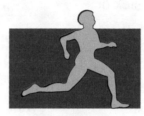

**Medical Decisions**

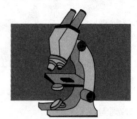

**Medical Exams & Tests**

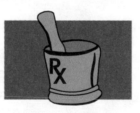

**Medications**

**Planning**

To learn more about topics covered in this Guide and other health issues, access the web site listed on the back cover of this book.

# Chapter 1. Stay Well

No matter what your age, good health habits are a big part of taking care of yourself. Practicing good health habits does not mean you will never get sick or that you will live longer. It can improve the way you feel and the quality of your life, though. It's not too late to follow good health habits. Even if you haven't exercised in years, now is the time to start.

## Stay Active with Exercise

Regular exercise has many benefits.

- It reduces stress, boredom, and depression.
- It improves skin and muscle tone.
- It improves blood circulation.
- It improves balance and flexibility.
- It helps manage appetite.
- It lowers blood pressure.
- It improves sleep.
- It helps reduce the risk for adult-onset diabetes (Type 2).

If you exercise on a regular basis, good for you! Keep it up! If not, it's never too late to start. Here is a list of exercise tips:

- Check with your doctor before you begin an exercise program.
- Choose one or more activities that you enjoy.
- Wear comfortable, cushioned, light-weight shoes with a strong arch support.
- Gradually ease into an exercise program. Start with 5 to 10 minutes a day.
- Find ways to increase your general activity.

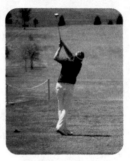

- Warm up before an exercise.
- Be careful when you exercise in hot or cold weather.
- Exercise indoors when outdoor temperatures are very hot or cold.
- Listen to your body. Rest when you need to.
- Drink plenty of water before, during, and after you exercise.
- Do not hold your breath when you exercise.
- Exercise to music.

### What Exercises Should You Do?

A recent study on twins showed that taking a brisk, half-hour walk just 6 times a month cut the risk of early death by 44%. Getting more fit is easier than you think. You can get active with:

- Exercise. (See "Types of Exercise" on page 13.)

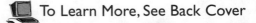 To Learn More, See Back Cover

- Recreation. Swim, golf, dance, etc.
- Active hobbies, such as working in the garden
- Chores, such as washing windows, walking the dog, etc.

## Types of Exercise

## 1. Aerobic Exercises

- Walking
- Swimming. This is good for those who have orthopedic problems or are obese. It reduces pressure on muscles and bones. Swimming may improve sleep and relaxation.
- Bike riding
- Rowing

**Walking Tips:**

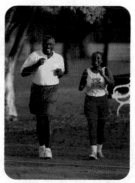

- Keep your head erect.
- Straighten your back.
- Point your toes forward.
- Swing your arms loosely.
- Wear cushioned, comfortable shoes.
- Don't race. Keep a comfortable pace.
- Walk with a friend or wear a headset for music.
- In bad weather, consider a morning mall walkers group.

- Make walking part of your daily routine.
- Find new routes.
- Set reasonable goals to increase time or distance.

When you do aerobic exercises, follow these three steps:

### A. Warm Up

The best warm up is to spend 5 to 10 minutes stretching different parts of your body. Extend each body part and hold it for 15 to 30 seconds. Doing this should not cause any pain. It should be a flowing, rhythmic motion that raises your heart rate a bit. Include all major muscle groups and parts of the body:

- Head and neck
- Shoulders, upper back, arms, and chest
- Rib cage, waist, and lower back
- Front and back of thighs
- Inner thighs
- Calf and Achilles tendon
- Ankles and feet

### B. Aerobic Activity

To be aerobic, the activity you choose should:

- Be steady and nonstop
- Use large muscles of the lower body (legs, buttocks)

- Last a minimum of 20 minutes. You can start out for shorter periods of time, many times a day. For example, do 5 minutes, 4 times a day. Progress to more minutes each time.

- Result in a heart rate of 60 to 80% of your maxi-mum heart rate. (See "Target Heart Rate Zone" box in next column.)

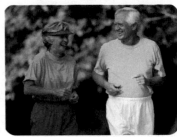

- Allow you to speak without gasping for breath

## C. Cool Down

The key is to cool down slowly. Choose a slower pace of the activity you were doing. For example, if you were walking briskly, walk slowly. Or stretch for about 5 minutes. Stretch all muscle groups. Stretch to the point of mild tension (not pain or burn). Hold for 10 to 30 seconds. Breathe in when the stretch is released. Breathe out when you begin to stretch.

## 2. Strengthening Exercises

- Lifting weights
- Push-ups and sit-ups

## Target Heart Rate

Your target heart rate is 60 to 80% of your maximum heart rate (MHR). This is the heart rate you should aim for during the aerobic phase of your activity.

To find your maximum heart rate (MHR):

**A.** Subtract your age from 220.

220 - _____ (your age)

= _____ (MHR)

**B.** Multiply your MHR by .60 and by .80.

_____ (MHR) x .60 = _____

_____ (MHR) x .80 = _____

**C.** Your 60-second heart rate should fall somewhere between these two numbers during the aerobic activity.

| Target Heart Rate Zone 60 to 80% of MHR | | |
|---|---|---|
| Age | Beats Per Minute | Beats Per 10 Seconds |
| 50 | 102 to 136 | 17 to 23 |
| 55 | 99 to 132 | 16 to 22 |
| 60 | 96 to 128 | 16 to 21 |
| 65 | 93 to 124 | 15 to 20 |

{**Note:** Consult your doctor before using this target heart rate range. Your range may need to be lower for medical reasons.}

 To Learn More, See Back Cover

These types of exercises:

- Let your muscles work longer before they get tired. (This is endurance.)
- Help you build muscle.
- Improve your bone density. This helps prevent osteoporosis and fractures.

### Guidelines

- Use weights or a stretch band. Try out different ones to find what's right for you. For strengthening, you should be able to do at least 2 sets and repeat these 8 times. The weight is too heavy if you can't. If you can easily do more than 3 sets, 12 times, use a heavier weight.
- Gives muscles a day to rest in between workouts. If you want to work out every day, do the upper body one day. Do the lower body the next day.
- Move slowly. Don't jerk the weights up. Don't drop them too fast.
- Always keep your knees and elbows slightly bent.
- Breathe properly during these exercises. Breathe out when you are at the hardest part of the exercise. Breathe in when you return to the starting position. Don't hold your breath.
- Work opposing muscles. For example, after you work the front of the arm (biceps), work the back of the arm (triceps).

- Talk to your doctor or a fitness consultant for a complete exercise program.

## 3. Stretching Exercises

These make your body more flexible. This helps you prevent injury during sports, exercise, and everyday activities. Stretching exercises should be done before and after every strengthening or aerobic workout.

### For stretching:

- Try slow, relaxing, stretches like those in yoga or tai chi.
- Try swimming. It builds flexibility.
- Stretch after exercise because muscles are warmed up.
- Stretch gradually.
- Do not bounce.
- Do not hold your breath. Exhale as stretching continues.

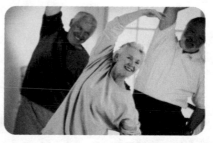

- Stretch every day, even if you're not physically active.
- Do not stretch areas when there is pain.

# Eat Well

- Build a healthy base. Use the Food Guide Pyramid, below.

- Drink 8 to 10 glasses of water a day.

- Choose a variety of grains daily, especially whole grains.

- Choose a variety of fruits and vegetables daily. Choose different kinds of fruits and vegetables to get essential vitamins and minerals, fiber, and other substances that are important for good health. Have 20 to 35 grams of dietary fiber per day.

- Keep foods safe to eat (see page 162).

- Choose a diet low in saturated fat and cholesterol and moderate in total fat. Limit animal fats, hard margarines, and partially hydrogenated shortenings. Use vegetable oils. Choose fat-free or low-fat dairy products, cooked dried beans and peas, fish, and lean meats and poultry. Eat no more than 300 milligrams of dietary cholesterol per day.

- Choose beverages and foods that limit your intake of sugar.

- Choose and prepare foods with less salt.

---

**The Food Guide Pyramid can help you make healthy choices.**

**Note:** Fat and added sugars come mostly from fats, oils, and sweets, but can be part of or added to foods from the other food groups as well.

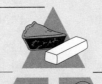

**Fats, Oils, & Sweets**
Use sparingly

**Milk, Yogurt, & Cheese Group**
2 to 3 servings per day

**Meat, Poultry, Fish, Dry Beans, Eggs, & Nuts Group**
2 to 3 servings per day

**Vegetable Group**
3 to 5 servings per day

**Fruit Group**
2 to 4 servings per day

**Bread, Cereal, Rice, & Pasta Group**
6 to 11 servings per day

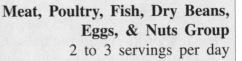

---

 To Learn More, See Back Cover

## Keep an Eye on Servings. What Counts as a Serving?

- Bread, Cereal, Rice, and Pasta Group
  - 1 slice of bread
  - About 1 cup of ready-to-eat cereal flakes
  - $1/2$ cup of cooked cereal, rice, or pasta
- Vegetable Group
  - 1 cup of raw leafy vegetables
  - $1/2$ cup of other vegetables (cooked or raw)
  - $3/4$ cup of vegetable juice
- Fruit Group
  - 1 medium apple, banana, or orange
  - $1/2$ cup of chopped, cooked, or canned fruit
  - $3/4$ cup of fruit juice

- Milk, Yogurt, and Cheese Group
  - 1 cup of milk or yogurt
  - $1^1/2$ ounces of natural cheese
  - 2 ounces of processed cheese
  - 1 cup of soy-based beverage with added calcium
- Meat, Poultry, Fish, Dry Beans, Eggs, and Nuts Group
  - 2 to 3 ounces of cooked, lean meat, poultry or fish
  - $1/2$ cup of cooked dry beans; $1/2$ cup of tofu; a $2^1/2$ ounce soyburger; 1 egg counts as 1 ounce of lean meat. Two tablespoons of peanut butter or $1/3$ cup of nuts count as 1 ounce of meat.

Some chronic health problems may require diet changes. Consult your doctor for advice. Changes in your diet are needed if these health problems exist:

- Diabetes
- High blood pressure
- Heart disease
- Osteoporosis
- Constipation
- Obesity

Some medications affect the diet. Certain drugs, for example, may affect metabolism. Others may alter the taste of foods or cause nausea (if inadequate food is taken with them). Some drugs dull the appetite. It may be hard to follow a well balanced diet. If you need help, ask you dietitian or doctor.

### For Information on Nutrition, Contact:

Consumer Nutrition Hotline
1-800-366-1655
www.eatright.org

## Vitamins & Minerals

Usually, a balanced diet provides all the vitamins and minerals needed. A variety of foods from the Food Guide Pyramid provide a balanced diet. Seniors, however, may be prone to certain deficiencies, such as vitamins $B_6$, $B_{12}$, C, and/or folic acid (a B vitamin). Here are good sources for these vitamins:

- Lean meats, chicken, fish, turnip greens, bananas, split peas for vitamin $B_6$

- Milk, eggs, and lean meats for vitamin $B_{12}$

- Citrus fruits, tomatoes, cantaloupe, strawberries, green peppers, broccoli, potatoes for vitamin C

- Green leafy vegetables, cantaloupe, orange juice, black-eyed peas, oatmeal for folic acid. Folic acid is now added to grain products.

You may need vitamin and/or mineral supplements if you:

- Have a hard time eating

- Have digestive problems

- Abuse alcohol

- Have heart disease. You may need vitamin E and/or folic acid supplements.

- Have or are prone to osteoporosis. You may need to take calcium and vitamin D supplements.

- Are at risk for cataracts. You may need a vitamin C supplement.

- Eat less than 1,500 calories a day. You may need a multivitamin and mineral supplement.

Ask your doctor if you need to take vitamin and mineral supplements. Find out which ones you should take and in what amounts.

{**Note:** Avoid large doses of vitamins and/or minerals. Do not take more than 10 times the RDI of any vitamin or mineral, unless your doctor tells you to.}

## Control Your Weight

A healthy weight is vital to wellness. Extra pounds cause strain on the heart and joints. As people age, less physical activity and a slower metabolic rate may make it hard to lose weight. To lose weight or to avoid gaining unwanted pounds, try these tips:

- Eat more slowly. Take 20 minutes to complete a meal.

- Reduce portion sizes. Use a smaller plate. Cut food into small servings.

- Say "No" to second helpings.

To Learn More, See Back Cover

- Avoid fatty foods. Increase high fiber foods.
- Cut back on sugar and products with sugar.
- Increase physical activity. Take a walk after a meal.
- Drink a glass of water before a meal. Take sips of water between bites.
- Start meals with a salad. Use nonfat dressings or lemon juice or vinegar.
- Leave some food on your plate.
- Never skip a meal. Meals keep your blood sugar levels even.
- Eat at least half your total food intake in the first half of the day.
- Trim all fat off meats. Take the skin off poultry before eating.
- Do not fry foods. Bake or broil them.
- Use nonfat cheeses, milks and other dairy products instead of ones with fat.

# Get Regular Dental Care

Overall health includes proper dental care and good oral hygiene.

- Brush your teeth once or twice a day. Brush after each meal, if you can.
- Brush or massage the gum area and the tongue, too.

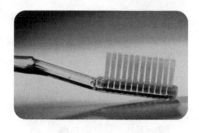

- Use a soft-bristled toothbrush. Replace it at least 3 times a year.
- Floss daily.
- See your dentist at least once a year for a cleaning and checkup. Go every 6 months, if you can.
- Eat less sugar, especially in hard or sticky candy.
- Use a fluoride toothpaste.
- Mouthwashes, such as Listerine, may help reduce plaque.

## If You Wear Dentures

To adjust to new dentures:

- Eat soft, non sticky foods at first.
- Cut food into small pieces.
- Be careful when eating hot foods.
- Watch for bones in food.
- Speak slowly if dentures click.
- Use a denture adhesive, if you must, but don't use too much. It can irritate your gums.

Additional tips:

- Keep dentures clean. Use a denture cleaner or toothpaste.

I. Stay Well

- Remove dentures for sleeping (6 to 8 hours per day). Soak them in a container with a denture cleaning product, such as Efferdent, Polident, etc.

- Keep dentures wet when not in the mouth.

- Replace them as advised by your dentist.

# Be a Nonsmoker

Wellness and smoking don't go together. If 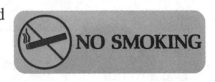 you smoke, quit. Quitting is not easy because nicotine is addictive, but it can be done. Here's how to begin:

- Consult your doctor for help. He or she may:

  - Tell you to wear a nicotine patch (i.e., Nicoderm or Nicotrol) or chew a gum like Nicorette. These help to reduce nicotine cravings.

  - Prescribe a nicotine nasal spray (i.e., Nicotrol NS), a nicotine inhaler (i.e., Nicotrol), or the medication Zyban. It reduces cravings for cigarettes.

- Get rid of all cigarettes. Hide smoking items, like matches or ashtrays.

- Practice deep inhales and exhales through the mouth.

- Keep your hands busy by holding something like a pen or binder clip.

- Try sugarless gum, mints, toothpicks, or coffee stirrers in place of cigarettes.

- Get plenty of sleep and exercise. Eat healthy foods.

- Drink plenty of water.

- Keep busy.

- Tell others you're quitting. Ask for their help.

- Think positive.

- Picture yourself as a nonsmoker.

- Wear a thick rubber band around your wrist. When a smoking urge occurs, snap it.

If you are not ready to totally quit smoking, cut back slowly. Here are some tips:

- Switch to a low tar, low nicotine brand.

- Don't smoke cigarettes all the way down.

- Take fewer draws on each cigarette.

- Reduce your inhaling. Don't inhale as deeply.

- Smoke fewer cigarettes each day.

- Refuse to smoke in front of anyone that you love.

## Use Alcohol Wisely

Alcohol slows down brain activity. It dulls alertness, memory, and judgment. It increases the risk of accidents. If you drink, do so in moderation. Follow these tips:

- Cut back on alcohol as you get older. If you drink, limit alcohol to 1 drink a day. These are examples of 1 alcoholic drink:
  - 4 to 5 oz. of wine
  - 12 oz. of beer
  - $1\frac{1}{2}$ oz. of 80 proof liquor
- After having one of these, have drinks without alcohol, or use the same amount of alcohol, but combine it with mixers to make more than one drink.
- Drink slowly. Don't gulp or guzzle alcohol.
- Find other ways to calm yourself.
- Don't drink on an empty stomach.
- Don't drink when you are alone.
- Don't drink and drive.
- Avoid problem drinkers.
- Set a strict limit for yourself.
- If you take medication, ask your doctor or pharmacist if it is safe for you to drink at all.
- Don't rely on black coffee, splashing water on your face, or fresh air to get sober.

## Manage Stress

- Try slow, deep breaths.
- Keep a sense of humor. Laugh often.
- Take a walk.
- Be more forgiving.
- Learn patience.
- Repeat positive self-statements.
- Take a warm bath or shower.
- Get moderate exercise.
- Listen to soothing music.
- Take time to relax.
- Don't compare yourself to others.
- Have someone massage your shoulders, neck, or back.
- Count your blessings.
- Think positive.
- Focus on the needs of others.
- Do something nice for your body. Take a nap.
- Eat something healthy.

# Stay Mentally Active

A key part of living "the good life" is staying mentally active. It is linked to good physical and mental health. There are many ways to remain mentally active:

- Find a labor of love. Even if you're retired, find some "meaningful" work. It can be paid or unpaid. People need to feel wanted and productive. Start a second career. Try part-time work.

- Get involved. Become a volunteer. Take a class. Join a group of walkers, a book club, or start a breakfast club. Become a mentor to a younger person.

- Get plenty of moderate to vigorous exercise. When you do this, the body releases endorphins, chemicals that make you feel good. {**Note:** Ask your doctor what exercises you should do.}

- Widen your circle of friends. Invite guests over, attend a meeting, travel, join a church or synagogue group. Call an old friend on the phone.

- Look for creative outlets. Paint, play a musical instrument, etc. Find ways to express yourself.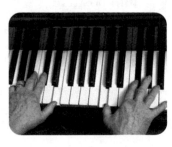

- Exercise your memory and mind. Continue to learn new things. Take a class at a local center or community college. Play along with TV game shows. Watch programs on public TV and other channels that show biographies, stories in history, medical news, etc. Do crossword and other puzzles. Work with computers.

- Get organized. Clean out clutter in all aspects of living.

- Read a newspaper or magazine daily.

- Listen to books on tape or read an enjoyable book. Look for large print books if it is hard for you to read small print.

- Accept invitations to new events. Keep a busy calendar.

- Eat well. This includes fresh fruits and vegetables, whole grain breads and cereals, lean meats, poultry and fish, and nonfat dairy products.

- Take vitamin and mineral supplements as advised by your doctor.

- Limit the use of alcohol.

- Check for mental side effects of medications. Some may cause fatigue. Report any side effects to your doctor.

To Learn More, See Back Cover

# Home Safety Checklist

Being safe in your home is a big part of staying well. Prevent accidents that can cause health problems. Follow these tips:

❑ Keep emergency phone numbers clearly posted.

❑ Stock first aid supplies. See "Your Home Pharmacy" on page 42.

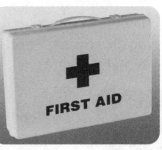

❑ Check your home for hazards every 6 months.

❑ Never smoke in bed or when you feel drowsy. Better yet, don't smoke at all!

❑ Install smoke alarms. Check them every 6 months. Keep a fire extinguisher in the kitchen.

❑ If you use a space heater, make sure it has an emergency shut off.

❑ Plan an escape route in case of fire.

❑ Keep flashlights handy.

❑ Use night lights.

❑ Keep lamp switches within easy reach from a bed.

❑ Keep stair areas well lit. Install a switch at the top and bottom of the stairs.

❑ Install handrails on both sides of the stairs.

❑ Keep stairs clear of clutter.

❑ Make certain carpet on stairs is nailed down securely.

❑ Install grab bars in the shower, tub, and toilet area.

❑ Use a shower bench that has rubber tips on the legs.

❑ Before getting in the tub, test the bath water. Make sure it is not too hot.

❑ Never lock the bathroom door.

❑ Use a bath mat with suction cups or use nonslip adhesive strips in the tub and shower.

❑ Don't use any loose area rugs.

❑ Arrange furniture so there is a clear path for walking.

❑ Test if furniture is sturdy enough to lean on.

❑ Clear away phone or electrical wires from walk paths.

❑ Only use step stools with sturdy handrails.

❑ Be alert to spills or wet floors.

❑ Have snow and icy patches cleared from the sidewalk and steps.

# Personal Safety Checklist

Not only in the home, but in all aspects of daily living, you need to guard against accidents and crime. Follow these tips:

❑ Ask your pharmacist or doctor which medicines make you unsteady or make driving difficult.

❑ Wear a medical alert tag to identify health concerns. Get one from a drug store or from: MedicAlert Foundation International 1-800-344-3226 www.medicalert.org

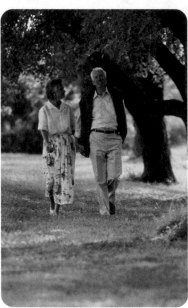

❑ Wear only snug-fitting shoes and slippers. Wear ones that are nonslip.

❑ Walk with a companion.

❑ Use a cane or walker if you feel more secure walking with one.

❑ Wear a helmet when riding a bike.

❑ Have eye exams on a regular basis.

❑ Never carry large amounts of cash.

❑ Carry credit cards or money in an inside pocket.

❑ Don't give your name or phone number to strangers.

❑ Use a peephole in the front door.

❑ Keep your doors locked.

❑ If you live alone, arrange for daily contact with a neighbor, mail carrier, or a relative.

❑ Don't get up too quickly after lying down, resting, or eating a meal. Low blood pressure can cause dizziness.

❑ Always wear a seat belt when in a car.

❑ Focus when you are driving. Don't do things, such as talking on a car phone, that could distract you.

❑ Don't drink and drive.

❑ Don't drive at night if you have limited night vision.

❑ Keep emergency supples in your car. These include a cellphone, flares, blankets, and bottled water.

**For Information on Safety Contact:**

The Federal Safety Hotline
1-888-252-7751
Safe USA
www.cdc.gov/safeusa

To Learn More, See Back Cover

## Choosing a Doctor

Your doctor is your partner in caring for your health. Choose doctors who will give you good care and who you can work well with.

- Look for a doctor who accepts your health insurance. If you have Medicare, find out if the doctor accepts what Medicare pays.

- If you belong to a managed care plan, get a list of doctors who work with the plan. Health Maintenance Organizations (HMOs) and Preferred Provider Organizations (PPOs) are two types of managed care plans. The doctor(s) you see now may be on your HMO or PPO list.

- Choose a primary care doctor to manage your medical needs. Internists and family practice doctors are good choices for a primary care doctor if your health is generally good. If you have a chronic illness, you may be better served having a geriatrician (a specialist in the care of older persons) as a primary care doctor. If your health plan allows it, you might want to use a specialist as your primary care doctor if you have a chronic condition, such as diabetes. If you are a member of an HMO, it will give you a list of doctors from which to choose a primary care doctor.

- If your primary care doctor cannot take care of your health problem, he or she can refer you to a specialist. In many plans, care by specialists is only paid for if you are referred by your primary care doctor. Find out how your plan covers specialists.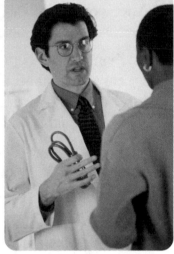

- Make a list of things you want in a doctor, such as location, gender, etc.

- Ask relatives and friends for doctors who have given them good medical care and whom they trust.

- Find out if the doctor is licensed by the state he or she practices in. Check with your local medical society. Find out, too, if the doctor is board-certified or board-eligible in the specialty in which he or she practices. To find out, call the American Board of Medical Specialists (ABMS) at 1-800-776-2378.

2. You & Your Doctor

**2. You & Your Doctor**

- Find out if a doctor is taking new patients. Check with your health plan or call the doctor's office.

- Look for a doctor whom you can relate to and who meets your needs of how medical decisions are made (the doctor alone, you alone, you and the doctor together).

- Ask about office hours to see if you can be seen when you need to be. Find out who you talk to if you can't speak with your doctor, and how calls are returned.

- Find out what other doctors serve as backups when the doctor is away. Ask who to contact after office hours.

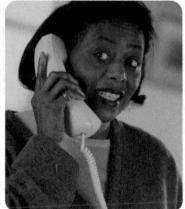

- Ask if your health plan or local hospital has a nurse advice telephone service. With this type of service, specially trained nurses can take your calls 24 hours a day and help you decide what to do.

- Ask what you should do if you need emergency care.

- Ask how costs are handled for visits and tests. Ask if you must pay a certain amount for your visit at that time or if you can be billed and pay later. Ask if the office staff bills your health plan or if you have to.

- Find out which hospital the doctor sends patients to. Ask if it accepts your health insurance.

- Ask if prevention services, such as exercise and nutrition programs, are covered by the health plan the doctor accepts.

To Learn More, See Back Cover

# Tell & Ask the Doctor Checklists

(Make copies as needed. Use the lines given to fill in the information.)

## Checklist 1 – Before You Call Or See Your Doctor

Be ready to **tell** your doctor these things:

❑ Your signs and symptoms. Be specific. If you have pain, be able to say where the pain is, how much it hurts, and if it is dull, aching, stabbing, throbbing, etc.
_____

❑ Results of home testing, such as your temperature, blood pressure, pulse rate per minute, etc. _____

❑ Medicines you take. Know the name(s), dose(s), etc. Include over-the-counter ones, vitamins, etc. See "Medicine Log" on page 46. _____
_____

❑ Allergies to medicines, food, etc. _____
_____

❑ Other medical conditions you have _____

❑ Medical conditions that run in your family _____
_____

❑ Your lifestyle: Eating, drinking, sleeping, exercising habits, etc. _____
_____

❑ Concerns you have about your health_____

❑ What you would like the doctor to do for you _____

❑ Your pharmacist's phone number _____

{**Note:** If needed, have your medical records, results of lab tests and x-rays, etc. from other health care providers sent to your doctor before your visit.}

2. You & Your Doctor

**2. You & Your Doctor**

## Checklist 2 – During the Doctor Visit Or Call

**A. Tell** the doctor what you wrote down in Checklist 1. (Take the list with you.) Make sure you have your eyeglasses and hearing aid, if you need them.

**B. Ask** your doctor these questions:

☐ What do you think the problem or diagnosis is? If you are confused by medical terms, **ask** for simple definitions. _____

_____

☐ Do I need any tests to rule out or confirm your diagnosis? If so, what tests do I need? Where do I go for the test(s) and how and when will I get the test results?

_____

☐ What do I need to do to treat the problem? How can I prevent it in the future?

_____

☐ Do I need to take any medicine? If so, what is it called, how often and for how long do I take it? What side effects should I let you know about? _____

_____

☐ When do I need to call or see you again? _____

☐ How are costs handled for this visit and for tests? _____

## Checklist 3 – After the Doctor Visit or Call

☐ Follow your doctor's advice. If you can't remember what to do, call the doctor's office. **Ask**, again, what you should do. _____

_____

☐ **Tell** your doctor if you feel worse, have additional problems, or have bad side effects from medicines your doctor told you to take. _____

_____

☐ Keep return visit appointments. If you need to cancel or reschedule an appointment, call your doctor's office at least 24 hours ahead of time.

 To Learn More, See Back Cover

## Gather Facts

Decisions you make about your health can affect both the length and quality of your life. Choose wisely. To do this, you need to gather facts. Use these sources:

- You. You know more about you than anyone else. Be in touch with how you feel, both physically and emotionally. Keep track of past and present health concerns. Fill in the "Medical History Chart" on page 37.

- Your doctor. Ask for his or her advice. Your doctor may also have written materials to give you on your condition.

- Medical resources. These include:

  - The Internet's world wide web. Look for credible sites, such as www.nih.gov, www.healthfinder.gov, and other web sites which end in .gov. Other credible sites are affiliated with hospitals, medical centers, medical associations and organizations. Most often, these sites end in .edu and .org. Web sites for specific health concerns are listed in many topics in Section II of this book. Beware of web sites that promote health fraud and quackery. Access www.quackwatch.com for information. Also, check with your doctor before you follow advice from a web site. The advice may not meet your particular needs.

- Not-for-profit groups. These include the American Cancer Society, the American Heart Association, and the American Diabetes Association. These groups can send information through the mail at your request by calling their toll-free numbers. These are listed in the topics "Cancer", "Coronary Heart Disease", and "Diabetes" in Section II. Most of these groups also have web sites.

- Government agencies. One is the National Institute on Aging (NIA), a division of the National Institutes of Health (NIH) at 1-800-222-2225 or www.nia.nih.gov on the world wide web. Another agency is the National Heart, Lung, and Blood Institute (NHLBI) at 1-800-575-WELL (575-9355) or www.nhlbi.nih.gov on the world wide web.

- Support groups for specific conditions, such as for breast cancer. Check local hospitals for lists of support groups near you or contact the National Self-Help Clearinghouse at 1-212-817-1822 or www.selfhelpweb.org on the world wide web.

Your job is to gather facts. Use the "Key Questions Checklist" and "Medical Comparison Chart" on the next pages to help you know what facts to look for. Once you have the facts, you and your doctor can make the medical decision(s) best suited to your needs.

# Key Questions Checklist

## 1. Diagnosis
- ❏ What is my diagnosis?
- ❏ Is my condition chronic or acute?
- ❏ Is there anything I can do to cure, treat, and/or prevent it from getting worse?
- ❏ Is my condition contagious or genetic?
- ❏ How certain are you about this diagnosis?

## 2. Treatment
- ❏ What is the recommended treatment?
- ❏ Is there a support group for my condition?

### *If you are discussing medications:*
- ❏ What will the medicine do for my particular problem?
- ❏ When, how often, and for how long should I take the medicine?
- ❏ How long before the medicine starts working?
- ❏ Will there be side effects?
- ❏ Will there be interactions with other medications I am taking?

### *If you are discussing a test:*
- ❏ What is the test called, and how will it help identify the problem?
- ❏ Will it give us specific or general information?
- ❏ Will more tests be necessary?
- ❏ How accurate and reliable is the test?
- ❏ How should I prepare for the test?
- ❏ Where do I go for the test?
- ❏ How and when will I get the test's results?

### *If you are discussing surgery:*
- ❏ Can I get a step-by-step account of the procedure, including anesthesia and recovery?
- ❏ Can you give me a list of others to contact who have had this surgery?

## 3. Benefits vs. Risks
- ❏ What are the benefits if I go ahead with the treatment?
- ❏ What are the possible risks and complications?
- ❏ Do the benefits outweigh the risks or vice-versa?

## 4. Success
- ❏ What is the success rate for the treatment?
- ❏ Are there any personal factors that will affect my odds either way?
- ❏ How long will the results of my treatment last?

## 5. Timing
- ❏ When is the best time to begin the treatment?
- ❏ When can I expect to see results?

## 6. Alternatives
- ❏ What will happen if I decide to do nothing?
- ❏ What are my other options?

## 7. Cost
- ❏ What is the cost of the recommended treatment?
- ❏ What related costs should I consider, i.e., time off work, travel, etc.?

## 8. Decision
- ❏ You can now make an informed decision.
- ❏ You have the right to choose or refuse treatment.

**3. Medical Decisions**

To Learn More, See Back Cover

# Medical Decision Comparison Chart

(Make copies as needed.)

Use this chart to help you compare medical options that are available to you.

Diagnosis _____

| | Option One | Option Two | Option Three |
|---|---|---|---|
| **Treatment** | | | |
| **Benefits** | | | |
| **Risks** | | | |
| **Success** | | | |
| **Timing** | | | |
| **Alternatives** | | | |
| **Cost** | | | |
| **Decision** | Yes ☐   No ☐ | Yes ☐   No ☐ | Yes ☐   No ☐ |

*(margin tab)* 3. Medical Decisions

# Patient Rights

What rights and privileges can you expect from a hospital when you become a patient? According to the American Hospital Association (AHA), there are specific standards of care that all patients are entitled to. The AHA has developed a voluntary code, The Patient's Bill of Rights, which presents guidelines for both staff and patients.

- You have the right to considerate and respectful care.

- You have the right to obtain from your doctor complete, current information concerning your diagnosis, treatment, and prognosis in terms you can reasonably be expected to understand.

- You have the right to receive from your doctor information necessary to give informed consent prior to the start of any procedure and/or treatment.

- You have the right to refuse treatment to the extent permitted by law, and to be informed of the medical consequences of your action.

- You have the right to privacy concerning your own medical care program, including all communications and records pertaining to your care.

- You have the right to expect that within its capacity a hospital must make a reasonable response to your request for services.

- You have the right to obtain information about any relationship of your hospital to other health care and educational institutions insofar as your care is concerned.

- You have the right to be advised if the hospital proposes to engage in or perform human experimentation affecting your care or treatment.

- You have the right to expect reasonable continuity of care.

- You have the right to examine and receive an explanation of your bill regardless of the source of payment.

- You have the right to know what hospital rules and regulations apply to your con- duct as a patient.

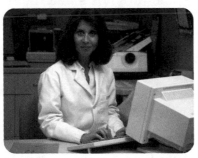

# Informed Consent

Informed consent is an ethical standard in medicine. It means that you agree to treatment only after it has been explained to you and that you understand it. You should know the nature of the treatment, its benefits and risks, and the likelihood of its success. You should also be told if your treatment is experimental in nature.

The physician should review any alternatives that are available in lieu of surgery or other procedures. There are no guaranteed outcomes in medicine, but informed consent enables YOU to make a rational and educated decision about your treatment. It also promotes greater understanding and joint decision making between you and your doctor.

With informed consent:

- You cannot demand services that go beyond what are considered "acceptable" practices of medicine or that violate professional ethics.

- You must recognize that you may be faced with some uncertainties or unpleasantness.

- You should, if competent, be responsible for your choices. Don't have others make decisions for you.

**3. Medical Decisions**

To Learn More, See Back Cover

# Advance Directives

There is a federal law called the Patient Self-Determination Act. It requires hospitals and nursing homes to give you information about your rights as a patient under their care. Advance directives are a legal way for you to declare your wishes to choose or refuse medical treatment. There are two types of advance directives:

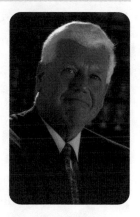

## Living Will

A document that spells out in writing what medical treatment you would want or not want if you were unable to state it yourself. A living will applies only when both of the following exist:

- You can't express your wishes on your own
- You suffer from a terminal illness or condition and aren't expected to survive.

In writing, you may choose or refuse:

- Measures to Support Life. Examples are cardiopulmonary resuscitation (CPR) and a respirator (a machine to breathe for you).

- Measures to Sustain Life. Examples are tube feedings and kidney dialysis (a machine that does the work of your kidneys).

- Measures to Enhance Life. These keep you comfortable without prolonging life. Examples are pain medications and hospice care.

## Durable Power of Attorney for Health Care

A document that names a person who would make treatment decisions for you if you are not able to make them yourself. Generally, it is a person who knows you and your values well and is in a good position to represent your wishes to your doctor. Your condition does not have to be terminal or irreversible to have someone speak on your behalf.

Most states have their own laws on advance directives. You can get forms for a living will and/or a durable power of attorney for health care from your local library or state representative's office.

After you fill them out, discuss your advance directives with your family and close friend(s). Talk to your doctor, too. Give him or her a copy to put with your medical records.

3. Medical Decisions

## Tests & What They Are For

The following tests can help detect health problems in early stages when they are easier to cure or treat.

**Blood Pressure Test** – Checks 2 kinds of pressure within blood vessels. The higher number gauges the pressure when your heart is pumping. The lower number gauges the pressure between heartbeats. High blood pressure may have no symptoms. It can lead to a heart attack and/or a stroke.

**Cholesterol Blood Test** – Checks cholesterol levels in the blood. High cholesterol levels are linked to heart disease.

**Diabetes Screening** – Checks for normal and abnormal blood sugar levels.

**Digital Rectal Exam** – Checks for early signs of colon, rectal, and/or prostate problems, including cancer

**Glaucoma Screening** – Checks for increased pressure within the eye. Glaucoma can result in blindness if not treated.

**Mammogram** – An X-ray to detect breast tumors or problems

**Pap Test** – Checks for early signs of cervical and uterine cancers, and genital herpes

**Professional Breast Exam** – A health care provider examines the breasts for abnormal signs.

**Prostate-Specific Antigen (PSA) Test** – A blood test that may help identify the presence of prostate cancer

**Sigmoidoscopy** – Checks for early signs of colon and rectal problems, including cancer

**Stool Blood Test** – Checks for early signs of colon and rectal problems, including cancer

**Vision** – Checks for marked changes or degeneration of the eyes

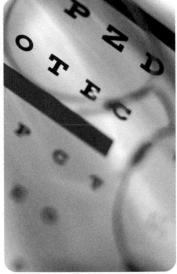

# Common Health Tests & How Often to Have Them*

| Test | | Ages 50 – 70 | Age 70 + |
|---|---|---|---|
| Physical Exam | | Every 1 to 2 years | |
| Blood Pressure | | At least every 2 years | |
| Vision/Glaucoma Screening | | Every 2 to 3 years | |
| Pap Test[1] | W | Every 1 to 3 years | Discuss with your doctor |
| Pelvic Exam | O | Every year | |
| Mammogram[2] | M | Every 1 to 2 years | |
| Breast Self-Exam[3] | E | Monthly | |
| Professional Breast Exam | N | Every year | |
| Testicular Self-Exam[4] | M | Monthly | |
| Prostate-Specific Antigen (PSA) | E N | Discuss with your doctor | |
| Digital Rectal Exam | | Every year | |
| Stool Blood Test | | Every year | |
| Sigmoidoscopy | | Every 3 to 5 years | |
| Cholesterol Blood Test | | Every 5 years | Every 5 years up to age 76 |
| Diabetes Screening | | Every 3 years or as advised | |
| Dental Checkup | | Every year | |

\* If you have an increased risk of a certain illness, you may need to have tests sooner or more often. Extra tests may also need to be done. Follow your doctor's advice. Also, check with your insurance company to see if and when tests are covered.

1. Pap tests should be given every year until tests are normal 3 years in a row. After that, pap tests should be given at least every 3 years. A woman should check with her doctor about the need for pap tests: If her cervix has been removed; or after age 65 (if all pap tests in the past were normal).

2. National Cancer Institute guidelines. Your doctor may advise that you get a mammogram every year.

3. See "Breast Self-Exam (BSE)" on page 339.

4. Call 1-800-4-CANCER or ask your health care provider for a step-by-step guide.

4. Medical Exams & Tests

# Immunizations

| Immunization | Age 50–60 | Age 65+ |
|---|---|---|
| Tetanus/diptheria (Td) vaccine | Every 10 years | |
| Influenza vaccine (flu shot) | Discuss with doctor | Every year |
| Pneumococcal (pneumonia) vaccine | Discuss with doctor | Once at age 65 * |

\* Some persons should get a second dose 5 or more years after the first dose

{**Note:** Ask your doctor or local health department if you need vaccines for Varicella (chickenpox), Hepatitis B, and /or Hepatitis A. Hepatitis A vaccine is recommended in selected U.S. states and/or other regions. Before you travel to other countries, find out if you need certain vaccines. Get information from the National Immunization Information Hotline at 1-800-232-2522 or at the www.cdc.gov/travel website. Discuss your needs with your doctor.}

# Immunization Record

| Immunization | Fill In Dates Given (Month and Year) | |
|---|---|---|
| Tetanus/diphtheria (Td) Vaccine | _____ | _____ |
|  | _____ | _____ |
| Influenza vaccine (flu shot) | _____ | _____ |
|  | _____ | _____ |
|  | _____ | _____ |
|  | _____ | _____ |
|  | _____ | _____ |
|  | _____ | _____ |
|  | _____ | _____ |
| Pneumococcal (pneumonia) vaccine | _____ | _____ |
| Other _____ | _____ | _____ |
| _____ | _____ | _____ |
| _____ | _____ | _____ |

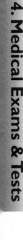

To Learn More, See Back Cover

# Medical History Chart

## A. Medical Conditions in Your Family
### (Father, mother, grandparents, brothers, sisters, aunts, uncles)

| Condition | Relative | Age of Onset | Age and Cause of Death |
|---|---|---|---|
| Allergies | | | |
| Arthritis | | | |
| Bowel Disorder | | | |
| Cancer | | | |
| Cataracts | | | |
| Diabetes | | | |
| Glaucoma | | | |
| Hearing Problems | | | |
| Heart Disease | | | |
| High Blood Pressure | | | |
| Pneumonia | | | |
| Stroke | | | |
| Thyroid Problems | | | |
| Smoker | | | |
| Other | | | |

## B. Your Medical History

| Condition | Date Diagnosed | Treatment to Date |
|---|---|---|
| | | |
| | | |
| | | |

| Surgeries | Date | Doctor/Hospital/Comments |
|---|---|---|
| | | |
| | | |
| Blood Type | | |
| Allergies | | |
| Drug Sensitivities | | |

4. Medical Exams & Tests

# Home Medical Tests

Home medical tests let you check for and monitor health conditions at home. Self-testing kits:

- Diagnose when conditions are or are not present. These include kits that test for blood cholesterol level and blood in the stool.

- Monitor an ongoing condition. These include kits that test for blood sugar levels and blood pressure readings.

The U.S. Public Health Service and the Food and Drug Administration (FDA) give tips for safe and proper use of self-testing kits. (Each of these does not necessarily apply to all tests.)

- Don't buy or use a test kit after the expiration date.

- Follow storage directions on the label.

- Study the package insert. First, read it through to get a general idea of how to perform the test. Then, go back and review the instructions and diagrams until you fully understand each step.

- Know what the test is meant to do and what its limitations may be. Tests are not always 100% accurate.

- Note special precautions, such as not eating certain foods before testing.

- If the test results rely on color comparison and you're colorblind, ask someone who is not colorblind to help you interpret the results.

- Follow instructions exactly.

- Don't skip a step.

- When you collect a urine specimen (unless you use a container from a kit), wash the container well and rinse out all soap traces. Use distilled water, if you can.

- When a step is timed, be precise. Use a watch with a second hand.

- Note what you should do if the results are positive, negative, or unclear.

- If something is not clear, don't guess. Call the "800" number on the package or call a pharmacist for information.

- Keep accurate records of results.

- As with medications, keep test kits that contain chemicals out of the reach of children. Throw away used test materials as directed.

Report any malfunction of a self-test to the manufacturer or to the:

U.S. Pharmacopeia Practitioner's Reporting Network, 12601 Twinbrook Parkway, Rockville, MD 20852
1-800-638-6725

## Safe Use of Medicines

### When Prescribed Medicine,

### Tell Your Doctor:

- All the medicines you take. This is both prescribed and over-the-counter (OTC) ones. If needed, put all your medicines, vitamins, etc. in a bag and take them with you. Keep them in their original containers.

- If you have medicine allergies, have had bad side effects from a medicine, or get side effects after you take a newly prescribed medicine.

- If it is hard for you to swallow pills, find out if pills can be cut in half, be crushed and mixed with food, or if there is a liquid form.

- If cost is a concern. There may be a generic or lower-cost medicine for you.

- If your health plan has a specific list (formulary) of medicines it uses. Your health plan provides a list. Take the list with you.

- If you can order 3 months of prescriptions by mail. Your doctor will have to write the prescription to cover 3 months.

- If you use alcohol, tobacco, or "street" drugs

- Any illnesses or problems another health care provider is treating you for

### Ask Your Doctor:

- The name of the medicine and what it is supposed to do

- If there is a generic equivalent

- How and when to take the medicine, how much to take, and for how long

- If you should stop taking the medicine if you feel better

- What food, drinks, other medicines, or activities you should avoid while taking the medicine. Examples are alcohol, grapefruit juice, sunlight, etc.

- If the medicine will interfere with other medicines you take

- What side effects the medicine may have and what to do if they occur

- If you can get a refill and how often

- About any terms or directions you do not understand

- What to do if you miss a dose

- If there is written information you can take home. You can ask the pharmacist for this, too.

- How to store the medicine

### Dos

- Throw away expired medicines.

- Keep all medicines out of the reach of children.

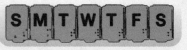

- Use the same pharmacy for prescribed and OTC medicines. This way, the pharmacist can be aware of all of the medicines you take and identify harmful combinations and food-and-medication interactions.

- Ask your pharmacist to clearly mark each container with all necessary instructions.

- Keep medicines in their original containers or in containers with sections 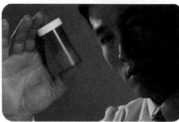 for daily doses (see box below).

- Try to reduce the need for medicines, such as sleeping pills. Take a warm bath to help you fall asleep at night. Check with your doctor for nonmedical ways to treat your problems.

**Don'ts**

- Don't stop taking medicines your doctor has prescribed, even if you feel better. Check with your doctor first.

- Don't drink alcohol while on a medicine if you don't know its effect. Some medicines, such as sedatives, can be deadly when used with alcohol. Read medicine labels for warnings on the use of alcohol with that medicine.

---

**Tips to Make Sure You Take Your Medicine(s)**

- Follow your treatment plan. Keep a current "Medicine Log" (see page 46). Check the log daily or as often as you need to.

- Ask family members or friends to remind you to take a dose and check that you did take a dose.

- Use products called compliance aids. Look for these products at your pharmacy or at a medical supply store:

  - Check-off calendars

  - Caps (or wristwatches) that beep when it is time to take a dose.

- Containers with sections for daily doses. Some have 4 separate sections for each day; one each for Breakfast, Lunch, Dinner, and Bedtime. This helps remind you to take each medicine at the time(s) prescribed.

- Talk to your doctor if you don't take your medicines as prescribed. Let him or her know why. It's okay to feel guilty or embarrassed. Don't let this stop you from talking to your doctor.

---

 To Learn More, See Back Cover

**5. Medicines**

- Never take someone else's prescribed medicine. Don't give your prescribed medicine to others.

- Don't take your medicines in the dark. Make sure the light is on so you can read the label. Wear your glasses or contact lenses, if you need to.

# Over-the-Counter (OTC) Medicines

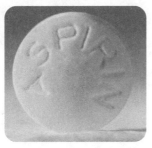

Over-the-counter (OTC) medicines are ones that you can get without a prescription. They are generally less potent than prescription medicines. When taken in large amounts, though, an OTC medicine might equal or exceed the dose of a prescription medicine. Follow the directions on the label or package insert.

### Use OTC Medicines Wisely

- Ask your doctor what OTC products you should avoid and which ones are safe for you to use. For example, find out what your doctor prefers you to take for pain and fever. (See "Pain relievers" in "Your Home Pharmacy" on page 43.)

- Do not exceed the dose on a label. Do not take OTC medicines on a regular basis unless your doctor tells you to.

- Ask your doctor if you should follow the instructions on the labels or take the medicine in a different way.

- Read warning sections on labels. These list the conditions under which the medicine should not be taken. Or, look up the name of the medicine in the *Physician's Desk Reference for Nonprescription Drugs*. Information and warnings listed can help you decide whether or not the product is safe for you to take. If you are unsure about taking an OTC medicine, check with your doctor or pharmacist.

- If you have an allergy to a medicine, check the list of ingredients on all OTC medicines to see if what you are allergic to is in them. Some labels will warn you not to take that medicine if you are allergic to a similar medicine.

- Before you take a medicine, check the expiration date. Discard ones that have expired. Replace items as needed.

- Be sure to store medicines in a convenient dry place. Store them out of children's reach.

- Don't ever tell children that medicine is candy.

**5. Medicines**

# Your Home Pharmacy

Read about the condition(s) in the "Common Uses" column before you take OTC medicine(s). Look in the index at the back of the book to find the pages the conditions are on. You may need to get medical care for the problem and not just use OTC medicines. Also, consult your pharmacist before you combine medicines. This includes OTC ones and prescribed ones.

| Medicines | Common Uses | Side Effects/Warnings |
|---|---|---|
| **Activated charcoal** | To absorb some poisons | Before using, call the Poison Control Center at 1-800-POISON1 (764-7661). |
| **Antacids** ex: Tums, Rolaids, Mylanta | Stomach upset, heartburn | Don't use for more than 2 weeks without your doctor's advice. Don't use high-sodium ones if on a low-salt diet. Don't use if you have chronic kidney failure. |
| **Antibiotic cream or ointment** ex: Neosporin | Minor skin infections, wounds | May result in local allergic reaction. |
| **Antidiarrheal medicine** ex: Kaopectate, Imodium A-D, Pepto-Bismol | Diarrhea | Pepto-Bismol can cause black stools. Don't give Pepto-Bismol to anyone under 19 years of age because it contains salicylates, which have been linked to Reye's Syndrome. |
| **Antihistamines** ex: Chlor-Trimeton, Benadryl | Allergies, cold symptom relief, relieves itching | May cause drowsiness, agitation, dry mouth, and/or problems with urinating. Don't use with alcohol, when operating machines, or when driving. Don't use if you have glaucoma or an enlarged prostate or problems passing urine. |

**5. Medicines**

To Learn More, See Back Cover

| Medicines | Common Uses | Side Effects/Warnings |
|---|---|---|
| **Cough suppressant** ex: Robitussin-DM or others with dextromethorphan | Dry cough without mucus | May cause drowsiness. People with glaucoma or problems passing urine should avoid ones with diphenhydramine. |
| **Decongestant** ex: Sudafed | Stuffy and runny nose, postnasal drip, allergies, fluid in the ears | Don't use if you have high blood pressure, diabetes, glaucoma, heart disease, history of stroke, or an enlarged prostate. |
| **Expectorant** ex: Robitussin or others with guaifenesin | Cough with mucus | Don't give with an antihistamine. |
| **Hydrocortisone cream** ex: Cortaid | Minor skin irritations, itching, rashes | May result in local allergic reaction. Do not use near the eyes. Do not use on burns or infections. |
| **Laxatives** ex: Ex-Lax, Correctol (stimulant-types), Metamucil (bulk-forming type) | Constipation | Long-term use of stimulant-type can lead to dependence and to muscle weakness due to potassium loss. |
| **Pain relievers** | {**Note:** If you have 3 or more drinks with alcohol per day, ask your doctor for advice on when and how you should take pain relievers.} | |
| **Acetaminophen** ex: Tylenol, Anacin-3, Datril | Pain relief, reduces fever. Does not reduce inflammation. | Gentle on stomach. Can result in liver problems in heavy alcohol users. Large doses or long-term use can cause liver or kidney damage. |

*Pain Relievers Continued on Next Page*

**5. Medicines**

| Medicines | Common Uses | Side Effects/Warnings |
|---|---|---|
| **Aspirin** ex: Bayer, Bufferin | Pain relief, reduces fever and inflammation. | Can cause stomach upset (which is made worse with alcohol use). May contribute to stomach ulcers and bleeding. Avoid if you: Take blood-thinning medicine; have an ulcer; have asthma and/or are having surgery within 2 weeks. High doses or prolonged use can cause ringing in the ears. |
| **Ibuprofen** ex: Advil, Medipren, Motrin **Ketoprofen** ex: Actron, Orudis KT **Naproxen Sodium** ex: Aleve | Pain relief, reduces fever and inflammation | Can cause stomach upset and ulcers. Take with milk or food. Can make you more sensitive to the effects of the sun. Don't use if you are allergic to aspirin. Don't use if you have ever had ulcers, blood clotting problems, or kidney disease. |
| **Syrup of Ipecac** | To induce vomiting for some poisons | Before using, call the Poison Control Center at 1-800-POISON1 (764-7661). |
| **Throat anesthetic** ex: Sucrets, Chloraseptic spray | Minor sore throat | Do not use anesthetics ending with "caine", such as benzocaine, if you are allergic to them. |
| **Toothache anesthetic** ex: Anbesol | Toothache and pain with dentures or other dental appliances | Do not swallow. Do not use if you are allergic to local anesthetics, such as benzocaine or other "caine" anesthetics. |

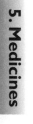
**5. Medicines**

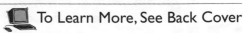
To Learn More, See Back Cover

## Basic Supplies that Can Help with Self-Care

| Supplies, Etc. | Common Uses |
| --- | --- |
| Adhesive bandages, sterile gauze, first aid tape, scissors | Minor wounds |
| Eye drops and artificial tears ex: Murine | Minor eye irritations |
| Heating pad/hot water bottle/heat pack; cold pack | Minor pains, strains, and injuries |
| Hemorrhoid preparation ex: Preparation H, Hemorid | Hemorrhoids |
| Humidifier, vaporizer (cool-mist) | Adds moisture to the air |
| Petroleum jelly ex: Vaseline | Chafing, dry skin |
| Rubbing alcohol | Topical antiseptic, used to clean thermometer |
| Sunscreen. Use one with a Sun Protection Factor (SPF) of 15 or more | Prevents sunburn, protects against skin cancer |
| Thermometer | Measure temperature |
| Tongue depressor, flashlight | Check for redness or infection in throat |
| Tweezers | Remove splinters |

{**Note:** The medicine cabinet in a bathroom is not a good place to store medicines. Dampness and heat can shorten the shelf life of some medicines. Store medicines in a cool, dry place, such as a top shelf of a closet. If there are children in the house, keep all medicines and vitamins locked in a high place, well out of their reach.}

## For Special Needs for Ongoing Health Conditions

1. Blood pressure cuff and stethoscope or self-measuring blood pressure kit
2. Blood sugar testing supplies
3. Urine test strips (many types)

5. Medicines

# Medicine Log

| Prescription Medicine Log | | | | | |
|---|---|---|---|---|---|
| (Make copies as needed.) | | | | | |
| Medicine Name/ Dose | Color/ Shape | Reason for Taking | Prescribed By | Date Started/ Stopped | Side Effects/ Notes |
| (Sample:) Precose 50 mg 3 x day | White/ round | Diabetes | Dr. Johnson | 5/98 to present | Take at start of each meal |
| 1. | | | | | |
| 2. | | | | | |
| 3. | | | | | |
| 4. | | | | | |
| 5. | | | | | |
| 6. | | | | | |

| Over-the-Counter Medicine Log | | | |
|---|---|---|---|
| (Make copies as needed.) List vitamins, minerals, herbs, too. | | | |
| Name/Dose | Reason for Taking | How Often | Side Effects/Notes |
| (Sample) Tums/500 mg | Get calcium | 1 tablet, 2 x day | None |
| 1. | | | |
| 2. | | | |
| 3. | | | |
| 4. | | | |
| 5. | | | |

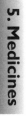
**5. Medicines**

 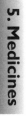 To Learn More, See Back Cover

## Planning for Health Care Coverage

Medical costs are expensive. Whether you are in your 50s, 60s, 70s, or older, now is the time to review how you cover them. Now is the time, too, to plan for how they will be paid for in the future. Health care costs the average older American about $3,000 a year. The average person over age 85 pays more than $5,000 a year. Without health insurance, some persons could lose all their assets if they had to pay for medical expenses.

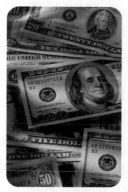

Like life insurance, health insurance can be hard to understand. Don't let it baffle you, though. Find out what you need to know to protect yourself and your assets. Don't find out you have too little coverage when it's too late. Use the "Health Insurance Checklist" on page 48 to keep track of your health care coverage.

## Medicare

Medicare is health insurance funded by the federal government. There is a lot to know about Medicare. For information, call the Medicare Choices Helpline at 1-800-MEDICARE (633-4227). Ask that a copy of the Medicare guide be mailed to you. You can also find out about Medicare on the Internet at www.medicare.gov.

To be "eligible" for Medicare means:

- You are 65 years or older. You must also be eligible for Social Security or Railroad Retirement Benefits, or

- You must be disabled for life and you have received Social Security Disability Insurance payments for at least 24 months, or

- You have end stage renal disease needing transplant or dialysis.

To apply for medicare, call the Social Security Administration. The number is 1-800-772-1213. You should call 3 months before you turn age 65. Don't wait any longer than 3 months after your 65th birthday to call. If you receive social security payments, you should automatically get a Medicare card, but don't take a chance. Call the Social Security Administration as mentioned above.

# Health Insurance Checklist

(Make copies of this form. Fill one out every year.)

Check off insurances that you have.

| Types of Insurance | Name of Plan | Who to Call |
|---|---|---|
| ❑ **Employer Insurance** | _____ | _____ |
| ❑ **Individual Policy** | _____ | _____ |
| ❑ **Medicare** | _____ | _____ |
| **Medicare Information** | | |
| Date called to apply for: | _____ | |
| {**Note:** Call 3 months before, or no later than 3 months after, you turn age 65.} | | |
| Effective Date | | |
|    Hospital Insurance: | _____ | |
|    Medical Insurance: | _____ | |
| Local Social Security | | |
|    Administration Number: | _____ | |
| Medicare Choices Helpline | 1-800-MEDICARE (633-4227) | |
| ❑ **Medicaid** | _____ | _____ |
| Case Load: | _____ | |
| ❑ **Medigap or Supplemental Insurance** | _____ | _____ |
| ❑ **Disability Insurance** | _____ | _____ |
| ❑ **Other** | _____ | _____ |

To Learn More, See Back Cover

## Disability Insurance

An accident or illness may make it impossible to work. This may mean a drastic drop in income. Disability insurance offers some protection. Benefits from these policies replace part of the wages lost.

If you're considering buying a disability insurance policy, ask the following:

- What percentage of your pre-tax salary is paid by the policy? (50 to 60% is average.)

- Is there a guarantee that the policy can be renewed?

- How long will benefits be paid? Months, years, a lifetime?

- How are benefits paid out? Are payments the same or greater in the first few months?

- Are pre-existing or chronic conditions included?

- Do you still pay premiums if you are disabled?

- Can you get disability insurance from your place of work? How much will this cost you? Group policies may be more flexible on chronic conditions.

## Long-Term Care Insurance

Long-term care insurance is meant to cover the cost of nursing home care and long-term home health care. Medicare and private health insurances do not cover these costs. This kind of insurance is not government regulated. In general, long-term care insurance is for persons whose net worth is between $100,000 to $1.5 million. You may want to purchase this for yourself. Your children may want to purchase it for you to protect themselves from having to pay for your long-term care or to protect their future inheritance.

Tips on buying long term care insurance:

- Get quotes from at least 3 companies. Call "Long Term Care Quote". The number is 1-800-587-3279. They will check out 15 top-rated providers and give you details on 3 policies that will fit your needs. This service only applies to carriers listed with the service. Check out independent agents, too.

- In general, look for a policy with a 3-year term. Long-term care is usually needed for 2 years.

**6. Planning**

- Consider a policy that starts paying on the 90$^{th}$ day instead of day 1. The difference in price can be 30%. Do this only if you can afford the long-term care center's cost for the first 3 months on your own.

- Check Moody's and Standard & Poors at your local library. Look for insurers rated "A" or better.

- Read a copy of the complete policy coverage. Consult an attorney or knowledgeable person to review it with you.

- Pay premiums, by check, directly to the insurance company. Never pay in cash.

- Fill out the policy application yourself or with a friend or relative. Don't allow someone to do it for you.

- Be cautious of companies advertised by celebrities.

- Insist on coverage that does not require a hospital stay before going to a nursing home.

- Resist high pressure insurance agents or claims that their long-term care insurance is endorsed by the government.

Be cautious before you purchase a policy. Ask the following questions:

- Will the policy cover home health care? Does this include "aides" or housekeeping coverage or just "skilled" care?

- Does the policy cover Alzheimer's disease, specifically?

- Must you be medically ill to receive benefits? What about custodial care?

- Does the coverage include nursing home custodial care, adult day care, or other community-based services?

- Does the policy require a prior hospital stay before entering a nursing home?

- Are there exclusions for "pre-existing" illnesses? Are there waiting periods?

- How long is a stay in a nursing home covered? (The average stay is just under 4 years.)

- How much will the nursing home be paid on a daily basis from this policy? What is the daily charge of the nursing home? You will have to pay the difference between the insurance coverage and what the nursing home charges.

- If premiums are being paid, is there a guarantee that the policy can be renewed?

- Is the policy one that can't be canceled?

- Will your coverage keep up with inflation?

- Are premiums waived while getting benefits?

# Cutting Health Care Costs

Good self-care lowers the need for expensive medical care. Learn more about self-care. See Section II of this book.

## For a Doctors' Care:

- Always get a second opinion when surgery is proposed. Check if your insurance plan covers a second opinion.

- Get a physical exam every 1 to 2 years after age 50.

- Keep doctors' bills organized. Use a filing system. Have services itemized whenever possible. Keep them in order of date. Check for duplicate testing and billing errors.

- Visits to an optometrist cost less than visits to an ophthalmologist. An "optometrist" examines eyes, prescribes lenses, and detects vision problems. "Ophthalmologists" are MDs who do everything optometrists do. They may also write prescriptions and do surgery. If you have no medical problems with your eyes, save money and see an optometrist.

- Quit smoking. You'll reduce visits to the doctor and save money.

- Use the emergency room only for real emergencies. A doctor's office is cheaper to take care of problems that do not need emergency care.

## For Medicines:

- Ask your doctor for samples before paying for a new prescription. You can try the drug first.

- Find out if your insurance plan has a mail order prescription service. In general, medicines are given in a 3-month supply. You pay 1 month's co-pay instead of 3.

- Ask about using generic drugs. These have the same chemical formula as brand name drugs. They may cost up to 40% less.

- Prices vary widely. Call several drug stores to get prices. Also, ask your pharmacist the cheapest way your doctor can prescribe the medicine(s) you need. Some medicines come in more than one dose, "are scored," and can be easily broken into halves. For example, it may cost less for you to get a prescription for 15 tablets that contain 100mg than for 30 tablets that contain 50mg . Instead of taking a 50mg tablet each day, you would take $1/2$ of a 100mg tablet each day.

6. Planning

Avoid buying "combination" cold pills. They cost more. You may not need both an antihistamine and a decongestant.

Many drug companies have "free" prescription plans. They are for low income people. A doctor's written request is needed. Call 1-800-762-4636 (Pharmaceutical Manufacturer's Association).

Do not buy drugs that claim to be miracle cures. They are costly and rarely work.

## For Medical Tests:

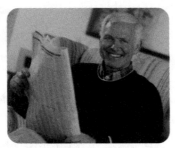

Attend free and low-cost medical screenings. Call your local health department. Check the newspaper, too, for dates, locations, and times.

Avoid taking the same medical tests more than needed. Keep a record of dates of x-rays, for example.

## For Health Insurance:

Consider a managed care plan, such as an HMO or PPO. Costs to you are less than with traditional health plans.

If you are healthy, raise your deductible. It will lower your insurance premium.

Read your policy carefully. Know what is and is not covered.

Check all benefits and payments on the insurance statement. Mistakes are made. Get an itemized list of services.

## For Saving Money in the Hospital:

Choose outpatient services whenever you can. Many diagnostic tests and surgeries can be done for less money as an outpatient. You avoid the cost of an overnight stay in a hospital.

If you are told that you need surgery, get a second opinion. Medicare and many private health insurance companies will pay for a second opinion. Most Medicaid programs also pay for a second opinion.

As an inpatient, stay only the prescribed time that is necessary. Ask your doctor about home health care, which can provide a wide range of services at less cost than in a hospital.

Beware of duplication of tests. Be sure to ask the doctor about what blood tests, x-rays, and medical procedures you can expect.

Be sure you know when checkout time is and make plans to observe it; otherwise, you're likely to be charged for an extra day's stay.

To Learn More, See Back Cover

- If your health problem isn't an emergency, avoid being admitted to a hospital on a weekend. The hospital staff is reduced then, and testing will usually not begin until Monday.

- Keep a list of all services you receive. Ask for an itemized bill so you can make sure you are billed correctly.

## Housing Options

Some older people find the upkeep for a house too demanding. Health concerns may not allow some people to meet these demands. Consider other housing options:

- Condominium. This is a townhouse or apartment that is privately owned. A fee is charged to cover maintenance of items like the lawn, swimming pool, etc.

- Co-Operative. This is a housing facility where everyone owns a share. People live in unit apartments and vote on key issues.

- Rental. A landlord takes care of maintenance. Residents pay a monthly rental fee plus a security deposit.

- Retirement Community/Assisted Living Facility. Residents live independently, but have services available to them. These include recreation activities, meals served in a common area, transportation. Often a social worker or counselor is on site. There may be age restrictions.

- Federal Housing. This is independent living for those over 62 years old with low to moderate incomes.

- Group Housing/Adult Custodial Care Homes. These provide room and board for those in need of nonmedical care. Help with daily living makes this option well suited for Alzheimer's patients.

- Life Care at Home (LCAH). Service is offered in one's own home. An initial fee is charged along with a monthly charge. A manager personalizes a program of medical care, aides, and supplies to a client.

- Intermediate Care. This is a residence for those who should not live alone, but can manage simple personal care, like dressing. Meals are provided. Cleaning services and nursing care are offered on site.

- Nursing Homes. They are designed for people who require care 24 hours a day. They are used by people needing convalescence. Nursing homes are medically supervised.

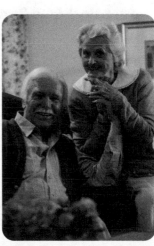

6. Planning

# Caregiver's Guide

Caregiving may be stressful. A caregiver's job is not easy, but it does not always have to be a burden. You will need to know the following things if you are thinking about being a caregiver or when you are a caregiver:

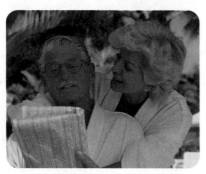

- The kind of care the person needs. This includes medical care, custodial care, home care, etc. Find this out from the person and from his or her health care providers, family, and friends.

- How the person's health care and living care expenses will be paid. Find out what assets and health insurance the person has and if these will cover the costs of his or her care.

- What support services are available. Call Eldercare Locator. The number is 1-800-677-1116. You will be put in touch with a local Area Agency on Aging which can provide a list of local organizations that can assist you and the person needing care.

For Alzheimer's Disease, contact:

1. The Alzheimer's Association 1-800-272-3900

2. The Alzheimer's Disease Education and Referral Center (ADEAR) 1-800-438-4380

- If there are any caregivers' support groups that you can join

- Good books about caregiving that you can read. Call the National Institute on Aging for a list. The number is 1-800-222-2225.

- How to get respite care for the person. Locate persons and/or places that provide this in your area.

- How much you can truly handle on your own and when the person you are caring for needs residential care.

- That it is necessary that you take care of your own health and needs, too. Eat well, exercise regularly. Get enough sleep. Get regular health exams and tests. See "Common Health Tests & How Often to Have Them" on page 35.

# Hospice Care

Hospice care is for people with a terminal illness. To enter a hospice program (and to receive Medicare benefits), a doctor's diagnosis is required stating that life expectancy is no more than about 6 months. Attention is given to "care, not cure." No efforts are made to prolong life or to hasten death. The patient is kept comfortable and pain free. Hospice eases the process of dying. The focus is on a peaceful setting where comfort is the first concern.

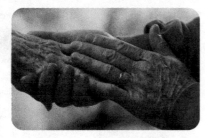

Most referrals for hospice come from doctors. Hospice care may be provided in:

- The home (80% of persons enrolled in hospice are cared for at home.)
- A hospital
- A nursing home
- A hospice facility

The bulk of care, especially with home hospice, is usually given by family members and friends. It is supported by a hospice care team which includes doctors, social workers, therapists, volunteers, clergy, nurses, and family members. The team plans care that ensures quality of life.

Most health insurance plans include the option of hospice care. Medicare and Medicaid cover the costs if the facility or hospice organization is certified by them. Under Medicare, the length of stay is two 90 day benefit periods. This may be followed by a 30 day period. Extensions are available. The patients must be certified to be terminally ill at the start of each period.

Sometimes patients are charged if they do not qualify for reimbursement. Hospice care is based on need. No one is rejected for lack of finances.

Some advantages to hospice care include:

- Availability of 24 hour a day, 7 day a week assistance. This is true for hospice care in hospitals, nursing homes, and hospice facilities. Find out if the home hospice program offers this service. It usually does.
- Respite for family caretakers when care is given in the home
- Emotional comfort and support by trained hospice staff and volunteers
- Bereavement counseling

For further information, contact the *National Hospice Organization* at 1-800-658-8898.

**6. Planning**

# SECTION II

## Common Health Problems

### Introduction

All these health care costs are going up:

- Doctor office and health clinic visits
- Prescriptions
- Tests
- Health insurance and Medicare copays, deductibles, etc.

You have to make decisions when you get sick:

- Should you wait and see if the problem gets better? Can you take care of it yourself?
- What things can you do to take care of yourself?
- Should you call your doctor?
- Should you go to the emergency room?

This section can help with these questions. It presents health problems in 3 parts:

- Facts about the problem: What it is, signs and symptoms, causes, and treatments
- Self-care measures to treat the problem
- Reasons to contact your doctor or to get help fast

This section can help you decide when to use self-care and when to get medical care.

**Eye Problems**

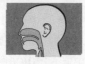
**Ear, Nose, & Throat Problems**

**Respiratory Conditions**

**Skin Conditions**

**Abdominal & Urinary Problems**

**Heart & Circulation Problems**

**Brain & Nervous System Conditions**

**Muscle & Bone Problems**

**Other Health Problems**

**Mental Health Conditions**

**Men's Health**

**Women's Health**

**Sexual Health**

**Dental & Mouth Problems**

# How to Use This Section

- Find the problem you are looking for in the index or the table of contents. The problems are listed in chapters. Each chapter covers certain concerns. Examples are "Eye Problems," "Ear, Nose, & Throat Problems," "Skin Problems," etc. The topics in each chapter are listed in order from A to Z.

- Read about the problem, what causes it (if known), its symptoms, and treatments.

- Use the information that tells you what to do. The headings and what they mean are listed below.

## Self-Care:

You can often take care of the problem yourself with self-care measures. Use the self-care tips that are listed in the topic. Read beyond the self-care section, too. You will find a list of symptoms for which self-care, alone, is not enough. You may need to contact your doctor. In rare instances you may need to get immediate care.

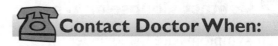

## Contact Doctor When:

If your symptoms are listed under this heading, call your doctor. State the problem. You will get advice on what to do.

The term "doctor" can be used for a number of health care providers:

- Your doctor
- Your Health Maintenance Organization (HMO) clinic, primary doctor, or other health care provider
- Walk-in clinic
- Physician's assistants (P.A.s), nurse practitioners (N.P.s), or certified nurses (C.N.s) who work with your doctor
- Home health care provider
- Your psychiatrist
- Your dentist

Write down phone numbers for your health care providers on page 1 of this book.

To learn more about topics covered in this Guide and other health issues, access the web site listed on the back cover of this book.

## Contact Counselor When:

If your symptoms are listed under this heading, call your mental health counselor. You will get advice on what to do.

The term "counselor" can be used for a number of mental health care providers:

- Your counselor or therapist, if you already have one
- A mental health professional provided by your Employee Assistance Program (EAP) at work
- A mental health center
- A clinical psychologist
- A social worker with a master's degree (M.S.W.)
- Another health care provider in the mental health field, such as a psychiatric nurse

{**Note:** Your primary care doctor may be able to provide some counseling, too, or help you by making a referral to another mental health care provider. If you belong to a Health Maintenance Organization (HMO) or other managed health care plan, you may need a referral from your primary care doctor for services to be covered. Also, a counselor may have you join a self-help/support group.}

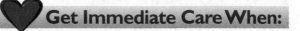

## Get Immediate Care When:

If your symptoms are listed under this heading, you should get help fast. See "Recognizing Emergencies" on page 380. It lists warning signs of a medical emergency. For one or more of these signs, go to a hospital emergency department if you can do so safely. If not, call 911, your local rescue squad, or an ambulance. Don't call 911 or use a hospital emergency department if symptoms do not threaten life. Get immediate care by calling your doctor right away or going to an "urgent care" center. Some hospital emergency departments have a "Prompt Care" area to treat minor injuries and illnesses. An example is a sprained ankle. Ask your doctor ahead of time where you should go for a sprained ankle or similar type of problem that needs prompt care, but not emergency care.

Find out, now, how your health insurance covers medical emergencies. Then you'll know what to do if one occurs.

Make sure you know phone numbers for emergency medical help. Write them down near your phone and on the "Emergency Phone Numbers" list on page 1 of this book. Call 911 where the service is available. If your HMO prefers that you use a certain ambulance service, find out their number and write it on page 1.

# Chapter 7. Eye Problems

## 1. How Aging Affects the Eyes

Growing older does not always mean you see poorly. But you may not see as well as you did before. Common changes that affect your eyes are:

- "Aging Eyes". The medical term for this is **presbyopia** (prez-bee-OH-pea-ah). This comes on slowly after age 40. Close objects or small print are harder to see.

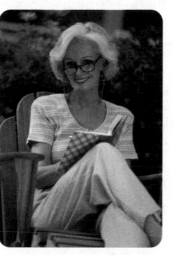

You may have to hold reading materials at arm's length. You may get headaches or "tired eyes" while you read or do other close work. Presbyopia can be corrected with glasses or contact lenses.

- The need for more light in order to see clearly. With aging, the pupil in the eye is unable to open as wide or to adapt to light as fast as it did before. This can make it harder to see in the dark. It can make it harder to tell one color from another. Blues can look like different shades of gray. To help with this, add more and brighter lights in places around the house, such as at work counters, stairways, and favorite reading places. This may help you see better and can sometimes prevent accidents. Also, don't wear tinted glasses or sunglasses at night, especially when you drive.

## 2. Eye Problems Chart

| Signs & Symptoms | What It Could Be | What to Do |
|---|---|---|
| Sudden loss of all or part of vision, especially in one eye with sudden weakness or numbness on one side | Stroke | Get immediate care. See "Stroke" on page 228. |
| Vision loss after head or eye injury. Sudden vision loss or blurred vision, and seeing dark spots, or flashes of light all of a sudden. | Detached or torn retina | Get immediate care. |

*Eye Problems Chart Continued on Next Page*

7. Eye Problems

## Eye Problems Chart, Continued

| Signs & Symptoms | What It Could Be | What to Do |
|---|---|---|
| Severe pain in and above the eye. Eye redness, swollen upper eyelid. Dilated and fixed pupil. Very blurred vision, halos around lights. | Angle-closure glaucoma | Get immediate care. See "Glaucoma" on page 67. |
| Object or chemical in the eye | Eye irritation or injury | See "Eye Irritations & Injuries" on page 63. |
| Gradual loss of side vision. Blurred vision. Halos around lights. Poor night vision. | Open-angle or chronic glaucoma | See "Glaucoma" on page 67. |
| Dark or blind spot in center of vision. Blurred or cloudy vision. Straight lines look wavy. | Macular degeneration | See "Macular Degeneration" on page 69. |
| Cloudy, fuzzy, foggy, or filmy vision. Halos around lights. Problems with glare from lamps or the sun. | Cataract | See "Cataracts" on page 61. |
| Pus discharge from the eye; the white of the eye and eyelid are red; crusting of the eyelid in the morning; feeling of sand in the eye | Conjunctivitis ("Pinkeye") | See "Pinkeye" on page 71. |
| Firm lump on eyelid or tender pimple on the edge of the eyelid | Sty | See "Sties" on page 72. |
| Seeing spots, specks, wavy lines, or streaks of light | Floaters and/or Flashes | See "Floaters and Flashes" on page 66. |
| Blurred vision when you look at close objects; headaches; eyestrain | "Aging Eyes" or presbyopia (see page 59) | Call eye doctor for appointment and advice. |

{**Note:** For information and help for eye problems see organizations listed in the box on page 73.}

# 3. Cataracts

A cataract is a cloudy area in the lens or lens capsule of the eye. A cataract blocks or distorts light entering the eye. Vision gradually becomes dull and fuzzy, even in daylight. Most of the time, cataracts occur in both eyes. Only one eye may be affected, though. If they form in both eyes, one eye can be worse than the other, because each cataract develops at a different rate. During the time cataracts are forming, vision can be helped with frequent eyeglass changes.

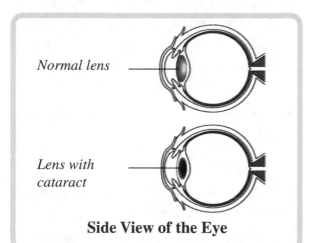

*Normal lens*

*Lens with cataract*

**Side View of the Eye**

## Prevention

- Limit exposing your eyes to x-rays, microwaves, and infrared radiation.

- While outdoors, wear sunglasses with UV block and wear a hat with a brim. Avoid overexposure to sunlight.

- Wear glasses or goggles that protect your eyes whenever you use strong chemicals, power tools, or other instruments that could result in eye injury.

- Don't smoke. Avoid heavy drinking.

- Eat foods high in beta-carotene and/or vitamin C, which may help to prevent or delay cataracts. Examples are: carrots, cantaloupes, oranges, and broccoli.

- Keep other illnesses, such as diabetes, under control.

## Signs & Symptoms

- Cloudy, fuzzy, foggy, or filmy vision

- Pupils which are normally black appear milky white

- Sensitivity to light and glazed nighttime vision. This can cause problems when driving at night.

- Double vision

- Halos may appear around lights

- Changes in the way you see colors

- Seeing glare from lamps or the sun

- Better vision for awhile, only in far-sighted people

Vision with Cataracts

7. Eye Problems

*Cataracts, Continued*

## Causes, Risk Factors & Care

- The most common form of cataracts come with aging due to changes in the chemical state of lens proteins. About half of Americans ages 52 to 64 and most persons over age 75 have cataracts.

- Cataracts can also result from damage to the lens capsule due to trauma; from ionizing radiation or infrared rays; from taking corticosteroid medicines for a long time; and from chemical toxins. Smokers have an increased risk for cataracts. So do persons with diabetes and glaucoma.

Treatment includes eye exams, corrective lenses, cataract glasses, and cataract surgery, when needed.

A person who has cataract surgery usually gets an artificial lens at the same time. A plastic disc called an intraocular lens is placed in the lens capsule inside the eye.

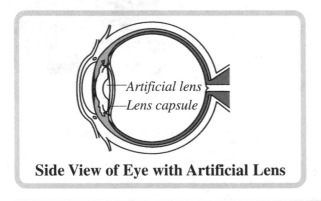

—Artificial lens
—Lens capsule

**Side View of Eye with Artificial Lens**

It takes a couple of months for an eye to heal after cataract surgery. Experts say it is best to wait until your first eye heals before you have surgery on the second eye if it, too, has a cataract.

### Self-Care:

- Be careful about driving at night. Night vision can be one of the first thing affected by cataracts. Let someone else drive if you can't see well.

- Wear sunglasses with UV block.

- When indoors, don't have lighting too bright or pointed directly at you. Install dimmer switches so you can lower the light level. Use table lamps, not ceiling fixtures.

- Use soft, white (not clear) light bulbs.

- Arrange to have light reflect off walls and ceilings.

- Read large print items. Use magnifying glasses, if needed.

- Schedule an eye exam every 2 years or as advised by your doctor.

- Wear your prescribed glasses.

### Contact Doctor When:

You have signs and symptoms of cataracts listed on page 61.

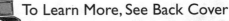 To Learn More, See Back Cover

# 4. Eye Irritations & Injuries

As you age, your eyes can get irritated more easily because they make less tears. Poorer vision increases the risk for eye injuries.

## Prevention

- Wear safety glasses for activities that expose your eyes to sawdust, etc.

- When using harsh chemicals, wear rubber gloves and protective glasses. Don't rub your eyes if you've touched harsh chemicals. Turn your head away from chemical vapors.

- To help prevent dry eyes, use a humidifier and limit exposure to smoke, dust, and wind. Avoid alcohol.

- Use artificial tear drops with your doctor's okay.

- Don't stare directly at the sun, especially during a solar eclipse.

- Wear sunglasses that block UV rays.

- Don't use eye makeup when an allergy or chemical irritant bothers your eye(s)

## Signs & Symptoms

You feel burning, dryness, itching, and/or pain and swelling in one or both eyes.

## Causes & Care

**For Eye Irritation:**

Causes include particles in the eye; too much sun exposure, low humidity; strong wind; and scratches from contact lenses. Allergies, infections, and diseases that make your eyes dry can also cause eye irritation.

**For Eye Injuries:**

Causes include a physical blow to the eye; harsh chemicals; and a foreign body that is stuck in the eye.

Mild eye irritations and injuries can be treated with self-care. More serious problems need medical care.

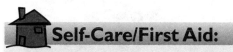

## Self-Care/First Aid:

**To Ease the Discomfort of Dry Eyes:**

With your doctor's okay, use over-the-counter artificial tear drops, such as Ocu-Lube. Read the label. If there are no preservatives, keep the solution refrigerated. Wash your hands before using.

**To Treat an Insect Bite Without a Severe Allergic Reaction:**

- Wash the eye(s) with warm water.

*Continued on Next Page*

7. Eye Problems

## Eye Irritations & Injuries, Continued

### Self-Care, Continued

- Take an antihistamine if okay with your doctor.

### To Remove a Foreign Particle On the White of the Eye or Inside the Eyelids:

- Do not remove an object imbedded in the eye, a metal chip, or a foreign body over the colored part of the eye. (See "First Aid for Foreign Body Sticking Into the Eye" on this page.)

- Wash your hands.

- If the foreign object is under the upper lid, have the person look down and pull the upper lid away from the eyeball by gently grabbing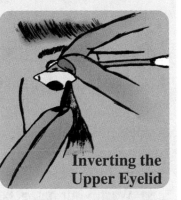
**Inverting the Upper Eyelid**
the eyelashes. Press a cotton-tipped swab down on the skin surface of the upper eyelid and pull it up and toward the brow. The upper lid will invert. Touch and remove the debris with the tip of the tissue.

- Twist a piece of tissue, moisten the tip with tap water (not saliva) and gently try to touch the speck with the tip. Carefully pass the tissue over the speck, which should cling to the tip.

- Do not rub the eye or use tweezers or anything sharp to remove a foreign object.

- Gently wash the eye with cool water.

### To Treat a Bruise from a Minor Injury that Surrounds the Eye but Does Not Damage the Eye Itself:

- Put a cold compress over the injured area right away. Keep doing this for 15 minutes, every hour, for 48 hours.

- Take an over-the-counter medicine for the pain and inflammation. (See "Pain relievers" in "Your Home Pharmacy" on page 43.)

- After 48 hours, put a warm compress over the injured area.

- Seek medical attention if these measures do not help.

### First Aid for Foreign Body Sticking Into the Eye Before Immediate Care:

- Do not remove the object.

- Don't press on, touch, or rub the eye.

*Continued on Next Page*

To Learn More, See Back Cover

*Eye Irritations & Injuries, Continued*

### Self-Care, Continued

- Cover the injured eye with a paper cup or other clean object that will not touch the eye or the foreign object. Hold the paper cup in place with tape without putting pressure on the eye or the foreign object.

- Gently cover the uninjured eye with a clean bandage and tape, too, to keep the injured eye still.

### First Aid for Harmful Chemicals in the Eye(s) Before Immediate Care:

- Flush the eye(s) with water immediately!

- Hold the injured eye open with your thumb and forefinger.

- At the faucet or with a pitcher or other clean container, flush the eye with a lot of water. Start at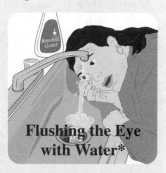

**Flushing the Eye with Water***

the inside corner and pour downward to the outside corner. This lets the water drain away from the body and keeps it from getting in the other eye.

- Keep pouring the water for 10 to 30 or more minutes. Flush the eye with water until you get medical help.

- If both eyes are injured, pour water over both eyes at the same time or quickly alternate the above procedure from one eye to another. Or, place the victim's face in a sink or container filled with water. Tell the victim to move his or her eyelids up and down and remove the face from the water at intervals in order to breathe. Use this method on yourself if you are the victim and are alone.

- Loosely bandage the eye with sterile cloth and tape. Don't touch the eye.

## ☎ Contact Doctor When:

You have any of these problems:

- Eye pain with eye irritation
- An eye that is red and/or swollen
- Yellow-green pus is under the eyelid or drains from the eye.

## ♥ Get Immediate Care When:

- Harmful chemicals have gotten into the eye(s). {**Note:** Before you get immediate care, give "First Aid for Harmful Chemicals in the Eye(s) Before Immediate Care" on this page.}

7. Eye Problems

*Eye Irritations & Injuries, Continued*

- A foreign body sticks into the eye. {**Note**: See "First Aid for Foreign Body Sticking Into the Eye Before Immediate Care" on page 64.}

- Any of these problems occurs with a blow to the eye or other eye injury:

  • Loss of vision

  • Blurred or double vision

  • Blood in the pupil

- A cut to the eye or eyelid occurs.

## 5. Floaters & Flashes

### Signs & Symptoms

- Floaters are specks, dots, cobwebs, or wavy lines that seem to fall within your line of sight. They rarely affect your eyesight. They are more visible against a plain or dark background.

- Flashes are streaks of light that "flash" across your field of vision. They can happen when your eyes are closed or when you are in extreme darkness.

## Causes, Risk Factors & Care

When you age, the middle portion of the eye, called the vitreous, becomes less solid and more liquid. This allows particles (floaters), which have always been in the eye, to begin to move around. Flashes can occur when the vitreous shrinks and pulls on the retina of the eye. This is common. On rare occasions when the vitreous detaches from the retina, it can rip or tear the retina. This may lead to retinal detachment. The retina peels away from the eye wall, causing sight loss. Risk factors for floaters and flashes are:

- Eye diseases or injuries

- A tear in the retina. Aging and cataract surgery increase the risk for this.

- High blood pressure

- Migraine headaches

- Nearsightedness

Self-care is enough to treat floaters and flashes unless they are due to another medical condition.

### Self-Care:

- Move your eyes up and down (not side to side) several times.

*Continued on Next Page*

To Learn More, See Back Cover

*Floaters & Flashes, Continued*

*Self-Care, Continued*

- Don't focus on or stare at plain, light backgrounds, such as a blank pastel wall or the light blue sky.

- You may notice flashes less if you avoid moving suddenly, don't bend over, and don't get up quickly from sitting or lying down.

## ☎ Contact Doctor When:

- A large red floater disturbs your vision.

- You have any of these problems with floaters or flashes:

  - A loss of side vision

  - A sudden appearance of a cloud of dark floaters with bright light flashes

  - A rapid increase in the number of floaters or sudden shower of many floaters

  - Bleeding in the eye

  - The floaters don't move as you look at them.

  - A history of migraine headaches or high blood pressure

  - The floaters or flashes last 10 to 20 minutes in both eyes.

# 6. Glaucoma

Glaucoma is a common major eye disorder in people over the age of 60.

## Signs & Symptoms

There are 2 types of glaucoma:

### Chronic (Open-Angle) Glaucoma

This type takes place gradually, usually causes no pain and has no symptoms early on. When symptoms begin, they are:

- Loss of side (peripheral) vision

- Blurred vision

In the late stages, symptoms include:

- Vision loss in larger areas (side and central vision), usually in both eyes

- Blind spots

- Seeing halos around lights

- Poor night vision

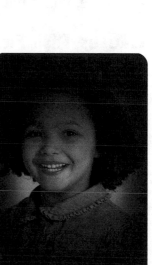

**Vision with Glaucoma**

- Blindness, if not treated early enough

**7. Eye Problems**

*Glaucoma, Continued*

### Acute (Angle-Closure) Glaucoma

This type can occur suddenly. It is a medical emergency! Symptoms include:

- Severe pain in and above the eye
- Severe throbbing headache
- Fogginess of vision, halos around lights
- Redness in the eye, swollen upper eyelid
- Dilated pupil
- Nausea, vomiting, weakness

## Causes, Risk Factors & Care

Glaucoma occurs when the pressure of the liquid in the eye gets too high and causes damage. It tends to run in families. The risk of getting glaucoma increases with age. It can also be triggered or aggravated by some medicines, like antihistamines and antispasmodics.

Glaucoma may not be preventable, but the blindness that could result from it is. Get tested for glaucoma when you get a regular vision checkup. If pressure inside the eyeball is high, an eye doctor will prescribe eye drops and perhaps oral medicines.

Medicines used for acute glaucoma are prescribed for life. If medicines do not control the pressure, ultrasound, laser beam surgery, or other surgical procedures may need to be done.

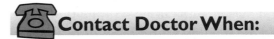 **Self-Care:**

- Do not take any medicine, including over-the-counter ones, without first checking with your doctor or pharmacist. Most cold medications and sleeping pills, for example, can cause the pupil in the eye to dilate. This can lead to increased eye pressure.
- Avoid getting upset and fatigued. These can increase pressure in the eye.
- Don't smoke.

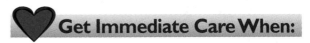 **Contact Doctor When:**

Symptoms of chronic (open angle) glaucoma are present (see page 67).

**Get Immediate Care When:**

Symptoms of acute (angle-closure) glaucoma, listed on this page, are present.

To Learn More, See Back Cover

# 7. Macular Degeneration (AMD)

Macular degeneration is a progressive eye disorder. Known as age-related macular degeneration (AMD), it is the most common cause of central vision loss in older Americans. The central part of the retina (the macula) deteriorates. This results in the loss of central, or straight-ahead, vision. One or both eyes may be affected. In many cases, the small vessels of the eye can become narrowed and hardened due to atherosclerosis. With this, the macula doesn't get the blood supply it needs so it wastes away. This is called the dry form. In the wet form, tiny blood vessels leak blood or fluid around the macula. The wet form is less common than the dry.

## Prevention

To reduce the risk for AMD:

- Don't smoke. If you smoke, quit.
- Follow a balanced diet.
- Protect your eyes from the sun's ultraviolet rays. Wear sunglasses with UV block. Wear a hat with a brim.
- Take measures to control high blood pressure (see page 203) and coronary artery disease (see page 199).
- Get your vision checked every year.

## Signs & Symptoms

Macular degeneration is painless. It usually develops gradually, especially the dry form. With the wet form, symptoms can occur more rapidly. Symptoms for both forms are:

- Blurred or cloudy vision
- Seeing a dark or blind spot at the center of vision
- Distorted vision, such as straight lines that look wavy
- Hard time reading or doing other close-up work

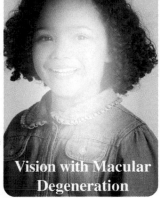

**Vision with Macular Degeneration**

- Hard time doing any activity, such as driving, that needs sharp vision
- Complete loss of central vision. Side vision is not affected.

## Causes, Risk Factors & Care

The exact cause of AMD is not known. Risk factors for AMD are:

- Advancing age
- Cigarette smoking

**7. Eye Problems**

*Macular Degeneration, Continued*

- Family history of the condition
- Having light-colored eyes
- Exposure to ultraviolet light
- Poor diet

If you have the wet form, laser-beam therapy may help to slow the progress of AMD. This therapy should be done before a lot of damage is done to the eyesight. Most dry form cases are not treatable. Your eye doctor may prescribe special eyeglasses.

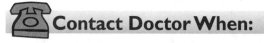

### Self-Care:

Use "Prevention tips" in this topic and:

- Wear the special eyeglasses and use other vision aids, such as magnifying devices, as advised by your doctor.
- Have your vision checked as advised by your doctor.

### Contact Doctor When:

- You have symptoms of AMD listed on page 69, especially when symptoms come on quickly.

- You look at the center dot in the grid below, and you see blurry, curvy, or distorted lines, or empty spots. Cover one eye when you look at the grid. Repeat, covering the other eye.

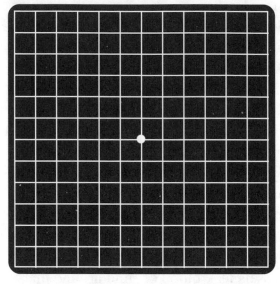

The grid below shows how the lines might look with macular degeneration.

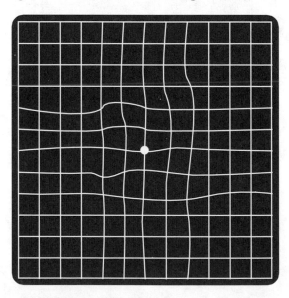

To Learn More, See Back Cover

# 8. Pinkeye

Pinkeye is an inflammation of the conjuctiva (conjunctivitis). The conjunctiva is the covering of the inside of the eyelids and the whites of the eyes.

It is called pinkeye when the cause is a bacterial or viral infection. This is because the white part of the eye looks pinkish-red. Conjunctivitis can also be due to an allergic reaction.

## Pinkeye Chart

| Signs & Symptoms | Cause | Treatment |
|---|---|---|
| Redness of the whites of the eyes. Yellowish-green, puslike discharge from the eye. Crusting on the eyelashes when you wake up. Feels like you have something in your eye. | Bacterial infection (very contagious) | Antibiotic eyedrops or ointment. Usually starts to clear up in 2 to 3 days. Take eyedrops as long as prescribed. |
| Redness of the whites of the eyes. Watery or puslike discharge from the eye. Feels like you have something in your eye. May have crusting on the eyelashes, runny nose, and sore throat. | Viral infection (very contagious) | Most infections are viral but antibiotic eyedrops are often prescribed. It is hard to tell a viral from bacterial infection because symptoms for both are the same. Can take 14 to 21 days to clear up. |
| Burning, itching, and watery eyes. May feel like you have something in the eye. | Allergic reaction (not contagious). Common irritants are cosmetics, contact lenses, dust, mold, pollen, and smoke. | Avoid the allergen. Use over-the-counter eyedrops, and/or artificial teardrops. Ask your doctor if it is okay to take an over-the-counter antihistamine. |

**7. Eye Problems**

*Pinkeye, Continued*

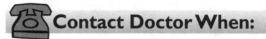

## Self-Care/Prevention:

**For Pinkeye:**

- Wash your hands often. Don't share towels, washcloths, etc. with others.

- Avoid contact with other people as much as you can the first 3 days you have pinkeye. Some places of work request employees with pinkeye to stay away from work for 3 days so they don't spread the infection.

- Don't touch the eye area with your fingers. Use a tissue instead.

- With your eyes closed, apply a washcloth soaked in warm (not hot) water to the affected eye 3 to 4 times a day for at least 5 minutes at a time. Use a clean washcloth each time.

- Throw away any makeup that could be contaminated. Don't wear eye makeup until the infection is all cleared up. Don't share makeup with others.

- Don't share eyedrops with others.

- Don't cover or patch the eye. This can make the infection grow.

- Don't wear contact lenses while your eyes are infected. Disinfect contact lenses before re-using.

**For Allergic Conjunctivitis:**

- Avoid things you know you are allergic to.

- Use over-the-counter eyedrops to soothe irritation and help relieve itching.

- Apply a washcloth rinsed in cold water to the eyes, several times a day.

- Use protective eyewear when you work with chemicals and fumes.

## Contact Doctor When:

- A puslike discharge with redness and irritation occurs.

- Your vision is affected and/or your eye(s) hurt a lot.

- You have tried self-care for a week and symptoms get worse.

- You have frequent bouts of conjunctivitis.

# 9. Sties

A sty is an infection in a tiny gland of the eyelid.

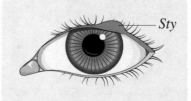

Sty

*Sties, Continued*

## Signs & Symptoms

- Red, painful bump or sore on an eyelid
- Watery or tearing eye that burns and itches
- The red bump may form a head and appears yellow if it contains pus. This usually drains on its own within days.

## Causes & Care

Sties form from clogged oil glands at the base of an eyelash.

Most sties respond well to self-care and don't need further treatment.

### Self-Care/Prevention:

- Wash your hands often.
- Don't touch your eyes with your fingers. Use a tissue instead.
- Use clean washcloths and towels each time you wash your face.
- Don't share washcloths, towels, makeup, or eyedrops with others.
- Don't expose your eyes to excessive dust or dirt.

### To Relieve the Discomfort of a Sty:

- Apply warm (not hot), wet compresses to the affected area 3 to 4 times a day for 5 to 10 minutes at a time. Use a clean washcloth each time.
- Don't poke or squeeze the sty.
- If the sty drains on its own, gently wash the pus away with a clean, wet cloth. Apply an antibiotic ointment with a cotton-tipped swab.

### Contact Doctor When:

- A sty makes it hard for you to see.
- Redness and swelling haven't drained within 1 or 2 days.
- Many sties come at the same time.
- You get one sty right after another.

### For Information On Eye Problems Contact:

American Foundation for the Blind
1-800-232-5463
www.afb.org

Lighthouse International
1-800-829-0500
www.lighthouse.org

National Eye Care Project Help Line
1-800-222-EYES (3937)

## 10. Earaches

### Earaches Chart

| Signs & Symptoms | What It Could Be | What to Do |
|---|---|---|
| Severe pain with swelling, bruising, or bleeding in the ear canal following a recent ear or head trauma. | Ear injury | Get immediate care. |
| Ear pain with stiff neck, high fever, drowsiness, <u>and</u> vomiting. | Meningitis | Get immediate care. |
| Ear pain with some hearing loss, blood or other discharge from ear (especially after sticking an object in the ear or exposure to extremely loud noises). | Ruptured eardrum | Contact doctor. |
| Ear pain, fever, chills, discharge of pus or blood from the ear. Blocked or full feeling in the ear. | Ear infection | Contact doctor. |
| Ear pain with blocked or full feeling in the ear. Ringing in the ear. Temporary, partial hearing loss. | Earwax | See "Earwax" on page 77. |
| Ear pain with jaw pain, headache, and a clicking sound when you open and close your mouth. | Temporomandibular Joint Syndrome (TMJ) | Contact doctor. |
| Ear pain and/or feeling of fullness in the ears during or after flying. | Airplane ears | See "To Open Up the Eustachian Tubes and Help Them Drain" on page 76. |

*Earaches Chart Continued on Next Page*

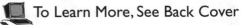 To Learn More, See Back Cover

*Earaches, Continued*

| Earaches Chart, Continued | | |
|---|---|---|
| **Signs & Symptoms** | **What It Could Be** | **What to Do** |
| Pain when you touch or wiggle your earlobe. Discharge from the ear (watery, yellow, or foul-smelling). Blocked feeling in the ear. Itchy, flaky skin by the opening of the ear. (Symptoms usually come after swimming in polluted water.) | Swimmer's ear | See "For a Mild Case of Swimmer's Ear" on page 77. Contact doctor if you still have symptoms after 4 to 5 days of self-care. |

## Prevention

- When you blow your nose, do so gently, one nostril at a time.

- Don't smoke. Avoid secondhand smoke.

- Heed the old saying, "Never put anything smaller than your elbow into your ear". This includes cotton-tipped swabs, bobby pins, your fingers, etc. Doing so could damage your eardrum.

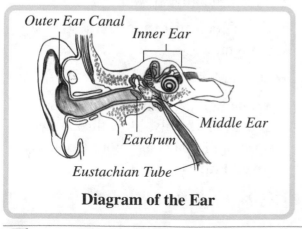

*Outer Ear Canal*
*Inner Ear*
*Middle Ear*
*Eardrum*
*Eustachian Tube*

**Diagram of the Ear**

## Causes & Care

The most common cause of earaches is plugged Eustachian tubes. These tubes go from the back of the throat to your middle ear. When they get blocked, fluid gathers, causing pain. Things that make this happen include an infection of the middle ear, colds, sinus infections, and allergies. Other things that can cause ear pain include changes in air pressure in a plane, something stuck in the ear, too much earwax, tooth problems, and ear injuries.

Self-care treats mild cases of "Swimmers's Ear," "Airplane Ears" and mild ear pain.

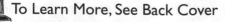

*8. Ear, Nose, & Throat Problems*

## Earaches, *Continued*

Very bad ear pain should be treated by a doctor. Treatment depends on the cause and includes pain relief, an antibiotic for an infection, and/or methods to dry up or clear the blocked ear canal.

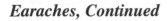 **Self-Care:**

### To Reduce Pain:

- Place a warm washcloth or heating pad (set on low) next to the ear. Some doctors advise putting an ice bag or ice in a wet washcloth over the painful ear for 20 minutes.

- Take an over-the-counter pain reliever. (See "Pain relievers" in "Your Home Pharmacy" on page 43.)

- Chew gum or suck on hard candy. When you do this, you have to swallow often; every time you do, you automatically force small amounts of air into your Eustachian tubes, reducing pain. This action also helps fluid drain from your ears.

### To Open Up the Eustachian Tubes and Help Them Drain:

(Use these tips for "Airplane Ears.")

- Sit up.

- Prop your head up when you sleep.

- Yawn. This helps move the muscles that open the eustachian tubes.

- Chew gum or suck on hard candy. This tip is especially helpful during pressure changes that take place during air travel, but can also be useful during the middle of the night if you wake up with ear pain.

- Stay awake during take-offs and landings.

- Take a decongestant. Don't use a nasal spray decongestant for more than 3 days, though, unless directed by your doctor. Take a decongestant:

  • At the first sign of a cold if you have gotten ear infections often after previous colds

  • One hour before you land when you travel by air if you have a cold or think your sinuses will block up

- Take a steamy shower.

- Use a cool-mist vaporizer, especially at night.

- Drink plenty of cool water.

- While holding both nostrils closed, gently, but firmly, blow through your nose until you hear a pop. Do this several times a day.

*Continued on Next Page*

To Learn More, See Back Cover

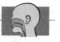

*Earaches, Continued*

## Self-Care, Continued

### For a Mild Case of "Swimmer's Ear":

The goal is to clean and dry the outer ear canal without doing further damage to the top layer of skin.

- Shake your head to expel trapped water.

- Dry the ear canal. Use a clean tissue. Twist each corner into a tip and gently place each tip into the ear canal for 10 seconds. Repeat with the other ear, using a new tissue.

- Use an over-the-counter product, such as Swim-Ear. Follow package directions.

- Do not remove earwax. This coats the ear canal and protects it from moisture.

### To Avoid Getting "Swimmer's Ear":

- Wear wax or silicone earplugs.
- Wear a bathing cap.
- Don't swim in dirty water.
- Swim on the surface of the water instead of underneath the water.

### For an Insect in the Ear:

Shine a flashlight into the ear. Doing this may make the insect come out. Contact your doctor if the insect does not come out.

# 11. Earwax

Earwax coats and protects the lining of the ear canal. It filters dust and helps keep the ears clean. Normally, earwax is soft and drains by itself. Sometimes it hardens and forms a plug.

## Prevention

- Wear earplugs when exposed to excessive dust or dirt.

- Don't use cotton swabs in the ear. They tend to pack the earwax down more tightly.

- Don't push objects into the ear canal.

## Signs & Symptoms

Signs and symptoms of earwax buildup are:

- Blocked or plugged feeling in the ear
- Partial hearing loss (temporary)
- Ringing in the ear
- Ear discomfort or pain

*Earwax, Continued*

## Causes, Risk Factors & Care

- Exposure to excessive dust or dirt
- A family history of earwax buildup

Simple earwax build-up can be treated using self-care. If self-care doesn't take care of the problem, a doctor can clear the earwax with a special vacuum, scoop, or water-pik-like device.

### Self-Care:

{**Note:** Use only if you know that your eardrum is not ruptured or infected. See signs of a ruptured eardrum and ear infection under "Contact Doctor When:" on this page and on page 79.}

- Use an over-the-counter product, such as Murine Ear Drops, Debrox, etc. Follow package directions.
- Hold a warm, wet washcloth on the blocked ear or, take a warm shower. Let the water gently flow into the ear. Use the tip of a warm washcloth to remove the softened wax. Don't use cold water. This may cause dizziness.

- Lie on your side or tilt your head sideways. Using a clean medicine dropper, carefully squeeze a few drops of lukewarm water into your ear. Leave the water there for about 10 minutes. Tilt your head to let the water drain out of the ear. After several minutes, do the same thing again. If the ear wax has not cleared in 3 hours, repeat this entire procedure. {**Note:** Instead of just warm water, you can use a mixture of 1 part warm water and 1 part hydrogen peroxide. Keep the drops in the ear for 3, not 10 minutes, though.}
- Rest a hot water bottle on the affected ear for a few minutes. Afterward, use a washcloth to remove the softened wax.
- Don't try to scrape out earwax. You could put a hole in your eardrum or damage the skin of your ear canal.

### 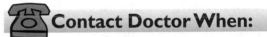Contact Doctor When:

- You have sudden or total hearing loss in one or both ears.
- You have signs of a **ruptured eardrum**:
  - Ear pain
  - Blood or other ear discharge

*Earwax, Continued*

- • Partial hearing loss
- • Ringing or burning in the ear
- ■ You have ear pain with any of these signs of an **ear infection**:
  - • Feeling of fullness in the ear that leads to ear pain
  - • Fever of 101°F or higher
  - • Blood, pus, or fluid from the ear
  - • Temporary hearing loss
  - • Redness and swelling of the skin of the ear canal
  - • Nausea, vomiting, and/or dizziness
- ■ Earwax has not cleared after using self-care for several days.

# 12. Hay Fever

The medical term for hay fever is "allergic rhinitis." Hay fever is most common in spring and fall when there is a lot of ragweed in the air. Some people have hay fever all year, though.

## Signs & Symptoms

- ■ Itchy, watery eyes
- ■ Runny, itchy nose
- ■ Congestion
- ■ Sneezing

## Causes & Care

Hay fever has nothing to do with hay or fever. It is a reaction of the upper respiratory tract to anything which you may be allergic to. Talk to your doctor if self-care measures do not help. He or she may prescribe:

- ■ Antihistamines. For best results, take the antihistamine 30 minutes before going outside. {**Note:** Some over-the-counter antihistamines may cause more drowsiness than prescription ones. Also, care should be taken when driving and operating machinery since antihistamines can make you drowsy.}
- ■ Decongestants, nasal sprays, and other medicines, like cromolyn sodium or corticosteroids
- ■ Skin tests to find out what things you are allergic to
- ■ Allergy shots

It is best to take what your doctor advises instead of testing over-the-counter products on your own.

*Hay Fever, Continued*

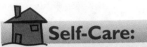 **Self-Care:**

Stay Away From Things That Give You Hay Fever:

- Let someone else do outside chores. Mowing the lawn or raking leaves can make you very sick if you are allergic to pollen and molds.

- Keep windows and doors shut and stay inside when the pollen count or humidity is high.

- Avoid tobacco smoke and other air pollutants.

- To limit dust, mold, and pollen:
  - Use rugs that can be washed often. Don't use carpeting.
  - Dust and vacuum often. Wear a dust filter mask when you do.
  - Use drapes and curtains that can be washed often.
  - Add an electronic air filter to your furnace or use portable air purifiers.
  - Put a plastic cover on your mattress.
  - Do not use a feather pillow.
  - Stay away from stuffed animals. They collect dust.

- Don't dry sheets and blankets outside. Pollen can get on them.

- Shower or bathe and wash your hair following heavy exposure to pollen, dust, etc.

- Put an air conditioner or air cleaner in your house, especially in your bedroom. Clean the filter often.

- Don't have pets. If you have a pet keep it outside the house, if possible.

**Contact Doctor When:**

- You have hay fever symptoms plus symptoms of an infection (fever; nasal discharge or mucus that is green, yellow, or bloody-colored; headache; or muscle aches).

- Hay fever symptoms interfere with your daily activities.

- Hay fever symptoms persist even when you avoid hay fever triggers.

**Get Immediate Care When:**

You have severe breathing difficulties or severe wheezing.

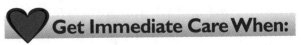

# 13. Hearing Loss

People over age 50 are likely to lose some hearing each year. The decline is usually gradual. About 30% of adults age 65 through 74 and about 50% of those age 85 and older have hearing problems.

Hearing problems can get worse if they are ignored and not treated. Some persons will not admit to a hearing problem. This is often due to fear, vanity, or just not knowing what to do. People with hearing problems may withdraw from others. They do this because they may not be able to understand what others say. Hearing loss can cause an older person to be labeled "confused" or "senile."

## Signs & Symptoms

- Words are hard to understand.
- Another person's speech sounds slurred or mumbled. This worsens when there is background noise.
- Certain sounds are overly loud or annoying.
- Hearing a hissing or ringing background noise. This can be constant or it can come and go.
- Concerts, TV shows, etc. are less enjoyable because much goes unheard.

## Causes & Care

There are many causes. Common ones are:

- **Presbycusis** (prez-bee-KU-sis), a gradual type of hearing loss, is common with aging. With this, you can have a hard time understanding speech. You may not tolerate loud sounds. You may not hear high pitched sounds. Hearing loss from presbycusis cannot be corrected, but it does not cause deafness. Hearing aids and self-care can be helpful.
- Ear wax that blocks the ear canal
- A chronic middle ear infection or an infection of the inner ear
- Medicines. Examples are aspirin and some medicines for arthritis. These can cause ringing in the ears, too.
- Blood vessel disorders, such as high blood pressure
- Acoustic trauma, such as from a blow to the ear or from excessive noise
- **Ménière's disease**, which causes excess fluid in canals of the inner ear.

If you have hearing loss, consult your doctor to find out the cause. Rare causes include tumors, which must be found early for optimum treatment. Your doctor may send you to an ear specialist or a certified audiologist, who tests and treats persons with hearing related problems.

**8. Ear, Nose, & Throat Problems**

*Hearing Loss, Continued*

Treatment for hearing loss includes:

- Earwax removal by a health care provider
- Hearing aid(s), to make sounds louder
- Speech reading, to learn to read lips and facial expressions
- Auditory training, to help you with your specific hearing problems
- Surgery, if the problem requires it

## Self-Care:

### For Gradual, Age-Related Hearing Loss (Presbycusis):

- Ask people to speak clearly, distinctly, and in a normal tone.
- Look at people when they are talking to you. Watch their expressions to help you understand what they are saying. Ask them to face you.
- Try to limit background noise when speaking with someone.
- In a church or theater, sit near, but not in the front row. Sit in the 3rd or 4th row with people sitting around you.

- Install a flasher or amplifier on your phone, door chime, and alarm clock.
- See a certified audiologist for an evaluation. He or she can decide if you need a hearing aid and show you ways to "train" yourself to hear better.
- If a hearing aid is prescribed, learn to use and wear it properly.

### To Hear Sounds Better:

- Use a hearing aid.
- Use listening devices made to assist you in hearing sounds.
- Use special audio equipment that can be installed in your phone.
- Use portable devices made especially to amplify sounds. These can be used for movies, classes, meetings, etc.

### To Clear Earwax:

See "Self-Care" in "Ear Wax" on page 78.

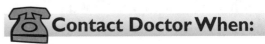 ## Contact Doctor When:

- You have any of these problems with hearing loss:
  - Discharge from the ear
  - Earache
  - Dizziness or feeling that things are spinning around you

To Learn More, See Back Cover

**8. Ear, Nose, & Throat Problems**

*Hearing Loss, Continued*

- Recent ear or upper respiratory infection

- Feeling that the ears are blocked or filled with wax

- You are not able to hear a regular (nondigital) watch ticking when you hold it next to your ear.

- You have a ringing sound in one or both ears all of the time.

- Hearing loss after recent exposure to loud noises (airplanes, machines, etc.) has not improved.

- Hearing loss occurs after taking a new medicine.

- Sudden hearing loss occurs in one ear.

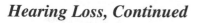
### Get Immediate Care When:

- All of these symptoms occur: Sudden hearing loss, ear pain, dizziness, blood or other discharge from the ear, and ringing sounds.

- A recent head or ear injury occurs with hearing loss with one or more of these problems:

  - Swelling or bruising behind the ear

  - Blood in the ear canal

  - Earache

## For Information Contact:

American Speech – Language Hearing Association
1-800-638-8255
www.asha.org

Better Hearing Institute
Hearing Help Line
1-800-327-9355
www.betterhearing.org

# 14. Laryngitis

Laryngitis is when your larynx (voice box) is irritated or inflamed.

## Signs & Symptoms

- Hoarse, husky, and weak voice or loss of voice

- Cough

- Sore throat, fever, and/or trouble swallowing (sometimes)

## Causes, Risk Factors & Care

- Irritants, such as smoke and air pollution

- Bacterial or viral infections

- Allergies

- Strained vocal cords

- Tumors or growths on the vocal cords or nerve damage to the vocal cords

- Thyroid disease

**8. Ear, Nose, & Throat Problems**

*8. Ear, Nose, & Throat Problems*

***Laryngitis, Continued***

Smoking, drinking alcohol, breathing cold air, and continuing to use already distressed vocal cords can make the problem worse.

Self-care treats most cases of laryngitis. If necessary, your doctor may prescribe an antibiotic for a bacterial infection.

## Self-Care:

- Don't talk if you don't need to. Instead, use a notepad and pencil to write notes. If you must speak, do so softly, but don't whisper.

- Use a cool-mist humidifier in your bedroom.

- Drink a lot of fluids. Drink warm drinks, such as weak tea, and/or hot water with honey and/or lemon juice.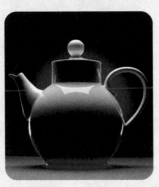

- Gargle every few hours with warm salt water ($1/4$ teaspoon of salt in a $1/2$ cup of warm water).

- Let hot water run in the shower or bath to make steam. Sit in the bathroom and breathe the moist air.

- Don't smoke. Avoid secondhand smoke.

- Suck on cough drops, throat lozenges, or hard candy.

- Take an over-the-counter medicine for pain and/or inflammation. (See "Pain relievers" in "Your Home Pharmacy" on page 43.)

## Contact Doctor When:

- You have a fever or cough up yellow, green, or bloody-colored mucus.

- You have hard, swollen lymph glands in your neck or you feel like you have a "lump" in your throat.

- Hoarseness has lasted more than a month.

- You have symptoms of low thyroid. (See "Thyroid Problems" on page 301.)

# 15. Nosebleeds

## Signs & Symptoms

- Bleeding from a nostril

- Bleeding from the nose and down the back of the throat

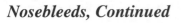

*Nosebleeds, Continued*

## Causes, Risk Factors & Care

Nosebleeds are often caused by broken blood vessels just inside the nose. Risk factors include:

- A cold or allergies
- Frequent nose blowing and picking
- Dry environment
- Using too much nasal spray
- A punch or other blow to the nose

A nosebleed is serious when heavy bleeding from deep within the nose is hard to stop. This type usually strikes the elderly. It can be caused by:

- Hardening of nasal blood vessels
- High blood pressure
- Medicines to treat blood clots
- A tumor in the nose

Self-care treats most nosebleeds. If they occur often, your doctor can order tests to diagnose the cause. Treatment for nosebleeds includes:

- Treating high blood pressure, if present
- Packing the nostril to stop the bleeding
- Cauterization. This seals the bleeding blood vessel.

### Self-Care:

- Sit with your head leaning forward.
- Pinch the nostrils shut, using your thumb and forefinger in such a way that

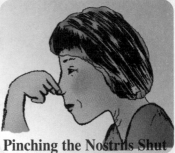

**Pinching the Nostrils Shut**

the nasal septum (the nose's midsection) is being gently squeezed.

- Hold for 15 uninterrupted minutes, breathing through your mouth.
- At the same time, apply cold compresses (such as ice in a soft cloth) to the area around the nose.
- For the next 24 hours, make sure your head is elevated above the level of your heart.
- Also, wait 24 hours before blowing your nose, lifting heavy objects, or exercising strenuously.

### Contact Doctor When:

- A nosebleed lasts 15 or more minutes.
- A nosebleed started after taking newly prescribed medicine.
- Nosebleeds happen often.

8. Ear, Nose, & Throat Problems

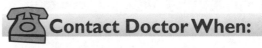

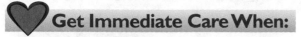

**8. Ear, Nose, & Throat Problems**

*Nosebleeds, Continued*

## ♥ Get Immediate Care When:

- A nosebleed followed a blow to another part of the head.
- A nosebleed occurs in a person taking blood-thinning medicine.

# 16. Sinus Infections

Your sinuses are behind your cheekbones and forehead, and around your eyes.

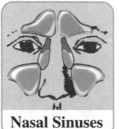

**Nasal Sinuses**

Healthy sinuses drain almost a quart of mucus every day. They keep the air you breathe wet. Your sinuses can't drain right if they are infected and swollen.

## Signs & Symptoms

- Fever
- Greenish-yellow or bloody colored nasal discharge
- Severe headache which doesn't get better when you take an over-the-counter pain reliever
- Headache that is worse in the morning or when you bend forward
- Pain between the nose and lower eyelid
- A feeling of pressure inside the head
- Eye pain, blurred vision, or changes in vision
- Cheek or upper jaw pain
- Swelling around the eyes, nose, cheeks, and forehead
- Foul-smelling or tasting postnasal drip

## Causes, Risk Factors & Care

Your chances of getting a sinus infection increase if you smoke, have hay fever, a nasal deformity, or an abscess in an upper tooth. Chances also increase if you sneeze hard with your mouth closed or blow your nose too much when you have a cold.

A sinus infection is treated with an antibiotic, a decongestant, and nose drops. Severe cases may require surgery to drain the sinuses.

You may have sinus congestion without an infection. With this, the drainage is clear and there is no fever. This does not require an antibiotic. A decongestant can help, though.

To Learn More, See Back Cover

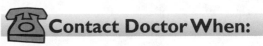
*Sinus Infections, Continued*

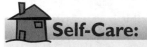 **Self-Care:**

- Use a cool-mist humidifier.

- Put a warm washcloth, warm compress, or cold compress over the sinus areas of your face. Use the one that better helps with the pain.

- Drink plenty of fluids.

- Take an over-the-counter pain reliever. (See "Pain relievers" in "Your Home Pharmacy" on page 43.)

- Take an over-the-counter oral decongestant, but only with your doctor's okay. You may find it easier to take an over-the-counter product that has both a pain reliever and a decongestant, such as Tylenol Sinus. {**Note:** Decongestants with antihistamines can cause urinary problems in older men.}

- Use nose drops for only the number of days prescribed. Repeated use of them creates a dependency. To avoid picking up germs, don't borrow nose drops from others. Don't let anyone else use yours. Throw the drops away after treatment.

**Contact Doctor When:**

You have 2 or more signs and symptoms of a sinus infection listed on page 86.

## 17. Sore Throats

Sore throats range from a mere scratch to pain so severe that it hurts to swallow saliva.

## Signs & Symptoms

- Dry, irritated throat
- Cough
- A hard time swallowing or pain with swallowing
- Swollen glands in the neck

**Symptoms of Strep Throat:**

- Fever
- The back of the throat looks bright red or has patches of pus.
- The tonsils and/or neck glands are swollen.

## Causes, Risk Factors & Care

- Smoking
- Breathing dust or harmful fumes
- Dry air
- Not drinking enough fluids

## Sore Throats, Continued

- Postnasal drip
- Upper respiratory infection
- Infection from bacteria, such as strep throat, or from a fungus

Self-care treats most sore throats. Your doctor may take a throat culture to see if strep or another type of bacteria is the cause. If so, he or she will prescribe an antibiotic. Be sure you take all of the antibiotic. An antifungal medicine is used to treat a fungal infection.

### Self-Care:

- Gargle every few hours with a solution of $1/4$ teaspoon of salt dissolved in $1/2$ cup of warm water or with hot or cold, double strength tea.
- Drink plenty of fluids, such as warm tea (with or without honey), and broth. If you are on a sodium-restricted diet, use low-sodium broth.
- For strep throat, eat and drink cold foods and liquids, such as frozen yogurt, popsicles, and ice water.
- Rest your voice, if this helps.
- Avoid eating spicy foods.

- Let hot water run in the shower. Sit in the bathroom when you do this. The steam will moisten your throat.
- Use a cool-mist vaporizer in the room where your spend most of your time.
- Don't smoke. Avoid secondhand smoke.
- Suck on a piece of hard candy or throat lozenge every so often.
- Take an over-the-counter pain reliever. (See "Pain relievers" in "Your Home Pharmacy" on page 43.)
- Take an over-the-counter decongestant for postnasal drip, if okay with your doctor.

### Contact Doctor When:

- You have any of these problems with a sore throat:
  - Fever
  - Swollen neck glands
  - The back of your throat or tonsils look bright red or have pus.
  - Ear pain
  - Bad breath
  - Skin rash
  - Dark urine
  - Diabetes

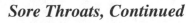

*Sore Throats, Continued*

- You have been in close contact with someone with strep throat over the last 2 weeks.

- The sore throat lasts for more than 3 weeks.

### ♥ Get Immediate Care When:

- You have a very hard time breathing with severe shortness of breath and can't say 4 or 5 words between breaths.

- You can't swallow your own saliva.

# 18. Tinnitus (Ringing in Ears)

Tinnitus is hearing ringing or other noises in the ears when no outside source makes the sounds. Almost everyone gets "ringing in the ears" at one time or another. This may last a minute or so, but then goes away. When hearing these sounds persists, suspect tinnitus. The noises can range in volume from a ring to a roar. Tinnitus affects nearly 36 million Americans, most of them older adults.

## Signs & Symptoms

- Ringing, buzzing, hissing, humming, roaring, or whistling noises in the ears, which can persist or come and go.

- Problems sleeping

- Emotional distress

- Hearing loss

Tinnitus can be quite disturbing. It can interfere with normal activities.

## Causes & Care

Exposure to loud noise which damages nerves in the inner ear is the most common cause. This can be from prolonged exposure or from one extreme incident.

Other causes include:

- Ear disorders, such as **labyrinthitis**, an inflammation of canals in the ear that help maintain balance

- Persistent allergies

- High blood pressure

- Reactions to drugs. These include: Aspirin; levodopa (for Parkinson's disease); quinidine (for irregular heartbeats); propranolol (for high blood pressure, etc.); quinine (for leg cramps); caffeine.

In some cases, no cause is found.

*8. Ear, Nose, & Throat Problems*

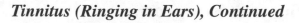

*Tinnitus (Ringing in Ears), Continued*

Treatment is aimed at finding and treating the cause of tinnitus. Treatment includes:

■ A hearing aid that plays a soothing sound to drown out the tinnitus

■ A tinnitus masker. Worn on the ear, it makes a subtle noise that masks the tinnitus without interfering with hearing and speech.

■ Sleeping pills, if needed

Also, support groups and clinics for tinnitus are available in most major cities.

### Self-Care:

■ Treat an ear infection right away.

■ For mild cases of tinnitus, play the radio or a white noise tape (white noise is a low, constant sound) in the background to help mask the tinnitus.

■ Use biofeedback or other relaxation techniques.

■ Exercise regularly. This promotes good blood circulation.

■ Limit your intake of caffeine, alcohol, nicotine, and aspirin.

■ Talk to your doctor if you use the drugs listed in "Causes & Care", on page 89.

■ Wear earplugs or earmuffs when exposed to loud noises. This can prevent noise-induced tinnitus.

■ If the noises started during or after traveling in an airplane, pinch your nostrils and blow through your nose. When you fly, chew gum or suck on hard candy to prevent the ear popping and ringing sounds in the ear. If possible, avoid flying when you have an upper respiratory or ear infection.

### Contact Doctor When:

■ You have 1 or more of these problems with tinnitus:

• Dizziness or vertigo

• Unsteadiness in walking or loss of balance

• Vomiting

• Sudden hearing loss

• Your sleep habits and/or daily activities are disrupted.

■ Tinnitus started after taking aspirin or other medicines that have salicylates, such as Trilisate or Disalcid.

### For Information Contact:

The American Tinnitus Association
1-800-634-8978
www.ata.org

To Learn More, See Back Cover

8. Ear, Nose, & Throat Problems

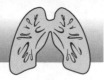

## 19. Asthma

Asthma is a disease that affects the air passages in the lungs. People with asthma have supersensitive airways (air tubes). Exposure to "triggers" (see "Asthma Attack Triggers" in next column) causes a response in the airways. This response is called an "attack" or "episode."

## Signs & Symptoms

- Shortness of breath
- Breathing gets harder and may hurt
- It is harder to breathe out than in
- Wheezing
- Tightness in the chest
- A cough that lasts more than a week. Coughing may be the only symptom. It may occur during the night or after exercising.

## Causes, Risk Factors & Care

What causes asthma is not yet known. You are more likely to have asthma if other members of your family have or had asthma and/or you have allergies.

Asthma is not caused by emotional problems. Strong emotions, whether happy or sad, can bring on an asthma attack, though.

### Asthma Attack Triggers

- Respiratory infections (colds, flu, bronchitis, sinus infections)
- Things you are allergic to, such as pollen, dust, molds, and animal dander
- Irritants, such as tobacco smoke, air pollution, fumes, and vapors
- Sulfites. These are additives found in wine and some processed foods.
- Cold air and changes in temperature and humidity
- Exercise, especially in outdoor cold air
- Some medicines, such as aspirin, beta blockers, and ACE inhibitors
- Showing strong feelings. This includes laughing and crying.
- Hormone changes, such as those that come with menopause

Asthma is too complex to treat with over-the-counter products. A doctor should diagnose asthma and keep track of how you are doing. He or she may prescribe:

- Anti-inflammatories. These drugs help with the swelling in the airways. They are taken as oral pills or inhaled medicines.

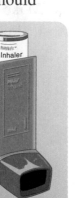

**Inhaler\***

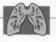

### Asthma, Continued

- Bronchodilators. These drugs relax the muscles of the airways and open up the air passages in the lungs. A metered-dose inhaler with a device called a spacer is a common way to take these drugs.

- Anti-leukotriene pills to help reduce chronic inflammation

- Peak flow meter to monitor your asthma at home

- Annual flu vaccine

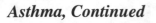 **Self-Care:**

- Drink 2 to 3 quarts of fluids a day to keep secretions loose.

- Avoid your asthma triggers.

- Don't smoke. Avoid secondhand smoke and air pollution.

- Make a special effort to keep your bedroom allergen-free.

  - Sleep with a foam, cotton, or other pillow that is made with an artificial fiber. Don't use a feather pillow. Wash pillows regularly. Replace pillows every 2 to 3 years.

  - Totally enclose your mattress, box springs, and pillows in allergen-proof covers.

- Wash mattress pads in hot water every week.

- Use throw rugs that can be washed or dry cleaned often. Don't use carpeting.

- Use drapes or curtains that can be washed often.

- Vacuum and dust often. Wear a dust filter mask when you do.

- Reduce clutter in your bedroom.

- Don't store things under the bed.

- Don't use bed ruffles and throw pillows on your bed.

- Put an air filter on your furnace or use portable air purifiers, such as ones with HEPA filters.

- Change and/or wash furnace and air conditioner filters on a regular basis.

- Stay out of the cold weather as much as you can.

- When you are outside in cold weather, wear a scarf around your mouth and nose. Doing so will warm the air as you breathe in and will prevent cold air from reaching sensitive airways.

- Stop exercising if you start wheezing.

- Don't take over-the-counter medicines unless your doctor tells you to.

*Continued on Next Page*

**9. Respiratory Conditions**

## Asthma, Continued

### Self-Care, Continued

- Take your medicines as prescribed.
- Use your inhaler the right way.
- Use your peak flow meter as advised. Keep records of results.
- Keep your asthma medicine handy. Take it at the start of an attack.
- During an asthma attack sit up; don't lie down. Keep calm. Focus on breathing slow and easy. Remove yourself from any stressors.

### Contact Doctor When:

- Changes occur in your asthma status: It is harder for you to breathe, you are short of breath more often than before, or you are breathing faster than usual.
- Your asthma attack does not respond to your medicines or they are not helping like they used to.
- With asthma, you have a fever, cold, the flu, and/or a cough with mucus.
- You have signs and symptoms of asthma listed on page 91. {**Note:** New onset of asthma symptoms in older adults may be a sign of heart disease.}

### Get Immediate Care When:

- You have severe shortness of breath or can't say 4 or 5 words between breaths or have purple lips or finger tips.
- You cough so much that you can't take a breath or have wheezing that doesn't stop.

## For Information Contact:

The Asthma and Allergy Foundation of America
1-800-7-ASTHMA (727-8462)
www.aafa.org

National Heart, Lung and Blood Institute (NHLBI)
1-800-575-WELL (575-9355)
www.nhlbi.nih.gov

# 20. Bronchitis

Acute bronchitis is inflammation of the air passages of the lung. Chronic bronchitis is inflammation and degeneration of the air passages of the lung.

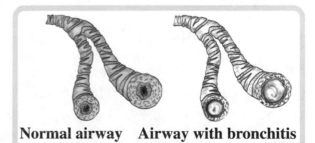

**Normal airway      Airway with bronchitis**

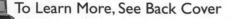
9. Respiratory Conditions

*Bronchitis, Continued*

## Signs & Symptoms

### For Acute Bronchitis:

- Cough with little or no sputum

- Chills, fever less than 101°F

- Sore throat and muscle aches

- Feeling of pressure behind the breast-bone or a burning feeling in the chest

### For Chronic Bronchitis:

- A cough with mucus or phlegm for 3 months or longer at a time and this occurs for more than 2 years in a row

- Shortness of breath upon exertion (in early stages)

- Shortness of breath at rest (in later stages)

Many people, most of them smokers, develop emphysema (destruction of the air sacs) along with chronic bronchitis. This is **chronic obstructive pulmonary disease (COPD)**.

## Causes & Care

### For Acute Bronchitis:

Causes are a viral or bacterial infection and pollutants, like smog.

These attack the mucous membranes within the windpipe or air passages in your respiratory tract, leaving them red and inflamed.

Acute bronchitis often develops in the wake of a sinus infection, cold, or other respiratory infection. It can last anywhere from 3 days to 3 weeks.

Treatment includes bronchodilators and an antibiotic.

### For Chronic Bronchitis:

Causes include:

- Cigarette smoking. This is the most common cause.

- Air pollution

- Repeated infections of the air passages of the lungs

Chronic bronchitis results in abnormal air exchange in the lungs and causes permanent damage to the respiratory tract. It's much more serious than acute bronchitis. Chronic bronchitis is not contagious.

Medical treatment is needed for airway infections and heart problems, if present. Supplemental oxygen is given when needed.

To Learn More, See Back Cover

**9. Respiratory Conditions**

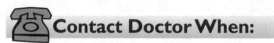

**Bronchitis, Continued**

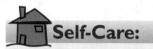

## Self-Care:

- Don't smoke. Avoid secondhand smoke.

- Reduce your exposure to air pollution. Use air conditioning, air filters, and a mouth and nose filter mask if you have to. If you develop bronchitis easily, stay indoors during episodes of heavy air pollution.

- Rest, when you must.

- Drink plenty of liquids.

- Breathe air from a cool-mist vaporizer. Note, though, that vaporizers can harbor bacteria, so clean them after each use. Inhaling bacteria-laden mist may aggravate bronchitis. Use distilled, not tap, water in the vaporizer.

- Take an over-the-counter medicine for fever, pain, and/or inflammation. (See "Pain relievers" in "Your Home Pharmacy" on page 43.)

- Instead of cough suppressants, use expectorants. Use bronchodilators and/or take antibiotics as prescribed by your doctor.

## Contact Doctor When:

- You have a fever of 101°F or higher.

- You cough up green, yellow, or bloody-colored mucus, or you vomit.

- You have an increase in chest pain.

- You have shortness of breath at rest and at non-coughing times.

## Get Immediate Care When:

You have severe shortness of breath and can't say 4 or 5 words between breaths or you have purple lips.

# 21. Common Cold

## Prevention

- Wash your hands often. Keep them away from your nose, eyes, and mouth.

- Try not to touch people or their things when they have a cold, especially the first 2 to 3 days they have the cold.

- Get regular exercise. Eat and sleep well.

- Use a handkerchief or tissues when you sneeze, cough, or blow your nose. This helps keep you from passing cold viruses to others.

- Use a cool-mist vaporizer in your bedroom in the winter.

To Learn More, See Back Cover

**9. Respiratory Conditions**

## Common Cold, Continued

- When you get a cold, check with your doctor about using zinc lozenges. They may shorten the duration of a cold and ease cold symptoms.

## Signs & Symptoms

- Runny, stuffy nose, and sneezing
- Sore throat
- Dry cough
- Fever of 101°F or less, if any

A cold usually lasts 3 to 7 days. In older persons, though, a cold can last longer. The cough that comes with a cold can last a few weeks after the other symptoms go away.

## Causes & Care

Colds are caused by viruses. You can get a cold virus from mucus on a person's hands when they have a cold, such as through a handshake. You can also pick up the viruses on towels, telephones, money, etc. Cold viruses also travel through coughs and sneezes.

Time and self-care usually treat a cold. Having a cold leaves you more open to getting a bacterial infection, though. If this occurs, you may need an antibiotic prescribed by your doctor.

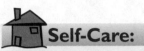

## Self-Care:

- Drink lots of liquids.
- Take an over-the-counter medicine for muscle aches and pains, and/or fever. (See "Pain relievers" in "Your Home Pharmacy" on page 43.)
- Use salt water drops for nasal congestion. Mix $1/2$ teaspoon of salt in 1 cup of warm water. Place in a clean container. Put 3 to 4 drops into each nostril several times a day with a clean medicine dropper.
- Use a cool-mist vaporizer to add moisture to the air.
- Have chicken soup to clear mucus.
- Check with your doctor about taking vitamin C. It seems to make some people feel better when they have a cold and may help prevent a cold, even though this has never been medically proven.

### For a Sore Throat:

- Gargle every few hours with a solution of $1/4$ teaspoon of salt dissolved in $1/2$ cup of warm water.
- Drink tea with lemon (with or without honey).
- Suck on a piece of hard candy or medicated lozenge every so often.

To Learn More, See Back Cover

## Common Cold, *Continued*

### 📞 Contact Doctor When:

Any of the following occur with a cold:

- Quick breathing, trouble breathing, or wheezing

- A temperature of 102°F or higher (101°F or higher in a person over age 60)

- You have any of these problems:
  - A bad smell from the throat, nose, or ears or an earache
  - A headache that doesn't go away
  - A bright red sore throat or sore throat with white spots

- You cough up mucus that is yellow, green, or gray.

- You have pain or swelling over your sinuses that gets worse when you bend over or move your head, especially with a fever of 101°F or higher.

- Symptoms get worse after 4 to 5 days or don't get better after 7 days.

- Symptoms other than a slight cough last for more than 14 days.

# 22. Coughs

Coughing clears the lungs and airways. Coughing itself is not the problem. What causes the cough is the problem.

## Signs & Symptoms

There are 3 kinds of coughs:

- Productive. This is a cough that brings up mucus or phlegm.

- Nonproductive. This is a dry cough.

- Reflex. This is a cough that comes from a problem somewhere else, like the ear or stomach.

## Causes & Care

Common causes are infections, allergies, tobacco smoke, and dry air. Other causes include having something stuck in your windpipe, acid reflux from the stomach, and certain medications, like some used to treat high blood pressure and congestive heart failure. Coughing is also a symptom of medical conditions, such as emphysema, congestive heart failure, tuberculosis, and lung cancer.

Self-care can treat most coughs. If the cause is due to a medical condition, treatment for that condition is needed.

**9. Respiratory Conditions**

*Coughs, Continued*

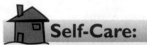 **Self-Care:**

### For Coughs that Bring Up Mucus:

- Drink plenty of liquids.

- Use a cool-mist vaporizer, especially in the bedroom. Put a humidifier on the furnace.

- Take a shower. The steam can help thin the mucus.

- Ask your pharmacist for an over-the-counter expectorant.

- Don't smoke. Avoid secondhand smoke.

### For Coughs that Are Dry:

- Drink plenty of liquids. Drink tea with lemon and honey.

- Suck on cough drops or hard candy.

- Take an over-the-counter cough medicine that has dextromethorphan.

- For postnasal drip, take a decongestant, if okay with your doctor.

- Make your own cough medicine. Mix 1 part lemon juice and 2 parts honey. Take 1 teaspoon 4 to 5 times a day.

**Other Tips:**

- Chew and swallow foods slowly so they don't "go down the wrong way".

- Stay away from chemical gases that can hurt your lungs.

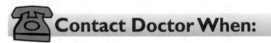 **Contact Doctor When:**

- You have wheezing, shortness of breath, rapid breathing, or swelling of the abdomen, legs, and ankles.

- You have a cough that starts suddenly and lasts an hour or more without stopping.

- You have an itchy, red splotchy rash with the cough.

- With a cough, you have a temperature of 102°F or higher (101°F or higher in a person over age 60).

- Your chest hurts only when you cough and the pain goes away when you sit up or lean forward.

- You cough up green, yellow, or bloody-colored mucus.

- With a cough, you lose weight for no reason, feel tired, and sweat a lot at night.

- Your cough lasts for more than 2 weeks without getting better.

To Learn More, See Back Cover

**9. Respiratory Conditions**

*Coughs, Continued*

##  Get Immediate Care When:

- With a cough, you have trouble breathing and can't say more than 4 or 5 words between breaths.

- You have sudden, severe pain in the chest wall followed by a cough and breathlessness without pain.

- You faint or cough up true red blood.

- You have a very sudden onset of coughing from inhaling a small object.

## 23. Emphysema

Emphysema is a chronic lung condition. With emphysema, the air sacs (alveoli) in the lungs are destroyed. The lung loses its elasticity and ability to take in oxygen.

When emphysema occurs with chronic bronchitis, it is called **chronic obstructive pulmonary disease (COPD)**.

## Prevention

- Don't smoke. Avoid secondhand smoke.

- Limit exposure to air pollution and lung irritants. Follow safety measures when working with materials that can irritate your lungs.

## Signs & Symptoms

Emphysema takes years to develop. When symptoms occur, they include:

- Shortness of breath on exertion. This gets worse over time.

- Wheezing

- Fatigue

- Repeated chest infections (colds and bronchitis)

- Slight body build with marked weight loss and a rounded chest that doesn't appear to expand when breathing in

## Causes, Risk Factors & Care

Emphysema is called "the smoker's disease." Most people with emphysema are cigarette smokers aged 50 or older.

Other causes include a genetic deficiency of a certain protein that protects the lungs from damage; repeated lung infections, chronic bronchitis, and asthma. Air pollution and exposure to lung irritants (workplace or other chemicals, including perfumed products, fumes, dust, etc.) can also cause emphysema.

By the time emphysema is detected, 50% to 70% of your lung tissue may already be destroyed. Treatment includes:

- A program, medication, and/or nicotine replacement to help you stop smoking

### *Emphysema, Continued*

- Physical therapy to loosen mucus in your lungs if you have chronic bronchitis

- Medicines, such as bronchodilators, corticosteroids, and antibiotics

- Flu and pneumonia vaccines

Emphysema can't be reversed. Prevention is the only way to avoid permanent damage.

## Self-Care:

- Don't smoke. If you smoke, quit. Avoid secondhand smoke.

- Use a cool mist vaporizer indoors.

- Drink plenty of fluids.

- Avoid dust, fumes, pollutants, etc.

- Do breathing exercises as advised by your doctor.

- Exercise daily as prescribed by your doctor or exercise therapist.

## Contact Doctor When:

- You have signs and symptoms of emphysema listed on page 99.

- With emphysema, your cough worsens.

- Your legs and ankles swell more than usual and/or you have a fever.

## Get Immediate Care When:

- Your skin is bluish or purple colored.

- You have severe shortness of breath or you can't say 4 or 5 words between breaths.

- You cough up true red blood.

# 24. Flu

Flu is short for "influenza." It is a virus that affects your nose, throat, breathing tube, and lungs. "Stomach flu" is stomach upset and diarrhea caused by a virus in the stomach and intestines. It is <u>not</u> true flu.

## Prevention

Aging itself, and a separate or recent illness can lower your resistance. To reduce your risk of getting the flu:

- Get a flu shot each fall if you are age 65 or older. You may be told to get a flu shot if you are younger than age 65 and have a chronic medical condition, such as diabetes, heart or lung disease, or if you are a caregiver. {**Note:** Persons allergic to eggs should not get a flu shot.}

- Stay away from persons with the flu.

- Wash your hands often and keep them away from your eyes, nose, and mouth.

- Eat well. Get plenty of rest. Exercise regularly.

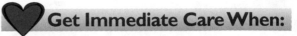 To Learn More, See Back Cover

**9. Respiratory Conditions**

*Flu, Continued*

## Causes, Risk Factors & Care

Flu is caused by certain viruses. Each year, different strains of types of viruses, such as type A and/or type B, cause the flu. The flu is picked up by hand-to-hand contact of the virus or by breathing in air droplets that contain the virus.

Each year, 20,000 people die from pneumonia and other complications of the flu. Older adults are especially at risk for flu complications if they are 65 or older, frail, and/or have:

- A chronic lung disease, such as emphysema or bronchitis

- Heart disease

- Anemia

- Diabetes

- A weakened immune system from an illness, chemotherapy, taking corticosteroids, etc.

When you get the flu, you are also more prone to bronchitis, sinus, and ear infections.

Most often, self-care treats the flu. Medical treatment may be needed for persons over 50, especially for those mentioned earlier, who are at risk of complications from the flu. Besides the annual flu shot, your doctor may prescribe:

- Medicines to relieve flu symptoms

| Signs & Symptoms | Flu | Cold |
|---|---|---|
| Fever, chills | Can last 3 to 4 days. Usual; can be high fever. | Low fever, if any |
| Headache | Usual | Rare |
| General aches and pains | Usual; often severe; affect the body all over | Mild, if any |
| Fatigue, weakness | Usual; often severe. Makes you want to stay in bed. | Mild, if any |
| Runny, stuffy nose | Sometimes | Common |
| Sneezing | Sometimes | Usual |
| Sore throat | Sometimes | Common |
| Cough | Common; can become severe. | Mild to moderate; hacking cough |

**9. Respiratory Conditions**

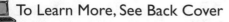

**9. Respiratory Conditions**

### *Flu, Continued*

■ Antiviral medicines. Examples are Relenza, Tamiflu, amantadine, and rimantadine. These medicines help make flu symptoms milder and help you recover sooner. Relenza and Tamiflu are effective for Type A flu and Type B flu. Amantadine and rimantadine are effective for only type A flu. {**Note:** Some antiviral medicines cause mental status changes in older persons and may be worse than the flu itself.}

■ An antibiotic, if a bacterial infection is also present

### Self-Care:

■ Rest and drink plenty of fluids.

■ Gargle with: Warm, strong tea; warm salt water ($^1/_4$ teaspoon of salt in 1 cup of water); or 1 tablespoon of hot water mixed with 1 tablespoon of mouthwash.

■ Take an over-the-counter medicine for fever and/or muscle aches. (See "Pain relievers" in "Your Home Pharmacy" on page 43.)

■ Suck on lozenges or hard candies to lubricate your throat.

■ Don't suppress a cough that produces mucus. Ask your pharmacist for an over-the-counter expectorant if this is all right with your doctor.

■ Avoid contact with others so you don't spread the flu.

■ Wash your hands often, especially after blowing your nose and before handling food.

### Contact Doctor When:

■ Your flu symptoms begin. Your doctor may prescribe an antiviral medicine, especially if you are at risk for complications from the flu.

■ You have: An earache, sinus pain, or thick mucus or phlegm.

■ You have chills or muscle aches with a fever of 101°F or higher.

■ Flu symptoms get worse or you have had the flu more than a week and not felt better using self-care.

■ You get bothersome side effects from prescribed or over-the-counter medicines.

To Learn More, See Back Cover

##  Get Immediate Care When:

- You have purple lips, severe shortness of breath, or wheezing.
- You cough up true red blood.

# 25. Lung Cancer

Lung cancer is the leading cause of death from cancer in men and women. It is especially deadly because the rich network of blood vessels that deliver oxygen from the lungs to the rest of the body can spread cancer very quickly. By the time it's diagnosed, other organs may be affected. The lungs are also a frequent site that cancer from other areas of the body spreads to.

## Prevention:

- Don't smoke. If you smoke, quit. Avoid secondhand smoke.
- Avoid or limit exposure to environmental pollutants and asbestos.

## Signs & Symptoms

Lung cancer does not usually cause symptoms when it first develops. When symptoms occur, they include:

- Chronic cough. This is the most common symptom.

- Hoarseness
- Blood-streaked sputum
- Shortness of breath, wheezing
- Repeated bouts of pneumonia or bronchitis
- Chest discomfort with each breath
- Appetite and weight loss
- Fatigue

## Causes, Risk Factors & Care

Cigarette smoking is the major cause. The more you smoke, the greater the risk. Also, the longer you smoke and the more deeply you inhale the smoke, the greater your risk of getting lung cancer. Other causes are exposure to secondhand smoke, asbestos, radon, and other cancer-causing agents

Treatment for lung cancer includes:

- Tests to determine the type of lung cancer present and the stage of the disease
- Lung surgery
- Respiratory therapy
- Radiation therapy
- Chemotherapy

**9. Respiratory Conditions**

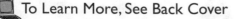

*Lung Cancer, Continued*

### Self-Care:

Follow "Prevention" tips in this topic and your doctor's treatment plan.

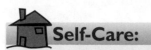

### Contact Doctor When:

- You have one or more signs and symptoms of lung cancer listed on page 103.
- You are age 45 or over and smoke heavily.
- You want advice on nicotine replacement, and/or programs and/or medication to help you stop smoking.

## For Information Contact:

Cancer Information Service
1-800-4-CANCER (422-6237)
www.nci.nih.gov

# 26. Pneumonia

Pneumonia is lung inflammation. It is one of the leading causes of death in the United States, especially in the elderly.

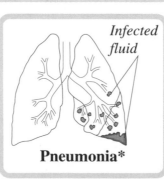

*Infected fluid*

**Pneumonia\***

## Prevention

- Get vaccines for influenza and pneumonia. (See "Immunizations" on page 36.)
- Don't smoke. If you smoke, quit. Avoid secondhand smoke.

## Signs & Symptoms

- Chest pain when breathing in
- Fever and chills
- Cough, often with bloody, dark yellow, green, or rust-colored sputum
- Shortness of breath
- Rapid breathing
- Appetite loss
- Fatigue, headache, nausea, vomiting
- Bluish lips and fingertips, if severe

## Causes, Risk Factors & Care

Viral or bacterial infections are the most common causes. Other causes are fungal infections and chemical irritants, like poisonous gases that are inhaled.

In general, elderly persons are at a greater risk for pneumonia than others because the body's ability to fight off disease lessens with age. Other factors are:

- Having had pneumonia before

## Pneumonia, Continued

- Being in the hospital for other conditions
- A suppressed cough reflex after a stroke
- Smoking
- Malnutrition, alcoholism, or drug use
- A recent respiratory infection
- Emphysema or chronic bronchitis
- Radiation treatments, chemotherapy, or any medications which wear down the immune system
- HIV/AIDS

Treatment for pneumonia will depend on its type (viral, bacterial, or chemical) and location. Treatment includes:

- Medicines, such as antibiotics for bacterial pneumonia; antiviral or anti-fungal medicines; nose drops, sprays, or oral decongestants; and cough medicines as needed
- Oxygen therapy, hospitalization, and removing fluid from the lungs, if needed

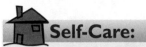

## Self-Care:

Any type of pneumonia is serious and can be life-threatening. With medical care, you may be advised to:

- Get plenty of rest. Rest in bed if you have a fever.
- Use a cool-mist vaporizer in the room or rooms in which you spend most of your time.
- Drink plenty of fluids.
- Take medicines as prescribed by your doctor. Take the medicine for pain and/or fever that your doctor advises. Over-the-counter pain relievers should be avoided for some types of bacterial pneumonia.

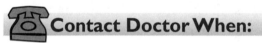

## Contact Doctor When:

- You have signs and symptoms of pneumonia.
- You need a flu or pneumonia vaccine.

## Get Immediate Care When:

- You have severe shortness of breath.
- You have blue or purple-colored lips and fingertips.

**9. Respiratory Conditions**

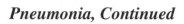

## 27. How Aging Affects the Skin

As you age, you may notice these changes in your skin:

- Your skin gets thinner.

- Your skin sags and loses its ability to snap back after being stretched

- Your skin bruises and tears more easily and takes longer to heal.

- You sweat less.

- Your skin gets dry and itches more easily. About 85 percent of older people develop "winter itch." The loss of sweat and oil glands with aging worsens dry skin.

- Your skin shows signs of sun damage over the years:
  - Wrinkled skin
  - Dry skin that feels leathery
  - Yellow or blotchy looking skin

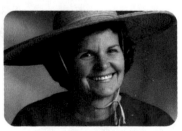

Sunlight is a major cause of the skin changes associated with aging. To keep your skin healthier and younger looking, protect it from the sun.

## 28. Age Spots

Age spots are skin blemishes that come with aging. All age spots are generally harmless. They are more a cosmetic issue than a medical one. It is important, though, to distinguish them from skin cancer. (See "Skin Cancer" on page 135.)

### Prevention

Reduce your exposure to the sun. When you are outdoors, use a sunscreen with a sun protection factor (SPF) of 15 or greater.

### Signs & Symptoms

- Small or large, flat, freckle-like marks that are different shades of brown (liver spots). These most often appear on the arms, backs of hands, back, face, or shoulders.

- Brown or yellow slightly raised spots (seborrheic warts)

- Red, pinpoint blemishes (cherry angiomas)

### Causes & Care

Age spots are due to aging and sun exposure. Aging skin is thinner and more sensitive to the sun's rays. Small, dark patches appear in response.

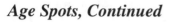

*Age Spots, Continued*

In general, age spots do not need medical treatment. A doctor can freeze an age spot with liquid nitrogen or remove it in a minor surgical procedure, if skin cancer is suspected.

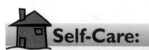

## Self-Care:

**To Help Make Age Spots Less Noticeable:**

- Avoid sun exposure.
- Try a bleaching cream.
- Apply lemon juice twice a day to age spots.
- Dab buttermilk on spots and lightly pat dry.
- Use fresh aloe gel on spots. Do this twice a day for a month.
- Use a mild, moisturizing make-up.

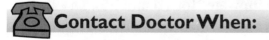

## Contact Doctor When:

- You suspect the spots are skin cancer. (See "Signs & Symptoms" of skin cancer on pages 136 and 137.)
- An age spot bleeds, itches, or tingles.

- You want advice on removing age spots; on creams with the medicine, Retin-A; or on chemical peels.
- You have bothersome age spots that resist fading after using self-care.

# 29. Animal/Insect Bites

The most common animal bites in the United States are from dogs, cats, and other humans in that order. Less common, but more dangerous, are bites from skunks, raccoons, bats, and other animals that live in the wild. These animals can have rabies, a serious and often fatal viral infection.

Most house pets are vaccinated for rabies. It's unlikely they carry the virus. Abandoned cats and dogs may be at risk, if not vaccinated.

Other bites can come from snakes, spiders, and deer ticks. Deer tick bites can cause **Lyme disease**, a bacterial infection.

## Prevention

- Get house pets vaccinated for rabies.
- Don't tease animals.
- Don't move suddenly or scream around an animal, or run from a strange dog.

**10. Skin Conditions**

*Animal/Insect Bites, Continued*

- Leave pet dogs and cats alone while they are eating or sleeping.

- Be careful when you handle your sick or injured pet.

- Don't keep wild animals as pets, and don't feed them with your hands.

- Wear heavy boots when walking in areas where snakes live.

### To Prevent Lyme Disease:

- Ask your doctor about a vaccine for Lyme disease

- Wear long pants, tucked into socks, and long-sleeve shirts when walking through fields or forests, etc. Wear light-colored, tightly-woven clothing. Inspect for ticks after these activities.

- Use an insect repellent that is approved for deer ticks.

## Signs & Symptoms

Depending on the animal/insect and how severe the bite is, symptoms include:

- Bleeding

- Infection

- Tissue loss, if the wound is disfiguring

- Skin rash (red bull's eye one with a white center around the bite) with Lyme disease. Fatigue, fever, and joint pain may also occur.

- Lockjaw. This is a painful, persistent stiffness of the jaw due to a toxin. Tetanus shots can prevent this . (See "Immunizations" on page 36.)

- Allergic reaction, such as with insect bites. Redness, swelling, and pain can occur at the site. A severe allergic reaction (see page 129) can also occur.

Self-care can be used for animal bites that cause superficial scratches and for insect bites that do not cause a severe allergic reaction.

### Self-Care/First Aid:

### For Dog and Cat Bites:

- Wash the bite area right away with soap and warm water for 5 minutes. If the bite is deep, flush the wound with water for 10 minutes. Dry the wound with a clean towel. Then get immediate care.

- If the wound is swollen, apply ice wrapped in a towel for 10 minutes.

*Continued on Next Page*

To Learn More, See Back Cover

10. Skin Conditions

## Animal/Insect Bites, Continued

### Self-Care, Continued

- Have the victim get a tetanus shot if his or her tetanus immunizations are not up-to-date. (See "Immunizations" on page 36.)

- If the bite hurts, take an over-the-counter pain reliever. (See "Pain relievers" in "Your Home Pharmacy" on page 43.)

- If you know the pet's owner, find out if the pet has been vaccinated for rabies.

- Report the incident to the animal control department.

### For Deer Tick Bites:

- Remove any ticks found on the skin. Use tweezers to grasp the tick as close to the skin as possible. Pull gently and carefully in a steady upward motion at the point where the tick's mouthpart enters the skin. Try not to crush the tick or grab it at the rear of its body. The contents may cause an infection.

- After removing ticks, wash the area and your hands with soap and water.

- Save one removed tick in a closed jar with rubbing alcohol. Ask your doctor if he or she would like to see it.

### For Human Bites Before Immediate Care:

- Wash the wound area with soap and water for at least 5 minutes, but don't scrub hard.

- Rinse with running water or with an antiseptic solution, such as Betadine.

- Cover the wound area with sterile gauze, taping only the ends in place.

### For Non-Poisonous Snake Bites:

- Wash the site with soap and water.

- Treat the bite as a minor wound. (See "Cuts, Scrapes & Punctures" on page 120.)

### Contact Doctor When:

- A bite over a joint causes pain when the joint is moved.

- Signs of infection (fever, increased redness or swelling, and/or pus) occur 24 or more hours after the animal bite.

- You have been bitten by a deer tick. (Take the removed tick in a jar to the doctor.)

- You have signs and symptoms of Lyme disease. (See "Skin Rash Chart" on page 139.)

**10. Skin Conditions**

## Animal/Insect Bites, Continued

### Get Immediate Care When:

- A bite caused severe bleeding and/or severely mangled the skin.

- A bite has punctured the skin.

- A bite was from a poisonous snake or any of these symptoms are present:

  - The skin discolors and swells quickly at the bite site.

  - Drowsiness, dizziness, nausea

  - Sweating or twitching skin

  - Double vision or slurred speech

  - Delirium, seizures, or tremors

- A bite was from a spider known to be poisonous or any of these symptoms are present:

  - Painful cramps and muscle stiffness in the abdomen or shoulders, chest, and back

  - Nausea, vomiting

  - Restlessness, dizziness, problems with breathing, convulsions

  - Fever, chills, heavy sweating

- A bite was from a pet that has not been immunized against rabies or from an animal known to carry rabies in your area. Check with your local health department if you are not sure.

- Signs of shock followed a bite. (See "Shock" on page 413.)

# 30. Athlete's Foot

Athlete's foot is a fungal infection. It usually affects the skin between the toes.

## Signs & Symptoms

- Moist, soft, red or gray-white scales on the feet, especially between the toes

- Cracked, peeling, dead skin areas

- Itching

- Sometimes small blisters on the feet

## Causes & Care

People usually pick up the fungus from walking barefoot over wet floors around swimming pools, locker rooms, and public showers.

Self-care treats most cases of athlete's foot.

### Self-Care:

- Wash your feet twice a day, especially between your toes. Dry the area well. Don't use deodorant soaps.

*Continued on Next Page*

10. Skin Conditions

*Athlete's Foot, Continued*

*Self-Care, Continued*

- Use an over-the-counter antifungal powder, spray, etc., between your toes and inside your socks and shoes.

- Wear clean socks made of natural fibers (cotton or wool). Change your socks during the day to keep your feet dry. Wear shoes, like sandals or canvas loafers, that allow ventilation.

- Alternate shoes daily to let each pair air out.

## Contact Doctor When:

- You have signs of athlete's foot, listed on page 110, and you are diabetic or have poor leg circulation.

- You have a fever and/or the infection is spreading or getting worse despite using self-care.

- You have recurrent episodes of athlete's foot.

# 31. Bedsores

Bedsores, also called pressure ulcers, are painful ulcers on the skin. Common sites are the head, back, buttocks, tailbone, knees, and ankles.

## Signs & Symptoms

- The skin may feel sore in areas where a bone is close to the skin. There may be no feeling at all.

- The skin gets irritated and red and then turns purple.

- The skin cracks and an open sore appears. The skin area can become infected.

## Causes, Risk Factors & Care

Bedsores are caused by constant pressure on the skin or frequent rubbing in one area.

Factors that increase the risk of bedsores include:

- Being confined to a bed or chair

- Urinary incontinence; poor bowel control

- Poor blood circulation and loss of sensation due to a stroke or spinal cord injury

Infected sores require antibiotics. Chronic or deep sores may also require antibiotics. If infected sores are left untreated too long, a blood infection that threatens life can result. This is rare, though. Bedsores may also need special dressings.

**10. Skin Conditions**

*Bedsores, Continued*

### Prevention/Self-Care:

A caregiver needs to assist with these.

- Change position every 2 hours if confined to a bed, every hour if confined to a chair.

- Check the skin daily for early signs of bedsores. Use mirrors for hard to see places. {**Note:** Redness is usually the earliest sign. Once the skin cracks or breaks down, seek medical attention.}

- Use a foam or sheepskin mattress cover.

- Use a waterbed or a bed with an air filled mattress, such as a ripple bed. This type of airbed has a small motor that creates a rippling effect by pumping air in and out of the mattress.

- If incontinent, wear absorbent pads or briefs.

- Clean the skin right away if there is contact with urine or stool.

- Keep the skin clean and dry. Use soft cloths, sponges, and mild soaps. Avoid hot water. Do not rub the skin.

- Apply cornstarch to the skin.

- Lift (do not drag or slide) an immobile person.

- Don't sit on donut-shaped cushions.

- Put pillows between knees and ankles so they don't touch.

- Use sheepskin under heels and buttocks.

- Don't massage bony body parts.

- Eat well and get adequate fluids.

- Ask your doctor about taking a vitamin C supplement.

- Handle a person with bedsores gently.

- Apply topical medication as advised.

### Contact Doctor When:

- The skin is cracked.

- Sores show signs of infection (fever; redness; pain; heat; pus; swelling).

- Sores have not improved after 2 weeks of self-care.

## 32. Boils

Boils are common, but usually minor, skin problems. They can occur on any skin area. Most often, they occur in areas where the skin becomes chaffed and where there are hair follicles. This includes the neck, buttocks, armpits, or genitals. A boil can range from the size of a pea to a ping pong ball.

To Learn More, See Back Cover

*Boils, Continued*

## Signs & Symptoms

- A round or cone-shaped lump or pimple that is red, tender, painful, or that throbs

- Pus may be visible under the skin's surface after several days.

- The boil usually bursts open on its own after 10 to 14 days.

## Causes, Risk Factors & Care

Boils are caused when a hair follicle or oil gland becomes infected with staph bacteria. Boils can be very contagious. Risk factors that make them more likely to occur include poor hygiene; overuse of corticosteroid medicine; diabetes; and short, curly hair that has a tendency to grow back down into the skin.

Self-care may be all that is needed to treat boils. If self-care is not enough, your doctor may need to lance and drain the boil and prescribe an antibiotic.

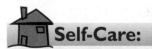

### Self-Care:

- Apply moist, warm compresses to the boil every 2 to 3 hours to help bring it to a head. Use compresses for 20 to 30 minutes each time.

- Put a hot water bottle over a damp washcloth and place it on the boil.

- Soak in a warm tub. Use an antibacterial soap. If boil is ready to burst open, take warm showers instead to lessen the risk of spreading the infection.

- Take an over-the-counter medicine for pain and swelling. (See "Pain relievers" in "Your Home Pharmacy" on page 43.)

- Wash your hands after contact with a boil. Keep clothing, etc. that was in contact with the boil away from others.

- Once the boil begins to drain, keep it dry and clean. Loosely cover the boil with a sterile gauze dressing and replace it if it gets moist.

- Wash bed linens, towels, or clothing in hot water. Do not share towels, athletic equipment, etc.

- Don't scratch, squeeze, or lance boils.

- Don't wear tight-fitting clothes over a boil.

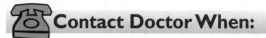

### Contact Doctor When:

- You have any of these problems with a boil:

  - A temperature over 101°F

  - Diabetes

**10. Skin Conditions**

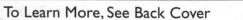

*Boils, Continued*

- Red streaks on the skin near the boil
- Pain from a boil that limits normal activity
- You have any of these problems:
  - Many boils that don't drain or heal
  - A boil on the lip, nose, ear, or eye
  - A boil larger than 1 inch
  - Boils occurred after taking antibiotics.
  - New boils occurred after 2 to 3 days of using self-care.
  - No relief after using 3 to 4 days of self-care

# 33. Bruises

Bruises are broken blood vessels under the skin. In areas where the skin is thin, like around the eyes, the bruise will show up more. Bruises on the head or shin tend to swell the most because the bones in these areas are very close to the skin.

## Signs & Symptoms

- Black and blue or red skin. As it heals, the skin turns greenish-yellow.
- Pain or tenderness
- Possible swelling
- A bruise usually lasts less than 2 weeks.

## Causes, Risk Factors & Care

Bruises are common. Most often, they occur after a fall or being hit by some force. They can, though, occur for no apparent reason.

The risk of getting bruises increases with:

- Taking certain medications, such as aspirin, blood thinners, corticosteroids, water pills, and drugs for arthritis
- Being female, middle aged, or elderly
- Being an alcoholic or drug user
- Having certain medical conditions. Examples are anemia, a blood platelet disorder, liver disease, and lupus.

Most small bruises need no treatment and will go away on their own. For some larger bruises, especially if there is pain or swelling, self-care can help. If bruises result from a medical condition, the medical condition needs to be treated.

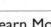 To Learn More, See Back Cover

10. Skin Conditions

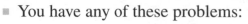

**_Bruises, Continued_**

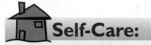 **Self-Care:**

- Apply a cold pack to the bruised area within 15 minutes of the injury. Keep the cold pack on for 10 minutes at a time. Apply pressure to the cold pack. Take it off for 30 to 60 minutes. Repeat several times for 2 days.
- Rest the bruised area.
- Raise the bruised area above the level of the heart, if practical.
- Two days after the injury, use warm compresses. Do this for 20 minutes at a time.
- Do not bandage a bruise.

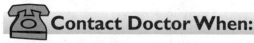 **Contact Doctor When:**

- You have any of these problems with a bruise:
  - Vision problems with a bruise near the eye
  - Signs of infection (fever; increased pain; redness, and/or swelling; pus)
  - Nosebleeds or excessive bleeding from cuts
  - Loss of weight and appetite
  - Joint pain, fever, or swollen lymph nodes

- You have any of these problems:
  - Bruising on the hip after a fall
  - Bruises appear often and easily.
  - Bruises take longer than 2 weeks to go away.
  - Over a year's time, more than 2 or 3 bruises appear for no apparent reason.

## 34. Burns

Burns can result from dry heat (fire), moist heat (steam, hot liquids), electricity, chemicals, or from radiation, including sunlight. The longer your skin is exposed to the burn source, the worse the burn can be.

### Signs, Symptoms & Causes

First-degree burns affect only the outer skin layer. The skin area appears dry, red, and mildly swollen. A first-degree burn is painful and sensitive to touch.

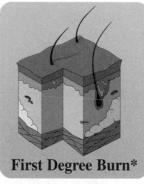

**First Degree Burn\***

Mild sunburn and brief contact with a heat source, such as a hot iron, cause first-degree burns. First-degree burns should feel better within a day or two. They should heal in about a week if there are no complications.

**10. Skin Conditions**

## Burns, Continued

Second-degree burns affect the skin's lower layers and the outer skin. They are painful, swollen, and show redness and blisters. The skin also develops a weepy,

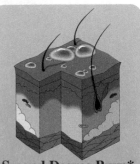

**Second Degree Burn***

watery surface. Causes of second-degree burns include severe sunburn, burns caused by hot liquids, and a gasoline flash. Self-care can treat many second-degree burns depending on their location and how much skin area is affected.

Third-degree burns affect the outer and deeper skin layers and any underlying tissue and organs. They appear black-and-white and charred. The skin swells, and underlying tissue is often

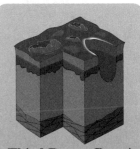

**Third Degree Burn***

exposed. Third-degree burns may have less pain than first-degree or second-degree burns. There can also be no pain when nerve endings are destroyed.

Pain may be felt around the margin of the affected area. Third-degree burns usually result from electric shocks, burning clothes, severe gasoline fires, etc.

## Care

Third-degree burns always require emergency care.

Second-degree burns need immediate care if the burn is on the face, hands, feet, genitals, or on any joint, or if the burn affects an area larger than 10 square inches.

Most first-degree burns and many second-degree burns can be treated with self-care.

### Self-Care:

**For First-Degree Burns:**

- Immerse the affected area in cold (not ice) water until the pain subsides. If the affected area is dirty, gently wash it with soapy water first.

- Do not apply ice or cold water for too long a time. This may result in complete numbness leading to frostbite.

- Keep the area uncovered and elevated, if possible. Apply a dry dressing, if necessary.

*Continued on Next Page*

To Learn More, See Back Cover

**10. Skin Conditions**

## Burns, *Continued*

### Self-Care, *Continued*

- Do not use butter or ointments, such as Vaseline. You can, though, apply aloe vera 3 to 4 times a day.

- Don't use local anesthetic sprays and creams. They can slow healing and may lead to allergic reactions.

- Take an over-the-counter pain reliever. (See "Pain relievers" in "Your Home Pharmacy" on page 43.)

**For Second-Degree Burns (that are not extensive and are less than 3" in diameter):**

- Immerse the affected area in cold (not ice) water until the pain subsides.

- Dip clean cloths in cold water, wring them out, and apply them to the burned area for as long as an hour. Blot the area dry. Do not rub.

- Don't use antiseptic sprays, ointments, and creams.

- Do not break any blisters. If the blisters break on their own, apply an antibacterial spray or ointment and keep the area wrapped with a sterile dressing.

- Once dried, dress the area with a single layer of loose gauze that does not stick to the skin. Keep it in place with bandage tape that is placed well away from the burned area.

- Change the dressing the next day and every 2 days after that.

- Prop the burned area higher than the rest of the body, if possible.

### ☎ Contact Doctor When:

- With second-degree burn, more than the outer skin layer has been affected; more than 3 inches in diameter of the skin has been burned, or blisters have formed.

- You have signs of an infection (fever; chills; or increased redness and swelling; and/or pus) at the burn site. This usually occurs after 48 hours.

- The burn does not improve after 2 days.

### ♥ Get Immediate Care When:

- You have a third-degree burn with little or no pain; charred, black-and-white skin; and exposure of tissue under the skin.

- You have a second-degree burn that is on the face, hands, feet, genitals, or on any joint (elbow, knee, shoulder, etc.) or that affects an area larger than 10 square inches.

**10. Skin Conditions**

# 35. Cold Hands & Feet

Many adults 50 and older complain of cold hands and feet. Often the cause is unknown and not serious.

## Signs & Symptoms

- Fingers or toes that turn pale white or blue, then red, in response to cold temperatures
- Pain when the fingers or toes turn white
- Tingling or numbness in the hands or feet

## Causes, Risk Factors & Care

- Poor circulation. This is most often due to diseased arteries.
- **Raynaud's disease**. This is a disorder that affects the flow of blood to the fingers and sometimes to the toes.
- Any underlying disease that affects the blood flow in the tiny blood vessels of the skin. Women who smoke may be more prone to this.
- Frostbite. (See "Frostbite & Hypothermia" on page 400.)
- Stress
- A side effect of taking certain medicines
- **Cervical rib syndrome**. This is a compression of the nerves and blood vessels in the neck that affects the shoulders, arms, and hands.

Treatment will depend on the cause. Emergency care is needed for frostbite. If a medical condition causes cold hands and/or feet, treatment for the condition helps treat cold hands and feet. Self-care can help most cases.

## Self-Care:

- Don't smoke. If you smoke, quit.
- Avoid caffeine.
- Don't handle cold objects with bare hands. Use ice tongs to pick up ice cubes, etc.
- Set your indoor thermostat at 65°F or higher.
- Wear mittens and wool socks to keep hands and feet warm.
- Don't wear tight-fitting footwear.
- Wiggle your toes. It may help keep them warm by increasing blood flow.
- Stretch your fingers straight out. Swing your arms in large circles, like a baseball pitcher warming up for a game. This may increase blood flow to the fingers. Skip this tip if you have bursitis or back problems.
- Meditate.

10. Skin Conditions

*Cold Hands & Feet, Continued*

##  Contact Doctor When:

- You have any pain, numbness, and tingling in the neck, shoulders, arms, and hands.

- With the feeling of coldness, you have weakness in the arms, hands, or feet.

- When exposed to the cold or when you are under stress, your hands or feet turn pale, then blue, then red, and get painful and numb.

## Get Immediate Care When:

You have signs and symptoms of frost-bite (see page 400).

# 36. Corns & Calluses

Corns and calluses are extra cells made in a skin area that gets repeated rubbing or squeezing.

## Signs & Symptoms

- Corns are areas of dead skin on the tops or sides of the joints or on the skin between the toes.

- Calluses are patches of dead skin usually found on the balls or heels of the feet, on the hands, and on the knees. Calluses are thick and feel hard to the touch.

## Causes & Care

Footwear that fits poorly and activities that cause friction on the hands, knees, and feet can lead to corns and calluses.

Self-care treats most cases. If not, consult a family doctor or foot doctor (podiatrist). He or she can scrape the hardened tissue and peel away the corn with stronger solutions. Sometimes warts lie beneath corns and need to be treated, too.

## Self-Care:

**For Corns:**

- Don't pick at corns. Don't use toenail scissors, clippers, or any sharp tool to cut off corns.

- Don't wear shoes that fit poorly or that squeeze your toes together.

- Soak your feet in warm water to soften the corn.

- Cover the corn with a protective, nonmedicated pad or bandage which you can get at drug stores.

*Continued on Next Page*

**10. Skin Conditions**

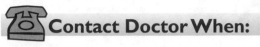

## Corns & Calluses, Continued

### Self-Care, Continued

- If the outer layers of a corn have peeled away, apply a nonprescription liquid of 5 to 10% salicylic acid. Gently rub the corn off with cotton gauze.

- Ask a shoe repair person to sew a metatarsal bar onto your shoe to use when a corn is healing.

### For Calluses:

- Don't try to cut a callus off.

- Soak your feet in warm water to soften the callus. Pat it dry.

- Rub the callus gently with a pumice stone.

- Cover calluses with protective pads. You can get these at drug stores.

- Check for poorly fitting shoes or other sources of friction that may lead to calluses.

- Wear gloves for a hobby or work that puts pressure on your hands.

- Wear knee pads for activities that put pressure on your knees.

## Contact Doctor When:

You have any of these problems with corns or calluses:

- Signs of infection (fever; swelling; redness; and/or pus)

- Circulation problems or diabetes

- Continued or worse pain after using self-care or no improvement after 2 to 3 weeks of self-care

# 37. Cuts, Scrapes, & Punctures

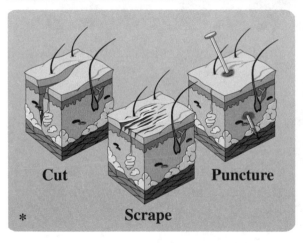

Cut          Puncture

\*          Scrape

- Cuts slice the skin open. Close a cut so it won't get infected.

- Scrapes hurt only the top part of your skin. They can hurt more than cuts, but they heal quicker.

### *Cuts, Scrapes, & Punctures, Continued*

- Punctures stab deep. They can get infected easily because they are hard to clean.

## Signs & Symptoms

Cuts, scrapes, and punctures can all result in pain and bleeding.

Blood clots after bleeding for a few minutes. The clotting slows down bleeding.

## Causes & Care

Causes include sharp objects, such as knives, opened can edges, nails that penetrate the skin, and falls that result in scraping the skin.

Most cuts, scrapes, and punctures can be treated with self-care. Emergency care is needed for heavy bleeding or severe injuries.

- Stitches are needed for cuts longer than an inch or for ones on areas of the body that bend, such as the elbow, knee, etc.

- If an infection occurs after a cut, scrape, or puncture, an antibiotic is usually prescribed.

- A tetanus shot may be needed after a cut, scrape, or puncture if your tetanus shots are not up-to-date. (See "Immunizations" on page 36.)

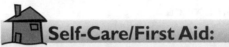

### Self-Care/First Aid:

**First Aid for Minor Cuts and Scrapes:**

- Clean the wound with soap and water.

- Press on the cut to stop the bleeding. Continue for up to 10 minutes, if needed. Use sterile, wet gauze or a clean cloth. Don't use dry gauze. It can stick to the wound. Don't use a bandage to apply pressure.

- Press on the cut again if it keeps bleeding. Get medical help if it still bleeds after 20 minutes. Keep pressing on it until you get help.

- Lift the part of the body with the cut higher than the heart, if practical.

- Apply a first-aid cream on the cut after it has stopped bleeding and when it is clean and dry.

- Put one or more bandages on the cut.
  - Put the bandage across the cut so it can help hold the cut together.
  - The sides of the cut should touch, but not overlap.

*Continued on Next Page*

**10. Skin Conditions**

## Cuts, Scrapes, & Punctures, Continued

### Self-Care/First Aid, Continued

- Don't touch the cut with your hand.
- Use a butterfly bandage if you have one.
- Use more than one bandage for a long cut.

**Bringing Cut Edges Together**

- For scrapes, make a bandage from gauze and first aid tape.
- Leave the bandage on for 24 hours. Change the bandage every day or two or more often if you need to. Be careful when you take the bandage off. If you have used gauze, wet it before you pull it off.
- Take an over-the-counter pain reliever. Don't take aspirin every day unless your doctor tells you to. Taking it too much can keep the blood from clotting. (See "Pain relievers" in "Your Home Pharmacy" on page 43.)

- Call your doctor or local health department if you have not had a tetanus shot in the last 10 years (5 years for a deep puncture).

### First Aid for Punctures that Cause Minor Bleeding:

- Let the wound bleed to cleanse itself.
- Remove the object that caused the puncture. Use clean, sterile tweezers. To sterilize them, hold a lit match or flame to the ends of the tweezers. {**Note:** Don't pull anything out of a puncture wound if blood gushes from it or if it has been bleeding badly. Get emergency care.}
- Clean the wound with warm water and soap.
- Soak the wound in warm, soapy water 2 to 4 times a day. Then dry it well and apply an antibiotic cream, such as Neosporin.

### Contact Doctor When:

- A cut or puncture is from dirty or contaminated objects, such as rusty nails or objects in the soil.
- A puncture goes through a shoe, especially a rubber-soled one.

To Learn More, See Back Cover

10. Skin Conditions

## Cuts, Scrapes, & Punctures, *Continued*

- A day or two after the injury, any signs of infection occur (fever; redness, swelling, tenderness at and around the site of the wound; increased pain; and/or general ill feeling).

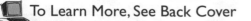

### Get Immediate Care When:

- Severe bleeding occurs or if blood spurts from the wound.

- Signs of shock (see page 413) are present.

- Severe bleeding continues after pressure has been applied to the wound for 10 or more minutes or bleeding continues after 20 minutes of applied pressure to what seems to be a minor cut.

- A deep cut or puncture appears to go down to the muscle or bone and/or is located on the scalp or face.

- A cut is longer than an inch and is located on an area of the body that bends, such as the elbow, knee, or finger. (Bending will put pressure on the cut.)

- Edges of a cut hang open.

## 38. Dry Skin

The skin naturally becomes drier with age. The body produces less oil and moisture. The skin also becomes thinner and less elastic.

### Signs & Symptoms

- Itchy skin. The skin can be red from scratching it.

- Chapped skin

- Skin that cracks, peels, and/or flakes

### Causes, Risk Factors & Care

Aging is only one cause. Other causes include:

- Cold winter weather

- Dry air or heat

- Harsh skin products

- Washing the skin often

- Some medications

- Allergies

- An underactive thyroid gland; diabetes; and/or kidney disease

- Other skin conditions, such as psoriasis

Dry skin is not a serious health risk. With self-care, it can be easily managed. When it is a symptom of a health condition, treating the condition treats the dry skin.

**10. Skin Conditions**

**Dry Skin, Continued**

### Self-Care/Prevention:

- Drink 8 or more glasses of water a day.

- Moisturize your skin daily. Use an oil-based lotion.

- Don't overexpose your skin to water, such as with washing dishes. Wear rubber gloves when you wash dishes.

- Take a shower instead of a bath. Use warm (not hot) water. Apply a moisturizing cream while your skin is damp. Use products with lanolin.

- If you prefer to bathe, bathe for only 15 to 20 minutes in lukewarm water. Pat yourself dry. Do not rub. Use a bath oil on your skin after bathing.

- Try sponge baths.

- Use a washcloth instead of soaping the skin directly.

- Use a mild liquid soap, like Cetaphil Lotion, or a fatted soap. Avoid deodorant, medicated, or alkaline soaps.

- Don't use moisturizers with fragrances, preservatives, or alcohol.

- Use a night cream for the face.

- Stay out of the strong sun.

- Do not use tanning salons.

- Use a sunblock with a sun protection factor (SPF) of at least 15.

- If you get symptoms of dry skin:

  - Don't scratch or rub the skin.

  - Apply oil-based moisturizers often.

  - Lessen exposure of the affected area to water.

### Contact Doctor When:

- You have any of these problems with dry skin:

  - Deep cracks on the hands or feet

  - Tight, shiny, or hardened skin

  - Itchy skin areas that are raised, have red borders, and are covered with large white or silver-white scales

- You have signs of an infection (fever; increased redness, swelling, pain, or tenderness; pus; blisters; red streaks from the affected area).

- You have diabetes and the dry skin is troublesome.

- You have symptoms of low thyroid (see page 301).

- You have dry skin without a rash and you itch all over.

- Severe itching keeps you from sleeping.

- Self-care brings no relief.

**10. Skin Conditions**

To Learn More, See Back Cover

# 39. Eczema

Eczema (atopic dermatitis) is a chronic skin condition. It usually appears on the scalp, face, neck, or creases of the elbows, wrists, and knees. It usually improves as you get older, but can be a lifetime problem.

## Signs & Symptoms

Patches of skin that are:

- Dry, red, and scaly
- Blistered and swollen
- Sometimes thick, discolored, or oozing and crusting

## Causes, Risk Factors & Care

Eczema tends to run in families. It is also more common in persons who have allergies or asthma. Contact with cosmetics, dyes, deodorants, skin lotions, permanent press fabrics, and other allergens can aggravate eczema; so can wool fabrics, stress, exposure to extreme weather conditions, and eating foods, such as eggs, milk, seafood, or wheat products.

Your doctor may prescribe antibiotics for skin infections and/or other medicines if self-care does not relieve symptoms.

## Self-Care:

- Don't scratch! This makes eczema worse. Your skin can get infected. Keep your fingernails cut short.
- Don't take baths too often. Add bath oil to the water. Sponge bathe in between tub baths. Take quick showers.
- Use warm (not hot) water when you take a bath or shower.
- Use a mild soap or no soap at all on the areas of eczema.
- Don't use wool clothes and blankets.
- Use a light, nongreasy and unscented lotion on your skin after you wash. Don't use lotions that have alcohol. They can dry the skin.
- Try to keep from sweating. For example, don't wear too many clothes for the weather.
- Wear rubber gloves when you do housework. Put talcum powder or cornstarch inside the gloves, or use latex gloves lined with cotton.
- Avoid foods, chemicals, cosmetics, and other things that make your eczema worse.

10. Skin Conditions

*Eczema, Continued*

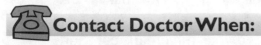
## Contact Doctor When:

- You have signs of an infection: Fever; and/or large amount of weeping or crusting skin areas.

- Your skin is red, you can't stop scratching, and this keeps you from sleeping.

- You get no relief from self-care.

# 40. Hair Loss

Most men and women have hair loss as they get older. Most men have some degree of baldness by age 60. After age 60, 50% of women do.

## Signs & Symptoms

- Thinning of hair on the temples and crown

- Receding hair line

- Bald spot on back of head

- Areas of patchy hair loss

## Causes & Care

Hair loss is due to one or more of these factors:

- Normal aging

- Family traits

- A side effect of some medicines, chemotherapy, and radiation therapy

- Crash dieting

- Hormonal changes, such as with menopause

- A prolonged or serious illness or major surgery. You may not notice the hair loss for several months.

- Medical conditions, such as lupus and thyroid disease (see page 301)

- **Areata**. This causes areas of patchy hair loss. It improves rapidly when treated, but can go away within 18 months even without treatment.

Treatment for hair loss includes:

- Medications. These include over-the-counter rogaine, prescription-strength Rogaine, propecia, and a topical steroid for areata.

- Surgical hair transplant operations

If a medical condition causes the hair loss, treating the condition may restore lost hair.

## Self-Care/Prevention:

- Try the over-the counter medication, Rogaine. This may help with some (not all) cases of hair loss.

*Continued on Next Page*

 To Learn More, See Back Cover

10. Skin Conditions

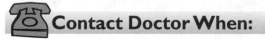

## Hair Loss, Continued

### Self-Care/Prevention, Continued

- Avoid (or don't use often) hair care practices that can damage your hair. These include bleaching, braiding, cornrowing, dyeing, perming, and straightening. Avoid hot curling irons and/or hot rollers.

- Air dry or towel dry your hair. If you use a hairdryer, set it on low.

- If your hair is damaged, change your hairstyle to one that needs less damaging hair care practices. Keep your hair cut short. It will look fuller.

- Use gentle hair care products.

- Don't be taken in by claims for vitamin formulas, massage oils, etc. that promise to cure baldness.

- If you take a medicine that has caused hair loss, ask your doctor if a substitute one is available without this side effect.

- When your head is exposed to the sun, wear a hat or use a sunscreen with a sun protection factor (SPF) of 15 or more on the bald parts of your head . The risk of sunburn and skin cancer on the scalp increases with baldness.

- To disguise hair loss, wear a hairpiece, wig, toupee, hat, etc.

## Contact Doctor When:

- You have sudden patches of hair loss or are not able to stop pulling out patches of your hair.

- You have signs of infection (redness; tenderness; swelling; and/or pain at the site of hair loss).

- You have hair loss with signs of low thyroid (see page 301).

- You lose hair only after you take prescribed medicine.

- You want information about hair implants, Rogaine, etc.

- You need a referral to a mental health care provider for help to manage anxiety.

# 41. Hives

Hives can be (but aren't always) an allergic response to something you touched, inhaled, or swallowed.

## Signs & Symptoms

- Red or pink, raised areas on the skin (weals). Each weal can range in size from less than $1/8$" to 8" or larger in diameter.

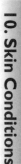

† *Reprinted with permission from the American Academy of Dermatology. All rights reserved.*

*Hives, Continued*

- Itching

- Hives often appear, sometimes in clusters, on the face, and trunk of the body. Less often, hives appear on the scalp or backs of the hands and feet.

- Swelling on the eyelids, lips, tongue, or genitals may occur.

- Hives can change shape, fade, then rapidly reappear.

- A single hive lasts less than 24 hours. After an attack, though, new ones may crop up for up to 6 weeks.

## Causes & Care

Common causes of hives are reactions to medicines, such as aspirin, sulfa, and penicillin and exposure to chemicals and things you are allergic to.

Sometimes it is not known what causes hives. To identify the triggers, keep a diary of when you get hives. List things you expect may have caused the hives.

In most cases, hives are harmless and go away on their own if you avoid what caused them. Self-care helps with symptoms. Prescribed medicines may be needed for severe hives or for attacks of hives that recur.

Your doctor may advise allergy testing if you have hives that last a long time or recur. Emergency medical care is needed for hives that are part of a severe allergic reaction. (See "Signs of a Severe Allergic Reaction" box on page 129.)

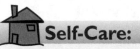
### Self-Care:

- Take a lukewarm bath or shower. Heat worsens most rashes and makes them itch more. Add an oatmeal bath product, such as Aveeno, or one cup of baking soda to the bath water.

- Apply a cold compress.

- Wear loose-fitting clothes.

- Relax as much as you can. Relaxation therapy may help ease the itching and discomfort of hives.

- Ask your doctor whether or not you should take an antihistamine and to recommend one. Antihistamines can help relieve itching and suppress hives. Take as directed by your doctor or by directions on the label.

- Use calamine lotion on itchy areas.

- Don't take aspirin, ibuprofen, ketoprofen, or naproxen sodium. These may make hives worse.

To Learn More, See Back Cover

**10. Skin Conditions**

*Hives, Continued*

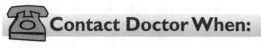 **Contact Doctor When:**

- You have constant and severe itching, and/or a fever with hives.

- Hives last for more than 6 weeks.

- Hives started after taking medicine.

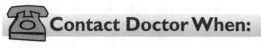 **Get Immediate Care When:**

Hives are present with signs of a severe allergic reaction (anaphylactic shock).

| Signs of a Severe Allergic Reaction |
|---|
| ■ A hard time breathing or swallowing |
| ■ Severe swelling all over, or of the face, lips, tongue, and/or throat |
| ■ Obstructed airway |
| ■ Wheezing |
| ■ Dizziness, weakness |
| ■ Shock (see page 413) |

# 42. Ingrown Toenails

An ingrown toenail digs into the skin next to the side of the nail. The most common site is the big toe. Other toes and even fingernails can be affected.

## Prevention

- Cut nails straight across. Don't cut the nails shorter at the sides than in the middle. {**Note:** If you have diabetes or circulation problems, follow your doctor's advise about clipping your toenails.}

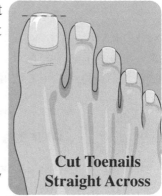

**Cut Toenails Straight Across**

- File the nails if they're sharp after you clip them.

- Wear shoes and socks that fit well.

## Signs & Symptoms

- Redness

- Tenderness

- Discomfort or pain

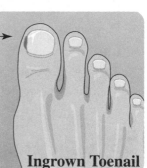

**Ingrown Toenail**

## Causes & Care

Causes include:

- Jamming your toes

- Wearing shoes or socks that fit too tight

- Clipping toenails too short. This can cause the corners to penetrate the skin as the nail grows out.

- Having wider-than-average toenails

10. Skin Conditions

## *Ingrown Toenails, Continued*

Self-care treats most ingrown toenails. If not, a physician or podiatrist may have to remove a part of the nail.

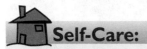

### Self-Care:

- Soak your foot in warm, soapy water, 5 to 10 minutes, 1 to 3 times a day.

- With the tip of a nail file, gently lift the nail away from the reddened skin at the outer corners.

- Soak a small piece of cotton in an antiseptic or topical antibiotic, such as Betadine. Place it just under the outer corners, if you can.

- Repeat the previous 3 steps daily until the nail begins to grow correctly and the pressure is relieved. Wear roomy shoes during this time.

### Contact Doctor When:

- You have signs of an infection (fever; pus; increased redness; tenderness, and/ or pain).

- You have an ingrown toenail and have diabetes or circulation problems.

- You get ingrown toenails often.

## 43. Insect Stings

Insects that sting include: Bumblebees, honeybees, hornets, wasps, yellow jackets, and fire ants.

### Prevention

Try to avoid getting stung.

- Keep food and drink containers tightly covered. (Bees love sweet things, like soft drinks.)

- Don't wear perfume, colognes, or hair spray when you are outdoors.

- Don't wear bright colors. Choose white or neutral colors, like tan.

- Wear snug clothing that covers your arms and legs.

- Don't go barefoot.

- If camping, look for insects in your shoes before you put them on.

- Wear insect repellants.

- Be careful when you work outdoors, pull weeds, mow tall grass, and work around shutters. Bees often build hives behind shutters.

- If an insect that stings gets in your car, stop the car. Put the windows down. Once the insect leaves, resume driving.

**10. Skin Conditions**

To Learn More, See Back Cover

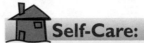

*Insect Stings, Continued*

## Signs & Symptoms

- Quick, sharp pain
- Swelling
- Itching
- Redness at the sting site
- Hives (see page 127)

Insect stings can even result in a severe allergic reaction. (See "Signs of a Severe Allergic Reaction" box on page 129.)

## Causes & Care

Insect stings come from bumblebees, honeybees, hornets, wasps, yellow jackets, and fire ants.

Self-care treats mild reactions to insect stings. A severe allergic reaction needs immediate care. Symptoms of a severe allergic reaction usually happen soon after or within an hour of the sting.

If you have had a severe allergic reaction to an insect sting, you should carry an emergency insect sting kit, prescribed by your doctor. You should also wear a medical alert tag that lets others know that you are allergic to insect stings. Persons who have had severe reactions to bee or wasp stings should ask their doctor about allergy shots.

### Self-Care:

- For a bee sting, gently scrape out the stinger as soon as possible. Use a blunt knife, credit card or a fingernail.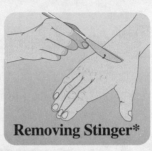

  **Removing Stinger***

  Yellow jackets, wasps, and hornets don't lose their stingers.

- Don't pull the stinger out with your fingers or tweezers. Don't squeeze the stinger. It contains venom. You could re-sting yourself.

- Clean the sting area with soapy water.

- Put a cold compress (ice in a cloth, etc.) on the sting. Don't put ice directly on the skin. Hold the cold compress on the site for 10 to 15 minutes.

- Keep the sting area lower than the level of the heart.

- Take an over-the-counter medicine for the pain. (See "Pain relievers" in "Your Home Pharmacy" on page 43.)

- Take an over-the-counter antihistamine, such as Benadryl, unless you have to avoid this medicine for medical reasons, such as glaucoma and prostate problems.

**10. Skin Conditions**

*Insect Stings, Continued*

##  Contact Doctor When:

You have hives and/or stomach cramps after you have been stung by an insect.

## ♥ Get Immediate Care When:

- You have signs of a severe allergic reaction (See "Signs of a Severe Allergic Reaction" box on page 127).

- The sting was in the mouth or on the tongue.

{**Note:** Before getting immediate care, give shot from emergency insect sting kit if there is one. Follow other instructions in the kit.}

# 44. Poison Ivy (Oak, Sumac)

Poison ivy, poison oak, and poison sumac are the most common plants that cause a skin rash. A sap, urushiol, that comes from these plants causes the rash. The sap is not really a poison, but can cause an allergic reaction in some people.

## Prevention

- Know what these plants look like and avoid them:

  - Poison ivy and poison oak both have 3 leaflets per stem. This is why you may have heard the saying, "Leaflets three, let them be".

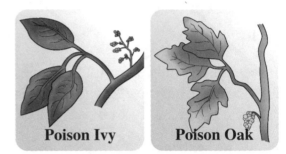

Poison Ivy    Poison Oak

  - Poison sumac has 7 to 11 leaflets.

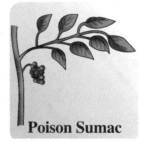

Poison Sumac

- Use an over-the-counter lotion (IvyBlock), which blocks skin contact with the sap. Use as directed.

To Learn More, See Back Cover

10. Skin Conditions

### Poison Ivy (Oak, Sumac), Continued

If you know you have come in contact with one of the plants, you may prevent an allergic reaction if you do the things below within 6 hours.

- Remove all clothes and shoes that have touched the plant.
- Wash your skin with soap and water.
- Apply rubbing alcohol or alcohol wipes to the parts of the skin that are affected.
- Use an over-the-counter product (Tecnu), that removes poison ivy sap.
- Rinse the affected area with water.

## Signs & Symptoms

One or 2 days after contact with the plant, skin rash symptoms can range from mild to severe. These include itching, redness, a burning feeling, swelling, and blisters.

## Causes & Care

You can get poison ivy, oak, or sumac when you touch one of these plants; touch clothing, shoes, items, or pets that have the sap on them; and/or come in contact with the smoke of these burning plants.

Self-care treats most cases of poison ivy, oak, and sumac. For severe cases, your doctor may prescribe corticosteroid medicine.

## Self-Care:

- Take a cold shower, put the rash area in cold water, or pour cold water over it. Use soap when you shower.
- Take an over-the-counter antihistamine, such as Benadryl, unless you have to avoid this medicine for medical reasons, such as glaucoma and prostate problems.
- For weeping blisters, mix 2 teaspoons of baking soda in 4 cups of water. Dip squares of gauze in this mixture. Cover the blisters with the wet gauze for 10 minutes, 4 times a day. Do not apply this to the eyes.
- Wash all clothes and shoes with hot water and a strong soap. Bathe pets that have come in contact with the plant. The sap can stay on pets for many days. Clean items used to wash clothing and pets. Wear rubber gloves when you do all these things.
- Keep your hands away from your eyes, mouth, and face.
- Do not scratch or rub the rash.
- Apply any of these to the skin rash:
  - Calamine (not Caladryl) lotion
  - Over-the-counter topical steroid cream, such as Cortaid.
  - A paste of 3 teaspoons of baking soda and 1 teaspoon of water.

*Poison Ivy (Oak, Sumac), Continued*

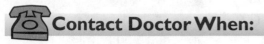

## Contact Doctor When:

You have any of these problems with poison ivy, oak, or sumac

- Skin that is very bright red
- Severe itching, swelling, or blisters
- Pus
- A rash on large areas of the body or the face
- A rash that has spread to the mouth, eyes, or genitals

# 45. Shingles

Shingles is a skin disorder triggered by the chicken pox virus which is thought to lie dormant in the spinal cord until later in life. Shingles most often occurs between the ages of 50 and 70 in both men and women.

## Signs & Symptoms

- Pain, itching, or tingling sensation before a rash appears
- A rash of painful red blisters which later crust over. Most often, the rash appears on one side of the torso or face.

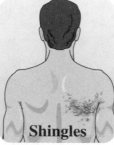

**Shingles**

- Though rare, fever and general weakness sometimes occur.
- After the crusts fall off, usually within 3 weeks, pain can persist in the area of the rash. This usually goes away within 1 to 6 months. Chronic pain (**post-herpetic neuralgia**) can last longer, even for years. The older you are, the greater the chance that this is the case. The recovery time may also take longer.
- Most cases of shingles are mild, but it can result in chronic, severe pain or blindness if it affects the eye.

## Causes, Risk Factors & Care

Herpes zoster virus causes shingles. To get shingles you must have had the chicken pox. You are more likely to get shingles after an illness or taking any medicines that suppress the immune system. Stress or trauma, either emotional or physical can also increase the risk for shingles.

Medical treatment can shorten the course of shingles and make symptoms less severe. Treatment includes:

- Prescribed medicines: Famvir, Valtrex, and Zovirax. The sooner one of these medicines is used, the better the results.
- Medicine for pain. Codeine may sometimes be prescribed.
- Other medicines as needed, such as antihistamines and corticosteroids

 To Learn More, See Back Cover

**10. Skin Conditions**

*Shingles, Continued*

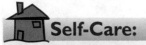

## Self-Care:

- Unless your doctor has given you prescription pain medicine, take an over-the-counter medicine for pain. (See "Pain relievers" in "Your Home Pharmacy" on page 43.)

- Keep sores open to the air. Until the blisters are completely crusted over, do not go near children or adults who have not yet had the chicken pox or others who have a condition which suppresses their immune system. Examples are cancer, HIV/AIDS, and chronic illnesses. They could get chicken pox from exposure to shingles.

- Don't wear clothing that irritates the skin area where sores are present.

- Wash blisters, but don't scrub them.

- To relieve itching, apply calamine lotion or a paste made of 3 teaspoons of baking soda mixed with 1 teaspoon of water to the affected area.

- Avoid drafty areas.

- Put a cool compress, such as a cold cloth dipped in ice water, on the blisters for 20 minutes at a time.

- Drink plenty of liquids.

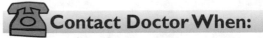

## Contact Doctor When:

- You first notice signs and symptoms of shingles listed on page 134.

- Shingles affects your eye, nose, or ear.

- You have any of these conditions with shingles:
  - A fever and/or general weakness
  - You are over 60 years of age.
  - You take medicines that suppress your immune system or have a chronic illness.

- The blisters itch uncontrollably or are very painful.

# 46. Skin Cancer

Skin cancer is the most common kind of cancer. When found early, skin cancer can be treated with success.

## Prevention

- Avoid exposure to midday sun (10 a.m. to 2 p.m. standard time, or 11 a.m. to 3 p.m. daylight savings time).

- Use a sunblock with a sun protection factor of SPF 15 or more as directed.

- Wear long sleeves, sun hats, etc. to block out the sun's harmful rays.

- Avoid sun lamps or tanning salons.

**10. Skin Conditions**

*Skin Cancer, Continued*

- Avoid unnecessary x-rays. Wear protective aprons when exposed to x-rays.

## Signs & Symptoms

There are 3 types of skin cancer:

1. Basal cell. More than 90% of all skin cancers in the United States are this type. It grows slowly. It seldom spreads to other parts of the body.

2. Squamous cell. This type of skin cancer spreads more often than the basal cell type. It is still rare for it to spread, though.

Basal and squamous cell cancers are found mainly on areas of the skin that are exposed to the sun. Examples are the head, face, neck, hands, and arms. Skin cancer can occur anywhere, though.

Early Warning Signs of These Cancers

- Small, smooth, shiny, pale, or waxy lump

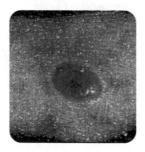

- Firm red lump

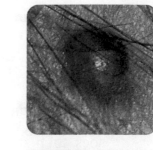

- A lump that bleeds or develops a crust

- A flat, red spot that is rough, dry, or scaly

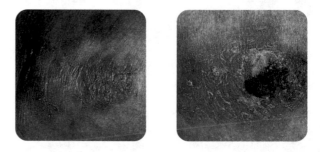

3. Melanoma. This is the most serious kind of skin cancer. It often spreads to other parts of the body. It can be fatal if it is not treated early.

Warning Signs of Melanoma

- Often, the first sign is a change in the size, shape, or color of an existing mole. It may also appear as a new, abnormal, or "ugly-looking" mole.

To Learn More, See Back Cover

**10. Skin Conditions**

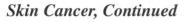

## Skin Cancer, Continued

- Think of "**ABCD**". These letters can help you think of what to watch for.

  **A.** Asymmetry. The shape of one half does not match the other.

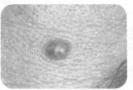 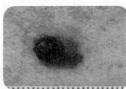

*Benign (normal) mole*    *Melanoma*

  **B.** Border. The edges are ragged, notched, or blurred.

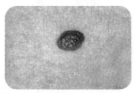 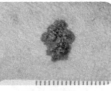

*Benign (normal) mole*    *Melanoma*

  **C.** Color. The color is uneven. Shades of black, brown, and tan may be seen. Areas of white, gray, red, or blue also may be seen.

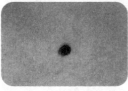 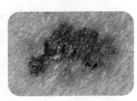

*Benign (normal) mole*    *Melanoma*

**D.** Diameter. There is a change in size. Also, melanoma lesions are often bigger than the diameter of a pencil eraser.

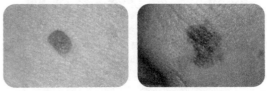

*Benign (normal) mole*    *Melanoma*

## Causes, Risk Factors & Care

- Recurrent sunburn from exposure to ultraviolet (UV) radiation from the sun is the main cause.

- Having had skin cancer or a family history of skin cancer

- Having fair skin that freckles easily, especially with red or blond hair and blue or light-colored eyes

- Aging

- Exposure to coal, arsenic, sun lamps and tanning booths

- Repeated exposure to medical or industrial x-rays

Treatment depends on the size and type and stage of the cancer. Treatment includes:

- Surgery. There are many types.

- Laser therapy

**10. Skin Conditions**

*Skin Cancer, Continued*

- Chemotherapy. One form is a cream or lotion with anticancer drugs that is applied to the skin. Other forms are given through an IV.
- Radiation therapy
- Interferon drugs
- Skin grafting may be needed to fill in the skin area and reduce scarring where the cancer was removed.

## Self-Care:

- Check for signs of skin cancer. Do a skin self-exam on a regular basis. The best time to do this self-exam is 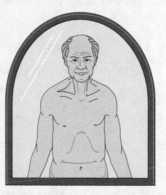 after a shower or bath. To check your skin, use a well-lit room, a full-length mirror, and a hand-held mirror
- Locate your birthmarks, moles, and blemishes. Know what they usually look like. Check for a change in the size, texture, or color of a mole. Check for a sore that does not heal.

- Check all areas.
  1. Look at the front and back of your body in the mirror. Then, raise your arms and look at the left and right sides.
  2. Bend your elbows and look carefully at the palms of your hands. Make sure to look at both sides of your forearms and upper arms.
  3. Look at the back and front of the legs. Look between the buttocks and around the genital area.
  4. Look at your face, neck, and scalp. Use a comb or a blow dryer to move hair so that you can see the scalp better.
  5. Sit and closely examine the feet. Look at the soles and the spaces between the toes.

## Contact Doctor When:

You notice any warning signs of basal cell or squamous cell cancer or melanoma listed and shown on pages 136 and 137.

## For Information Contact:

The Cancer Information Service
1-800-4-Cancer (800-422-6237)
www.nci.nih.gov

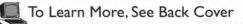 To Learn More, See Back Cover

10. Skin Conditions

# 47. Skin Rashes

## Skin Rash Chart

| Signs & Symptoms | What It Could Be | What To Do |
|---|---|---|
| Rash of deep red or purple spots with high fever, vomiting, headache, <u>and</u> stiff neck | Meningitis | Get immediate care. |
| Red or pink raised areas on the skin, sometimes with white centers. May come and go anywhere on the body. Itching.<br><br>May have swollen eyelids, lips, tongue, throat; wheezing, hard time breathing. | Hives. See picture of hives on page 127.<br><br>Severe allergic reaction (anaphylactic shock) | Get immediate care for a severe allergic reaction. See "Signs of a Severe Allergic Reaction" box on page 129 {**Note:** If you have an emergency kit for an allergy, give the shot from the kit and follow other instructions before immediate care.} See "Hives" on page 127. |
| Pink to red rash on the arms, legs, and palms of the hands. Often starts near the wrists and ankles, then spreads inward. Rash darkens in color, spreads, and can bleed. Also have fever and chills, headache, and delirium. | Rocky mountain spotted fever | Contact doctor right away. |
| Rash of painful red blisters (most often on only one side and in only one area of the body). Pain, itching, burning, or tingling feeling before the rash appeared. | Shingles. See illustration of shingles on page 134. | See "Shingles" on page 134. |

10. Skin Conditions

## Skin Rashes, Continued

### Skin Rash Chart, Continued

| Signs & Symptoms | What It Could Be | What To Do |
|---|---|---|
| A fever and red rash 3 days to 2 weeks after a deer tick bite. The rash has raised edges with pale centers. It fades after a few days. Joint pain may develop later. | Lyme disease | Contact doctor. See also "Treatment" and "Self-Care" sections for "Lyme Disease" in this topic. |
| Red rash with small, flat, round dots on the palms of the hands and soles of the feet. | Syphilis | Contact doctor. |
| Redness. Itchy, scaly patches of skin that are round with distinct edges. Moistness in the folds of the skin (under the breasts or in the groin area). | Tinea corporis. This is a fungal infection. It is also called body ringworm. | Contact doctor. |
| Dry, red, itchy patches of skin from direct contact with an irritant (plants, cleaning products, cosmetics, jewelry, etc.). | Contact dermatitis. <br><br> Poison ivy, † oak or sumac. | See "Treatment" and "Self-Care" sections for "Contact Dermatitis" in this topic. See "Poison Ivy (Oak, Sumac)" on page 132. |
| Scaly, oily rash with small, reddish-yellow patches. Areas affected are usually oily ones, such as around the edge of the scalp, the forehead, the nose, the eyebrows, the back, and the chest. | Seborrhea. This is a type of dermatitis when glands in the skin make too much oil. | See "Treatment" and "Self-Care" sections for "Seborrheic Dermatitis" in this topic. |

† *Reprinted with permission from the American Academy of Dermatology. All rights reserved.*

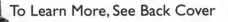 To Learn More, See Back Cover

**10. Skin Conditions**

## Skin Rashes, Continued

| Skin Rash Chart, Continued | | |
|---|---|---|
| **Signs & Symptoms** | **What It Could Be** | **What To Do** |
| Patches of skin that are dry, red, scaly, blistered, swollen, and sometimes thick, discolored, or oozing and crusting. | Eczema | See "Eczema" on page 125. |
| Red rash on the face. Red nose that looks swollen; puffy cheeks. May be pus-filled spots without blackheads or whiteheads. Often occurs with pinkeye (see page 71). | Rosacea. This is adult acne. | See "Treatment" and "Self-Care" sections for "Rosacea" in this topic. |
| Tiny red pimples that itch intensely. Common sites are the webs between the fingers; the wrists; elbows; armpits; and along the belt line. May see wavy lines in the skin up to an inch long. | Scabies. This is caused by skin parasites called itch mites. | See "Treatment" and "Self-Care" sections for "Scabies" in this topic. |
| Itchy, red patches covered with silvery-white flaky skin. Common sites are the scalp, elbows, forearms, knees, and legs. | Psoriasis. This is a chronic skin disease. | See "Treatment" and "Self-Care" sections for "Psoriasis" in this topic. |
| Rash with small red pimples, pink blotchy skin, and itching. Common sites are between skin folds (armpits, under the breasts, the groin). | Heat rash or chafing | See "Treatment" and "Self-Care" sections for "Heat Rash or Chafing" in this topic. |

† *Reprinted with permission from the American Academy of Dermatology. All rights reserved.*

**10. Skin Conditions**

*Skin Rashes, Continued*

# Care

## For Contact Dermatitis :

If self-care doesn't take care of the rash, your doctor may prescribe:

- A more potent hydrocortisone cream than one you can get over-the-counter
- Antihistamines
- An antibiotic if you have an infection
- Oral corticosteroid drugs

## For Seborrhea:

Your doctor may prescribe a more potent hydrocortisone cream than one you can get over-the-counter.

## For Rosacea:

If self-care doesn't take care of the rash, your doctor may prescribe an antibiotic. Examples are tetracycline and metronidazole, a topical gel.

## For Scabies:

Your doctor will prescribe a topical medicine with permethrin or pyrethrin. Ones with lindane are not good to use because this chemical can cause convulsions and other problems. Family members and others you have been in close contact with should be treated, too.

## For Psoriasis:

When self-care is not enough, treatment includes:

- Ultraviolet light treatments
- Prescribed creams or ointments, such as Dovonex and coal tar products
- Oral drugs. One example is methotrexate, an anticancer drug.

## For Lyme Disease:

Your doctor will prescribe an antibiotic. Medicines may be prescribed for arthritis symptoms.

## For Heat Rash or Chafing:

Your doctor will prescribe an antibiotic for a bacterial infection or an antifungal medicine for a fungal infection.

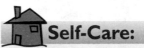 **Self-Care:**

### For Contact Dermatitis:

- Try to identify the irritant and avoid direct contact with it.
- Don't scratch the rash. This will make it worse. Wear gloves to keep from scratching. Keep your nails trimmed short. If you can't avoid scratching the rash, cover the affected area with a sterile dressing.

*Continued on Next Page*

To Learn More, See Back Cover

10. Skin Conditions

## Skin Rashes, Continued

### Self-Care, Continued

- Wash the area with a mild soap or cleaner that has no fragrance. Use warm (not hot) water.

- Add oatmeal or an oatmeal bath product, such as Aveeno, to bath water.

- Don't bathe longer than 30 minutes.

- Pat your skin dry. Don't rub.

- Apply petroleum jelly or a moisturizing lotion that is free of fragrance to dry skin. Use calamine lotion on an oozing rash.

- For severe itching, take an over-the-counter antihistamine as directed on the label. Heed the label's warnings.

- Apply a 0.5 to 1% hydrocortisone cream on the affected area.

- Wash new clothes and bedding before using them.

### For Seborrhea:

- Use an over-the-counter hydrocortisone product on the affected area.

- Use an antidandruff shampoo on the affected area.

- Handle the skin gently.

- Don't scratch. Don't use irritants, such as detergents.

### For Rosacea:

- Avoid hot and/or spicy foods.

- Avoid alcohol and caffeine.

- Don't rub or massage the face.

- Avoid strong sunlight.

### For Scabies:

- Wash clothes and bed linen thoroughly.

- Apply the prescribed cream as directed by your doctor.

### For Psoriasis:

- To prevent dryness, use a moisturizer.

- Use an over-the-counter hydrocortisone or coal tar cream or ointment.

- If psoriasis affects your scalp, use an antidandruff shampoo.

- Take a bath with mineral salts or an oatmeal bath product, such as Aveeno

- Limit exposure to cold temperatures.

- Try to prevent cuts and scrapes.

- Reduce stress.

- Avoid alcoholic beverages.

- Follow your doctor's advice about sun exposure.

*Continued on Next Page*

10. Skin Conditions

*Skin Rashes, Continued*

*Self-Care, Continued*

**To Protect Yourself from Lyme Disease:**

- When you walk through fields and forests, wear long pants, tucked into socks, and long-sleeve shirts. Light-colored, tightly woven clothing is best. Inspect for ticks after these outdoor activities.

- Apply an insect repellent with DEET to exposed skin areas or to clothing.

- Remove any ticks found on the skin. With tweezers, gently remove the tick by pulling it straight out. Try not to crush the tick because the secretions released may spread disease.

- After removing ticks, wash the wound area and your hands with soap and water.

- Save one removed tick in a closed jar with rubbing alcohol. Ask your doctor if he or she would like to see it.

**To Treat Heat Rash or Chafing:**

- Take a bath in cool water, without soap, every couple of hours.

- Let your skin air dry.

- Stay in a cool, dry area.

- Apply calamine (not Caladryl) lotion to the very itchy spots.

- Put cornstarch in body creases, such as elbow creases.

- Don't use ointments and creams that can block sweat gland pores.

## 48. Splinters

Splinters are pieces of wood, metal, or other matter that get caught under the skin.

### Prevention

- Wear shoes when you walk out-of-doors and on unfinished floors.

- Sand, varnish, and/or paint unfinished wood.

- Clean up all broken glass and metal shavings. Wear hard-soled shoes when you clean them up. Be careful when you handle broken glass.

- Wear work gloves when you handle things that can splinter, such as wood, plants with thorns, etc.

### Signs & Symptoms

Splinters tend to hurt if they are stuck deep under the skin. Those near the top of the skin are usually painless.

To Learn More, See Back Cover

**10. Skin Conditions**

*Splinters, Continued*

## Care

Self-care takes care of most splinters. A doctor may need to remove a splinter for a diabetic, or if it is deep in the skin.

### Self-Care:

- Remove splinters so they don't cause an infection.

- Wash your hands, but don't let the area around a wooden splinter get wet. A wooden splinter that gets wet will swell and be harder to remove.

- Sterilize tweezers. Place the tips in a flame. Wipe off the blackness on the tips with sterile gauze if you use a lit match for the flame.

- Use the tweezers to gently pull the part of the splinter that sticks out through the skin. It should slide right out. If you need to, use a magnifying glass to help you see close up.

- If the splinter is buried under the skin, sterilize a needle. Gently slit the skin over one end of the splinter. Use the needle to lift that end. Pull the splinter out with sterilized tweezers.

- Get all of the splinter out.

- If you still can't get the splinter out, soak the skin around the splinter in a solution made with 1 tablespoon of baking soda and 1 cup of warm water. Do this 2 times a day. After a few days, the splinter may work its way out.

- Once the splinter is removed, clean the area with soap and water. Blot it dry with a clean cloth or sterile gauze. Apply a sterile bandage.

- To remove a large number of close-to-the-surface splinters, such as cactus spines, apply a layer of hair removing wax or white glue to the skin. Let it dry for 5 minutes. Gently peel it off by lifting the edges of the dried wax or glue with tweezers. The splinter(s) should come up with it.

### Contact Doctor When:

- A splinter is deeply embedded in the skin, you cannot get it out (and it is painful), and/or you have diabetes.

- You have signs of an infection at the site of the splinter (pus, swelling, redness, etc.).

- Your tetanus shots are not up-to-date. (See "Immunizations" on page 36.)

10. Skin Conditions

*Splinters, Continued*

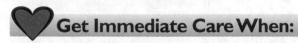

## ❤ Get Immediate Care When:

You have a fever, swollen lymph nodes and red streaks that spread from the splinter towards the heart.

## 49. Sunburn

You should never get sunburned! It leads to premature aging, wrinkling of the skin, and skin cancer.

### Prevention

- Avoid exposure to the midday sun (10 a.m. to 2 p.m. standard time or 11 a.m. to 3 p.m. daylight saving time).

- Use sunscreen with a sun protection factor (SPF) of 15 to 30 or more when exposed to the sun. The lighter your skin, the higher the SPF number should be. Make sure the sunscreen blocks both UVA and UVB rays. Reapply sunscreen every hour and after swimming.

- Use moisturizers, make-up, lip balm, etc. with sunscreen.

- Wear a wide-brimmed hat and long sleeves.

- Wear clothing with sunscreen protection or muted colors, such as tan. Bright colors and white reflect the sun onto the face.

- Wear sunglasses that absorb at least 90% of both UVA and UVB rays.

### Signs & Symptoms

- Red, swollen, painful, and sometimes blistered skin

- Headache

- Mild fever

- Chills, fever, nausea, and vomiting if the sunburn is extensive and severe

### Causes, Risk Factors & Care

Sunburn results from too much exposure to ultraviolet (UV) light from: The sun, sunlamps, and workplace light sources, such as welding arcs. Severe sunburn can occur even when the skies are overcast.

The risk for sunburn is increased for persons with fair skin, blue eyes, and red or blond hair and for persons taking some medicines. These include sulfa drugs, tetracyclines, some diuretics, and Benadryl, an over-the-counter antihistamine.

To Learn More, See Back Cover

**10. Skin Conditions**

### *Sunburn, Continued*

Self-care treats most cases of sunburn. Medical treatment is needed for a severe case of sunburn. Immediate care is needed if dehydration and/or a heat stroke is also present with the sunburn.

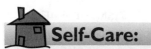

## Self-Care:

- Cool the affected area with clean towels or gauze dipped in cool water. Take a cool bath or shower.

- Take an over-the-counter medicine for pain and/or fever. (See "Pain relievers" in "Your Home Pharmacy" on page 43.)

- Apply aloe vera gel to the sunburned area 2 to 3 times a day.

- When you go in the sun again, wear sunscreen and cover sunburned skin so you don't get burned more.

- Rest in a cool room. Find a position that doesn't hurt the sunburn.

- Drink plenty of water.

- Don't use local anesthetic creams or sprays that numb pain, such as Benzocaine or Lidocaine. If you must use them, use only a little, because they cause allergic reactions in some people.

## Contact Doctor When:

You have a fever of 102°F or higher and/or severe pain or blistering with a sunburn.

## Get Immediate Care When:

You have signs of heat stroke. (See "Heat Exhaustion & Heat Stroke on page 405.)

## 50. Warts

Warts are small skin growths. Most are harmless and painless. They can appear on any part of the body.

### Prevention

- Don't touch, scratch, or pick at warts on yourself or others.

- When you shave, use an electric shaver instead of a razor blade, or use an over-the-counter hair remover cream or lotion.

- Wear plastic sandals or shower shoes in locker rooms or public pool areas.

- Change shoes often to air them out.

- Condoms should always be used with new or unknown sex partners to prevent genital warts, as well as some other sexually transmitted diseases.

10. Skin Conditions

*Warts, Continued*

## Signs & Symptoms

There are many kinds of warts.

- Common warts. These are firm and often have a rough surface. They are round or have an irregular shape. They are found on sites subject to injury, such as the hands, fingers, and knees. Common warts are flesh-colored to brown. They may spread, but are never cancerous.

- Flat warts. These are smooth and flesh-colored. They are found mainly on the hands and face. They may itch.

- Plantar warts. These occur on the soles of the feet. They look like corns or calluses and may have little black dots in the center. They can be painful.

- Digitate warts. These are threadlike warts that grow on the scalp.

- Filiform warts. These are long, narrow, small growths. They appear mainly on the neck, eyelids, or armpits.

- Genital warts. (See "STD'S Chart – Genital Warts" on page 364.)

## Causes, Risk Factors & Care

Warts are caused by any of the 60 related human papilloma virus types. The virus may enter the body through a cut or nick in the skin. Scratching or picking at warts may spread them to other sites. Some persons are more prone to getting warts than others. People who cannot fight off disease are also more at risk for warts. You cannot get warts from frogs or toads.

Treatment for warts depends on their location, type, and severity, as well as the length of time they have been on the skin. About 50% of warts go away in 6 to 12 months without treatment. An over-the-counter wart remover with salicylic acid can help get rid of some warts. When this and other self-care measures are not enough, medical care can treat some warts.

- A doctor can treat common warts with liquid nitrogen to freeze them or with other chemicals, which destroy the wart. New warts can sometimes develop around the edges of old ones.

- Plantar warts can be softened with a strong salicylic acid applied as a solution or plaster. Doctors may inject chemicals to destroy the warts.

To Learn More, See Back Cover

*10. Skin Conditions*

*Warts, Continued*

- Flat warts are often treated with peeling agents, such as retinoic or salicylic acid, which causes the warts to come off with the scaly skin.

- Genital warts can be removed with surgery or with topical medicine. Even with treatment, genital warts can recur.

## Self-Care:

- Never cut or burn a wart off.

- Try an over-the-counter wart remover with salicylic and lactic acids. {**Note:** Do not use these wart removers on the face or genitals. Follow package directions. Afterward you may need to use a pumice stone to remove the dead skin.}

- Apply an over-the-counter medicated wart pad or patch. Cut it to the size of the wart before you apply it.

- Ask your doctor about Retin A for flat warts.

- If you have plantar warts, put pads or cushions in your shoes. This can help the pain when you walk.

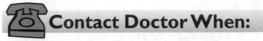

## Contact Doctor When:

- You have any of these problems with the wart:
  - It is near the genital or anal area.
  - It is painful.
  - It changed its shape or color.
  - Signs of infection (redness; swelling; pain; pus and/or drainage) occur at the wart site.

- The location of the wart limits normal movement.

- The wart is a new wart on a person over 45 years old.

- You have any of these problems:
  - The wart is bothersome and has not responded to home treatment.
  - The wart has been irritated or ripped off.
  - The wart is on the face and you want it removed.
  - Multiple warts are present.

**10. Skin Conditions**

## 51. How Aging Affects Digestion

Many people have few, if any, digestive problems due to aging itself.

As you age, though, your digestive muscles move slower. Your body makes less acid. Other things can hamper the digestive system, too. These include:

- Increased use of medicines

- Getting less exercise

- Changes in eating habits

- Dental problems

- Loss of muscle tone and elasticity. This could be a factor in hiatal hernias (see page 172) and diverticulosis (see page 158), which are common in persons as they get older.

This chapter covers common digestive and other abdominal conditions. It also covers problems that affect your urinary system.

## 52. Abdominal Pain

The abdomen is the body region between the lower ribs and the pelvis. Many vital organs make up this body region.

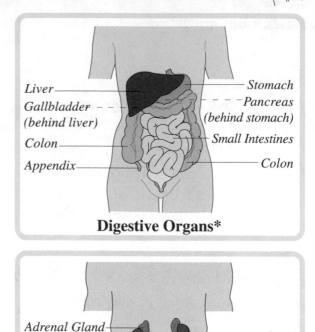

**Digestive Organs***

Liver — Stomach — Gallbladder (behind liver) — Pancreas (behind stomach) — Colon — Small Intestines — Appendix — Colon

**Urinary Tract Organs***

Adrenal Gland — Kidney — Ureter — Bladder — Prostate Gland (Males)

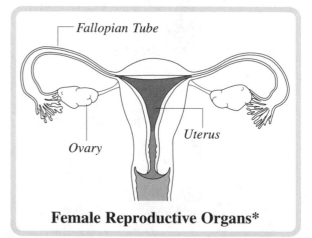

**Female Reproductive Organs***

Fallopian Tube — Uterus — Ovary

*Abdominal Pain, Continued*

## Signs & Symptoms

Abdominal pain can range from mild to severe. The pain can be dull or sharp. It can be acute or chronic. Acute pain is sudden pain. Chronic pain can be constant or pain that recurs over time. The type of pain, its location, and other symptoms that come with it point to the cause.

## Causes & Care

There are many causes for abdominal pain. The pain can be a symptom of a condition that affects any of the abdominal organs shown on page 150.

Constipation, heartburn, and infections, such as an intestinal virus or urinary tract infection are common causes.

What to do for abdominal pain depends on the cause. The key is knowing when it's just a minor problem like a mild stomach ache or when it's something worse. Pain that persists can be a sign of a medical condition or illness. Very severe abdominal pain usually requires immediate medical care.

### Self-Care:

**To Help Ease Pain:**

- Use a hot water bottle or a heating pad set on low.
- Find a comfortable position. Relax.
- Take an over-the-counter pain medicine. (See "Pain relievers" in "Your Home Pharmacy" on page 43.)
- Don't wear tight-fitting clothes.
- Don't do strenuous exercise.

**For Lactose Intolerance:**

- Avoid foods that are not easy for you to digest. Some people with lactose intolerance can tolerate certain dairy products if they have small portions at a time.
- Try foods that have had lactose reduced by bacterial cultures. Examples are buttermilk, yogurt and sweet acidophilus milks.
- Take over-the-counter products (drops or pills) with lactase when you have foods with lactose.
- If the above measures don't help, avoid products with milk, milk solids, and whey. Products marked "parve" are milk free.

*Continued on Next Page*

## Abdominal Pain, Continued

### Self-Care, Continued

See also "Self-Care" for:

- "Anxiety" on page 306
- "Constipation" on page 154
- "Diarrhea" on page 156
- "Flatulence (Gas)" on page 160
- "Heartburn" on page 166
- "Irritable Bowel Syndrome" on page 173
- "Urinary Tract Infections" on page 186
- "Vomiting & Nausea" on page 189

## ☎ Contact Doctor When:

- You have signs and symptoms of kidney stones (see page 176).
- You have any of these problems with abdominal pain:
  - The whites of the eyes or the skin looks yellow (jaundice)
  - A recent blow to the abdomen
  - Severe diarrhea
  - Constipation for more than a week
  - Sensitive skin or skin rash on the abdomen
  - Fever
- You have signs and symptoms of a urinary tract infection (see page 186).
- You are female and have any of these problems with abdominal pain:
  - Vaginal bleeding (not during a period) or after menopause
  - Vaginal discharge that is thick or watery, colored, or bad-smelling
  - Pain during sexual intercourse
- You are male and have any of these problems with abdominal pain:
  - Blood in the urine
  - Constant urge to urinate
  - Urinating often
  - Fever and chills
  - A discharge from the penis
  - Swelling or discomfort in the groin that is made worse by coughing or lifting heavy objects
- You have signs and symptoms of a hernia (see page 171).

*Abdominal Pain, Continued*

### ♥ Get Immediate Care When:

- You have "Heart Attack Warning Signs" (see page 202).

- The pain spreads to your back, chest, or right shoulder, and/or you feel a throbbing mass in your abdomen.

- The pain is very severe or hurts so bad that you can't move.

- You vomit true red blood or stuff that looks like coffee grounds.

- You vomit, have a fever and shaking chills, and have pain in one or both sides of the back.

- You have all of these symptoms of **appendicitis** and you have not had your appendix removed:

  • Pain and tenderness that usually starts in the upper part of the stomach or around the belly button and that moves to the lower right part of the abdomen. The pain can be sharp and severe.

  • Nausea, vomiting, or no appetite

  • Mild fever

- Blood in the stools or stools that are tarlike and black in color

# 53. Colon & Rectal Cancers

The colon and rectum form the large bowel. The colon is the upper 5 to 6 feet. The rectum is the last 6 to 8 inches.

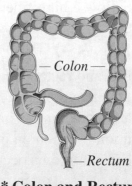

— Colon —

— Rectum

**\* Colon and Rectum**

When abnormal cells grow in the colon, a cancerous tumor may form. Colon tumors grow slowly. They may get big and block the bowel. If found early, a cure is possible.

## Prevention

- Early detection is the most important factor. Colon and rectal cancers are completely curable if found early. Have the following screening tests:

  • A digital rectal exam and a stool blood test every year starting at age 50

  • A sigmoidoscopy every 3 to 5 years starting at age 50 or at time intervals that your doctor advises

  {**Note:** You may need these or other tests, such as a colonoscopy sooner or more often if you have a family history of colon polyps or colon or rectal cancers.}

II. Abdominal & Urinary Problems

### *Colon & Rectal Cancers, Continued*

- Have colon polyps removed.
- Follow a high fiber, low-fat diet.

## Signs & Symptoms

Colon and rectal cancers can occur without clear symptoms. For this reason, yearly screening is important. (See "Prevention" section on page 153.)
When symptoms occur, they include:

- A change in bowel habits for 2 or more weeks or constipation or diarrhea for 1 or more weeks.
- Frequent gas pains, cramps, bloating, or feelings of fullness in the abdomen
- Red or dark blood in or on the stool or rectal bleeding
- Fatigue and/or iron deficiency anemia in men and older women
- Pencil thin stools
- A feeling that the bowel does not empty completely
- Weight loss for no known reason

## Causes, Risk Factors & Care

Risk factors for colon and rectal cancers:

- Polyps (benign growths that can become cancerous over time). Most colon and rectal cancers develop from polyps.
- Family history of colon or rectal cancers, chronic colitis, or colon polyps. Unless it is treated, an inherited condition called Familial Polyposis puts a person at a very high risk.
- Age. Colon and rectal cancers occur most often in people over age 50.
- Exposure to asbestos
- Eating a diet high in fat and low in fiber
- Physical inactivity

Finding and treating the cancer early is vital. Treatment is based on the size and location of the tumor and the stage of the disease. Age and general health are also factors in treatment. Treatment includes surgery, chemotherapy, and radiation therapy.

### Self-Care:

- Schedule and go to follow-up exams.
- Join a cancer support group.
- Follow a high fiber, low-fat diet. Eat whole grain breads and cereals. Have at least 5 servings of vegetables and fruits a day.

### Contact Doctor When:

- You have any symptoms of colon and rectal cancer listed on this page.

To Learn More, See Back Cover

*Colon & Rectal Cancers, Continued*

- You need to schedule screening tests for colon and rectal cancer. Follow the schedule your doctor advises.

## For Information Contact:

The Cancer Information Service
1-800-4-CANCER (422-6237)
www.nci.nih.gov

The American Cancer Society
1-800-227-2345
www.cancer.org

# 54. Constipation

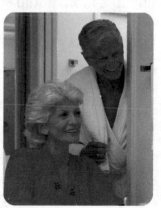

Constipation is when you have trouble having bowel movements. Older people report this problem more often than younger ones. "Regularity" does not mean that you need to have a bowel movement every day. Normal bowel habits range from 3 movements a day to 3 each week. What is more important is what is normal for you.

## Signs & Symptoms

- A hard time passing stool, not being able to pass stool, having very hard stools
- Straining to have a bowel movement
- Abdominal swelling or feeling of continued fullness after passing stool

## Causes & Care

Constipation is caused by:

- Drinking too few fluids and not eating enough dietary fiber
- Not being active enough
- Not going to the bathroom when you have the urge to pass stool
- Misusing laxatives
- A side effect of some heart, pain, and antidepressant medicines, as well as antacids, antihistamines, water pills, and narcotics
- Some chronic illnesses, such as diabetes, which slow the digestive tract

In persons 50 and older, the digestive system gets more sluggish. The abdominal and pelvic floor muscles become weaker. These, too, can help cause constipation.

Self-care treats most causes of constipation. You may also need to talk to your doctor about medications and health conditions that could be causing you to be constipated.

**11. Abdominal & Urinary Problems**

*Constipation, Continued*

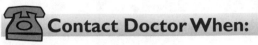

### Self-Care:

- Eat foods high in dietary fiber: Bran; whole-grain breads and cereals, and fresh fruits and vegetables.

- Drink at least $1\frac{1}{2}$ to 2 quarts of water and other liquids every day.

- Have hot water, tea, or coffee. These may help stimulate the bowel.

- Get plenty of exercise.

- Don't resist the urge to eliminate.

- Know that antacids and iron supplements can be binding. If you get constipated easily, discuss the use of these with your doctor.

- Ask your doctor about the use of stool softeners, like Colace, or fiber supplements, such as Metamucil. Take as directed by your doctor.

- Do not use "stimulant" laxatives, such as Ex-Lax, or enemas without your doctor's okay. Long-term use of them can:
  - Make you even more constipated
  - Lead to a mineral imbalance and reduce nutrient absorption
  - Make it harder for your body to benefit from medicines

### Contact Doctor When:

You have constipation with any of these problems:

- Blood seen in the stools

- Unrelieved abdominal pain, especially on the lower left side

- Fever and/or vomiting

- Very thin, pencil-like stools

- Symptoms that worsen or do not improve after 1 week of self-care

## 55. Diarrhea

Diarrhea occurs when body wastes are discharged from the bowel more often and in a more liquid state than usual.

### Signs & Symptoms

- Watery, loose stools
- Frequent bowel movements
- Cramping or pain in the abdomen

### Causes & Care

Common causes are infections that affect the digestive system, overuse of laxatives or alcohol, and taking some antibiotics, like tetracycline. Diarrhea is also a symptom of lactose intolerance, diverticulitis, irritable bowel syndrome, ulcerative colitis, or Crohn's disease.

*Diarrhea, Continued*

Self-care can be used for most bouts of diarrhea. If the diarrhea is caused by a medical condition, treatment for the condition treats the diarrhea.

### Self-Care:

- If vomiting is also present, treat for vomiting first. (See "Vomiting & Nausea" on page 189.)

- Follow your normal diet if there are no signs of dehydration (dry mouth; thirst; muscle cramps; weakness; etc.)

- If there are signs of dehydration, stop solid foods. Have around 2 cups of clear fluids per hour (if vomiting isn't present). Fluids of choice are:

  - Sport drinks, such as Gatorade.

  - Kool-Aid. This usually has less sugar than soda pop.

  - A mixture of 4 teaspoons of sugar, 1 teaspoon of salt, and 1 quart of water.

- Avoid having high "simple" sugar drinks, like apple juice, grape juice, gelatin, regular colas, and other soft drinks. These can pull water into the gut and make the diarrhea persist. Don't have boiled milk, either.

- Don't have just clear liquids for more than 24 hours.

- Start eating normal meals within 12 hours. Good food choices are:

  - Starchy foods, like rice, potatoes, cereals (not sugar-sweetened ones), crackers, and toast

  - Vegetables and soups with noodles, rice, and/or vegetables

  - Lean meats

  - Yogurt, especially with live active cultures of lactobacillus acidophilus

- Avoid fatty and fried foods.

- The B.R.A.T. diet: just having bananas, rice, applesauce, and dry toast is no longer the diet of choice for diarrhea. These foods are still okay to eat, though. Bananas are a good source of potassium.

- Don't exercise too hard until the diarrhea is gone.

- Try an over-the-counter antidiarrheal medicine, such as Imodium A-D, but wait at least 12 hours before you take this.

- Wash your hands after going to the toilet and before preparing food, especially if the diarrhea is from an infection in the GI tract. Use disposable paper towels to dry your hands.

11. Abdominal & Urinary Problems

*Diarrhea, Continued*

## ☎ Contact Doctor When:

- Severe abdominal or rectal pain occurs with diarrhea. (See your Doctor the same day.)

- You have any of these problems with diarrhea:

  - Fever

  - The diarrhea has lasted 48 hours or longer.

  - You have a chronic illness and had diarrhea more than 8 times a day.

  - You are taking medicines (this includes regular medicines that the body may not be absorbing due to the diarrhea, or prescribed, or over-the-counter ones that might be contributing to the diarrhea).

## ♥ Get Immediate Care When:

- Signs and symptoms of dehydration (see page 391) occur with diarrhea.

- There is blood in the diarrhea or its color is tarlike or maroon.

# 56. Diverticulosis & Diverticulitis

Sometimes small sac-like pouches protrude from the wall of the colon. This is called diverticulo-

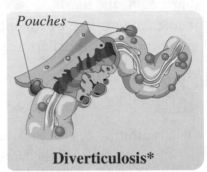

*Pouches*

**Diverticulosis\***

sis. The pockets (called diverticuli) can fill with intestinal waste, especially seeds. With diverticulitis, the intestinal pockets and areas around them get inflamed or infected.

## Signs & Symptoms

**For Diverticulosis:**

In most cases, there are no symptoms. When they occur, they are:

- Tenderness, pain, mild cramping, or a bloated feeling, usually on the lower left side of the abdomen

- Gas, nausea

- Constipation that alternates with diarrhea

📟 To Learn More, See Back Cover

*Diverticulosis & Diverticulitis, Continued*

### For Diverticulitis:

- Severe cramping in the abdomen, usually on the lower left side. The pain is made worse with a bowel movement.

- Tenderness over the abdomen

- Fever

- Nausea

- Blood in the stool

## Causes, Risk Factors & Care

Many older persons have diverticulosis. The digestive system becomes sluggish as a person ages. These things increase the risk for diverticulosis:

- Not eating enough dietary fiber

- Overuse of laxatives or continual use of medicines that slow bowel action, such as strong painkillers

- Having family members who have diverticulosis

- Having gallbladder disease

- Being obese

Diverticulitis needs medical treatment. This includes antibiotics, pain relievers, bed rest, and a stay in the hospital, if needed. Fluids and medicine may need to be given through an IV.

Diverticulosis can't be cured. You can, though, reduce the discomfort and prevent complications with self-care.

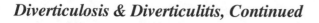 **Self-Care:**

- Eat a diet high in fiber throughout life. Good food sources are whole-grain breads and cereals, fresh fruits and vegetables, and legumes. Check with your doctor about adding wheat bran to your diet.

- Avoid corn, nuts, seeds, and foods with seeds, like raisins and figs. These seeds are easily trapped in the troublesome pouches. Avoid foods that bother you.

- Drink $1\frac{1}{2}$ to 2 quarts of water daily.

- Ask your doctor about taking bulk-forming laxatives, like Metamucil.

- Avoid the regular use of laxatives that make your bowel muscles contract, such as Ex-Lax.

- Try not to strain when you have bowel movements.

- Get regular exercise.

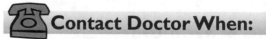 **Contact Doctor When:**

- You have blood in the stool or black or tarry stools. (See your doctor the same day.)

*Diverticulosis & Diverticulitis, Continued*

- You have changes in bowel habits that last longer than 2 weeks.
- Any signs and symptoms of diverticulosis last longer than 2 weeks

### Get Immediate Care When:

- You have very severe abdominal pain.
- You have signs of an intestinal obstruction:
  - You can't pass stool or even gas.
  - Mild fever and weakness
  - Abdominal cramps that come and go
  - Your abdomen gets more and more swollen with increasing pain
  - Hiccups that don't stop
  - Vomiting

# 57. Flatulence (Gas)

Flatulence is passing gas through the anus. For the average adult, this happens about 6 to 20 times a day.

## Signs & Symptoms

- Pressure or discomfort in the lower abdomen or anal area
- Passing gas
- Foul odor (sometimes)

## Causes & Care

Gas is caused by swallowing air and digesting foods. Eating high fiber foods, like beans, peas, and grains creates more gas than other foods. Dairy foods can create large amounts of gas in some people.

Gas may signal other problems, too. These include lactose intolerance, taking certain antibiotics, and abnormal muscle contractions in the colon

Self-care treats most cases of gas. If the gas is due to another medical condition, treating the condition treats the problem.

### Self-Care:

- Try not to swallow air at mealtimes. Avoid carbonated beverages and chewing gum. These things can cause more air to get into your stomach.
- When you add fiber to your diet, do so gradually.
- Release the gas when you need to. Don't try to hold it in. Go to another room if it will make you less self-conscious.

*Continued on Next Page*

*Flatulence (Gas), Continued*

### Self-Care, Continued

- Keep a list of all of the foods you eat for a few days. Note when and the number of times you have gas. Foods that often cause gas include apples; dairy products (for persons allergic to lactose); eggs; beans and peas; bran; onions; broccoli, brussels sprouts, cabbage, and cauliflower; popcorn; prunes and raisins; and sorbitol (an artificial sweetener). If you notice that you have excess gas after eating beans, for example, try cutting down on or eliminate them from your diet. See if the gas persists. Do the same for other foods that you think are causing you to have gas.

{**Note:** Eliminate or go easy on only the foods that affect you. Other than sorbitol, the foods listed provide nutrients, so should not be cut out altogether.}

- If you are lactose-intolerant, use lactose-reduced dairy foods or add an over-the-counter lactose-enzyme product, such as Lactaid.

- Try an over-the-counter medicine with simethicone, Mylicon or Gas-X. Your doctor can prescribe one, too.

- Beans, such as kidney beans, are a good source of dietary fiber. To lessen getting gas after eating them, use dry beans instead of canned ones. Cover them with water and let them soak overnight. Replace the water with fresh water. Cook the beans thoroughly. Also, try an over-the-counter product, such as Bean-O or Phazyme. Each of these may curb gas caused by eating some foods, such as baked beans.

## ☎ Contact Doctor When:

Gas occurs with any of these problems:

- Steady pain in the upper abdomen
- Nausea and vomiting
- Yellowing of the whites of the eyes or skin (jaundice)
- Excessive gas only after taking a prescribed antibiotic

# 58. Food Poisoning

Food poisoning comes from eating food that contains a harmful substance.

**11. Abdominal & Urinary Problems**

*Food Poisoning, Continued*

## Prevention

- Wash your hands before you handle food. Use clean utensils and clean surfaces when you prepare foods. Use antibacterial cleaners for your hands and surfaces you prepare food on.

- Wash your hands, knives, cutting boards, and utensils after handling uncooked foods.

- Instead of wooden cutting boards, use acrylic ones. Wash them in a dishwasher or in very hot, soapy water.

- Completely defrost poultry before cooking it. Defrost meats in the refrigerator or microwave. Cover poultry and meat when heating them in a microwave.

- Rinse all fruits and vegetables in clean, soapy water, to remove dirt and other particles that cling to the skins.

- Wash dirty eggs before using them. Wash your hands after touching raw eggs.

- Don't eat uncooked and rare meats.

- Throw out any canned goods with leaks or bulges.

- Keep party or picnic foods on ice or in coolers with ice or ice packs.

- Keep hot foods hot and cold foods cold. Hot foods should be kept higher than 140°F. Cold foods should be kept at 40°F or below. Do not eat these foods when kept for more than 2 hours between 40°F and 140°F.

- Don't eat foods after the expiration date printed on the package or foods that smell or look bad.

- Don't store foods or liquids in lead crystal containers or ceramic dishes with lead-based paints.

- "When in doubt, throw it out."

- When the news reports contaminated food products, avoid them.

## Signs & Symptoms

Signs of food poisoning vary. Symptoms may come on quickly or take up to 2 to 3 days to appear. Symptoms include:

- Nausea, vomiting, diarrhea
- Stomach pain
- Fever
- Shock or collapse

### For Chemical Food Poisoning:

- Sweating
- Dizziness, mental confusion
- Very teary eyes, watery mouth
- Stomach pain, vomiting, diarrhea

*Food Poisoning, Continued*

### For Botulism:

- Dry mouth
- Muscle fatigue or paralysis
- Breathing problems
- Difficulty speaking or swallowing
- Vision problems, such as blurry vision or drooping eyelids

## Causes, Risk Factors & Care

- Bacterial causes:

  - Staphylococcal poisoning is a common cause. It is linked with unrefrigerated meats and dairy products, and picnics or gatherings where food is not kept cold.

  - Listeria poisoning can come from eating uncooked meats and vegetables, or foods that get contaminated after processing. Examples are soft cheeses and cold cuts. The bacteria is also found in unpasteurized milk products. Persons more likely to become very ill with listeria are pregnant women, newborns, elderly persons and those with weakened immune systems.

  - E. Coli poisoning can come from eating undercooked meats or foods contaminated with animal feces.

- Salmonella poisoning can come from eating: Raw or undercooked eggs; undercooked poultry; and food that comes in contact with surfaces contaminated with salmonella.

- Viruses, such as ones in undercooked shellfish, like mussels, clams, or oysters or undercooked foods in contact with contaminated water

- Chemicals, such as ones in poisonous mushrooms, and foods that contain insecticides

- Toxic substances, such as:

  - Botulism, bacterial toxins that form when foods are not canned or preserved correctly

  - Mercury, found in some contaminated fish

  - Lead, found in some imported foods packed in lead-soldered cans. This can also occur when food is eaten off ceramic dishes (usually imported) that have lead in the paint.

Most cases of food poisoning can be treated at home with self-care. Emergency care is needed for botulism, chemical food poisoning, and some severe cases of bacterial food poisoning.

## Food Poisoning, Continued

### Self-Care:

- If you suspect chemical food poisoning, call your Poison Control Center.

- If vomiting, follow "Self-Care" in "Vomiting and Nausea" on page 189.

- If diarrhea is present, follow "Self-Care" in "Diarrhea" on page 157.

- It is best to check with your Doctor before you take over-the-counter antinausea and antidiarrheal medicines. If you do take one of these, wait 24 or more hours after the onset of symptoms. Let your body get rid of the food poisoning source.

### Contact Doctor When:

- You have any of these problems with diarrhea:
  - Severe vomiting
  - Temperature over 101°F
  - Blood-streaked stools
  - Pain that has lasted for several hours or pain that is getting worse

- Diarrhea is present after 2 days of using self-care or vomiting is present after 12 hours of eating only ice chips.

### Get Immediate Care When:

You have any of these problems:

- Botulism symptoms (see page 163)

- Chemical food poisoning symptoms (see page 162)

- Signs of dehydration (see page 391)

- You vomit bright red blood or material that looks like coffee grounds.

- You have bright red blood in diarrhea and/or you look and act very sick.

- You have a headache, stiff neck, confusion, and loss of balance or you have a convulsion.

## 59. Gallstones

The gallbladder stores bile, a substance used in the digestion of fats.

Gallstones are stone deposits that are found in the gallbladder or bile ducts, which carry bile to the small intestine. Gallstones contain a mixture of cholesterol, bilirubin, and protein. They can range in size from less than a pinhead to 3 inches across. When a stone gets trapped in one of the bile ducts, a "gallbladder attack" occurs.

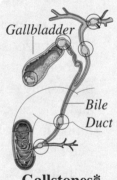

Gallbladder

Bile Duct

**Gallstones***

To Learn More, See Back Cover

*Gallstones, Continued*

## Prevention

- Get to and stay at your ideal body weight. If you are overweight, lose weight slowly (1 to $1^1/_2$ pounds per week). Do not follow a rapid weight loss diet, unless under strict medical guidance.

- Follow your doctor's advice to lower your cholesterol, if it is high.

- Follow a high fiber, low-fat, low cholesterol diet.

## Signs & Symptoms

- Feeling bloated and gassy, especially after eating fried or fatty foods

- Steady pain in the upper right abdomen lasting from 20 minutes to 5 hours

- Pain between the shoulder blades or in the right shoulder

- Indigestion, nausea, vomiting

- Severe abdominal pain with fever and sometimes yellow skin and/or eyes

## Causes, Risk Factors & Care

Doctors aren't sure why gallstones form, but some people are more prone to get them than others. Risk factors are:

- A family history of gallbladder disease

- Obesity and/or very rapid weight loss

- Eating a diet high in cholesterol

- Middle age

- Being female, having had many pregnancies, taking estrogen

- Having diabetes or diseases of the small intestine

Depending on their size and location, gallstones may cause no symptoms or may need medical treatment. {**Note:** Gallstone symptoms can be hard to tell apart from heart-related or other more serious conditions. A doctor should evaluate any new symptoms.} Once diagnosed, treatment for gallstones includes:

- A low-fat diet to reduce contractions of the gallbladder and limit pain

- Medicines to dissolve the stones

- Lithotripsy (the use of sound waves to shatter the stones)

- Surgery to remove the gallbladder. This is the most common treatment. The digestive system can still function without a gallbladder.

### Self-Care:

Self-care does not apply to gallstones. To reduce your risk of gallstones, see "Prevention" in this topic.

## Gallstones, Continued

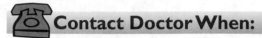

### Contact Doctor When:

You have any of the signs and symptoms listed in this topic, especially with any of these conditions:

- Temperature of 100°F or higher

- Diabetes or any illness or use of medicines that lower the immune system

- A history of gallstones

### Get Immediate Care When:

- You have symptoms of a heart attack that mimic symptoms of a gallbladder attack:

  - Sudden, severe pain in the upper right abdomen

  - Pain in the right shoulder and arm, especially if it started in the chest (See "Heart Attack Warning Signs" on page 202.)

- You have very severe abdominal pain or pain in the upper right abdomen that lasts more than 4 hours.

# 60. Heartburn

Heartburn has nothing to do with the heart. It involves the esophagus and the stomach. The esophagus passes behind the breastbone alongside the heart, so the

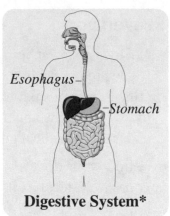

**Digestive System***

irritation that takes place there feels like a burning feeling in the heart.

## Signs & Symptoms

- Burning feeling behind the breastbone that occurs after eating

- Chest pain when you bend over or lie down

- Bitter, hot, or sour taste in the mouth

## Causes & Care

Gastric acids from the stomach splash back up into the lower portion of the esophagus. This causes pain. The medical term for this is **gastroesophageal reflex disease (GERD)**. The digestive acids don't harm the stomach, thanks to its protective coating. The esophagus has no such armor, though, which results in discomfort.

To Learn More, See Back Cover

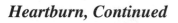

**II. Abdominal & Urinary Problems**

## Heartburn, Continued

Common heartburn triggers are:

- Taking aspirin, ibuprofen, naproxen sodium, arthritis medicine, or cortisone

- Eating heavy meals, eating too fast, or eating chocolate, garlic, onions, peppermint, tomatoes, or citrus fruits

- Smoking or lying down after eating

- Drinking alcohol or coffee (regular or decaffeinated)

- Being very overweight

- Wearing tight clothing

- Swallowing too much air

- Stress

- Hiatal hernia (see page 172)

Heartburn is common. Self-care can be used for most cases. Heartburn symptoms can be confused, though, for a heart attack or other medical conditions.

### Self-Care:

- Sit straight while you eat. Stand up or walk around after you eat. Bending over or lying down after you eat makes it too easy for gastric secretions to move up to the esophagus.

- Lose weight if you are overweight.

- If heartburn bothers you at night, raise the head of the bed. Put the head of your bed up on 6-inch blocks or buy a wedge especially made to be placed between the mattress and box spring. Don't just prop your head up with pillows. This makes the problem worse by putting pressure on your stomach.

- Avoid wearing tight-fitting garments around the abdomen.

- Eat small meals. Limit alcohol.

- Limit foods and drinks that contain air, such as whipped cream and carbonated drinks.

- Don't eat or drink for 2 to 3 hours before bedtime.

- If other treatments fail, take antacids, such as magnesium hydroxide or Tums. If these don't bring relief, take an over-the-counter acid controller, such as Pepcid AC, Tagamet HB, etc. These not only relieve heartburn, but can prevent it. {**Note:** Read labels before taking antacids or acid controllers. Check with your doctor, too. Adverse side effects are more likely and more severe in older persons who take some acid controllers, such as Tagamet HB.}

*Continued on Next Page*

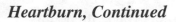

**11. Abdominal & Urinary Problems**

*Heartburn, Continued*

*Self-Care, Continued*

- Don't take baking soda. It may neutralize stomach acid at first, but when its effects wear off, the acid comes back to a greater degree, causing gastric-acid rebound.

- Don't smoke.

- If you do take aspirin, ibuprofen, naproxen sodium, or arthritis medicines, take them with food.

### ☎ Contact Doctor When:

- You have a hard time swallowing with heartburn symptoms.

- You have had symptoms often over 3 days and/or have tried self-care measures and found no relief.

### ♥ Get Immediate Care When:

- You have symptoms of a heart attack. (See "Heart Attack Warning Signs" on page 202.)

- You vomit bright red blood or material that looks like coffee grounds.

- Your stools are tarlike, maroon, or bloody in color.

- Pain goes through to your back or you have a gripping pain in the upper abdomen.

# 61. Hemorrhoids

Hemorrhoids are veins under the rectum or around the anus that are dilated or swollen.

## Signs & Symptoms

- Rectal bleeding

- Rectal tenderness and/or itching

- Uncomfortable, painful bowel movements, especially with straining

- A lump that can be felt at the anus

- Mucus passed from the anus

## Causes, Risk Factors & Care

Hemorrhoids are usually caused by repeated pressure in the rectal or anal veins, usually from repeated straining to pass stool.

The risk for getting hemorrhoids increases with constipation, a low dietary fiber intake, and obesity.

Hemorrhoids are common, but seldom a serious health problem. Most people have some bleeding from them once in a while.

🖳 To Learn More, See Back Cover

## Hemorrhoids, *Continued*

It is never wise, though, to assume that rectal bleeding is "just hemorrhoids." Unless you have had a recent evaluation by your doctor and have been told you have hemorrhoids, get any unexplained rectal bleeding diagnosed by your doctor.

If symptoms of hemorrhoids are not relieved with self-care or with time, medical treatment may be needed. This includes:

- Cryosurgery, to freeze the affected tissue
- A chemical injection into an internal hemorrhoid to shrink it
- Laser heat or infrared light to destroy the hemorrhoids
- Surgery. One type cuts out the hemorrhoid. Another type called ligation, uses rubber bands that are placed tightly over the base of each hemorrhoid, causing it to wither away.

### Self-Care:

- Drink at least $1^1/_2$ to 2 quarts of fluid per day.
- Eat foods with good sources of dietary fiber, such as whole grain or bran cereals and breads, and fresh vegetables and fruits.

- Eat prunes. Drink prune juice.
- If necessary, add bran to your foods. Add about 3 to 4 tablespoons per day.
- Lose weight if you are overweight.
- Get regular exercise.
- Pass a bowel movement as soon as you feel the urge. If you wait and the urge goes away, your stool could become dry and be harder to pass.
- Don't strain to pass stool.
- Don't hold your breath when trying to pass stool.
- Keep the anal area clean.
- Take warm baths.
- Use a sitz bath with hot water. A sitz bath is a basin that fits over the toilet. Get one at a medical supply or drug store.
- Use moist towelettes or wet (not dry) toilet paper after a bowel movement.
- Check with your doctor about using over-the-counter products, such as:
  - Stool softeners
  - Zinc oxide preparations, such as Preparation H
  - Medicated wipes, such as Tucks
  - Medicated suppositories

*Continued on Next Page*

*Hemorrhoids, Continued*

*Self-Care, Continued*

- Don't sit too much. This can restrict blood flow around the anal area. Don't sit too long on the toilet. Don't read while on the toilet.

- For itching or pain, put a cold compress on the anus for 10 minutes at a time up to 4 times a day.

## Contact Doctor When:

- You have unexplained rectal bleeding with or without bowel movements.

- A hard lump is felt where a hemorrhoid used to be.

- Rectal pain is severe or lasts longer than 1 week.

- The bleeding from a hemorrhoid lasts longer than 2 weeks despite using self-care.

## Get Immediate Care When:

You have severe rectal bleeding that is continuous or that occurs with weakness or dizziness.

# 62. Hernias

A hernia occurs when part of an internal organ "bulges" through a weak area or hole in a surrounding muscle. Often, this happens in the wall of the abdomen.

Common hernias include:

- Hiatal hernia, see page 172

- Inguinal hernia. A part of the intestine bulges through a muscle near the groin or scrotum.

- Incisional hernia, a bulge through a muscle at the site of a past surgical scar.

- Femoral hernia, a bulge in the top front of a thigh. This type is most common in obese women.

## Prevention

- Follow proper lifting techniques. (See the "Dos and Don't's of Lifting" in "Back Pain" on page 234.)

- Exercise to keep abdominal muscles strong. Follow your doctor's advice.

- Avoid constipation. (See "Self-Care" in "Constipation" on page 156.)

- Lose weight if you are overweight.

- Don't smoke. Avoid secondhand smoke.

*Hernias, Continued*

## Signs & Symptoms

- A bulge in the skin. The bulge may be more easy to see when you cough, lift, or strain or when you lie down flat on your back. The bulge may feel soft.

- Mild pain or discomfort at the hernia site. The pain may only be felt when you strain, lift, or cough.

- For an inguinal hernia, weakness, pressure, burning, or pain in the groin area

- Swelling of the scrotum

- Groin lump that shows when standing

- Extreme pain when the hernia bulges out and can't be pushed back in

## Causes, Risk Factors & Care

A weakness in the abdominal wall is often the cause. Some persons are born with such a weakness. Hernias can run in families. Other causes include:

- Lifting heavy objects; heavy coughing

- Obesity

- Straining to have a bowel movement, as with chronic constipation

- Abdominal surgery

- Being male or elderly

If the hernia can be positioned back into the body, surgery may not be needed. If not, outpatient surgery may be needed to repair it.

### Self-Care:

- Wear a weight lifting belt to support the back when lifting.

- Maintain a healthy diet.

- Avoid constipation. Don't strain when having bowel movements.

- When you do sit ups, keep knees bent and your feet flat on the floor.

- Wear a truss. This is a device that holds a hernia in place.

- For mild pain, take an over-the-counter medicine for pain. (See "Pain relievers" in "Your Home Pharmacy" on page 43.)

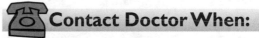

### Contact Doctor When:

You have any of these problems:

- A bulge or swelling in the abdomen or groin

- Mild groin pain lasts more than a week

- You suspect that you have a hernia.

**11. Abdominal & Urinary Problems**

*Hernias, Continued*

## ♥ Get Immediate Care When:

- You have sudden severe pain in the area of the hernia, groin, or scrotum.

- You are unable to pass gas or to have a bowel movement.

# 63. Hiatal Hernia

With hiatal hernia, a small part of the stomach bulges up through the diaphragm, the muscle that divides the stomach from the chest cavity. As a result, the normal mechanism that closes off the top of the stomach does not work well and food or stomach acids back up into the esophagus. This is known as **Gastroesophageal Reflux Disease (GERD)**.

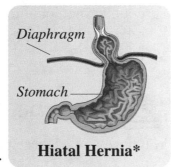

Diaphragm

Stomach

**Hiatal Hernia***

## Prevention

- Do exercises on a regular basis to keep abdominal muscles in shape.

- Stay at a healthy body weight. Lose weight, if you are overweight.

- Don't smoke. If you smoke, quit.

- Avoid spicy foods, alcohol, and caffeine.

## Signs & Symptoms

Many people have no symptoms with an hiatal hernia. Others have one or more of these problems:

- Acid reflux (bringing up stomach acid into the esophagus)

- Chest pain. {**Note:** Don't assume that chest pain is due to a hiatal hernia. See "Chest Pain" on page 194.}

- Pain in the esophagus; heartburn

- Hiccups; belching after meals

- A hard time swallowing

## Causes, Risk Factors & Care

Hiatal hernias are common in people over age 50. The actual cause is not known. Risk factors are obesity, being a woman, or being middle aged. Smoking, lifting, strong coughing, and straining during bowel movements also increase the risk. So does having spicy foods, alcohol, and caffeine.

Hiatal hernias are usually not serious and can often be treated with self-care. If not, surgery is an option.

To Learn More, See Back Cover

*Hiatal Hernia, Continued*

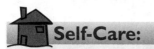

## Self-Care:

- Eat 5 to 6 small meals a day instead of 3 larger meals.

- Follow a low-fat diet. Avoid alcohol, caffeine, and spicy foods.

- Don't smoke. If you smoke, quit.

- Don't lie down after eating. Wait 2 to 3 hours.

- Raise the head of the bed 6 inches. Put 6 inch blocks under the legs of the head of your bed. Or put a 6 inch wedge between the mattress and box springs at the head portion of your bed. Don't prop your head up with pillows. Doing this applies pressure on your stomach area and can help force acid up into your esophagus.

- Don't strain during bowel movements.

- Take over-the-counter antacids or acid controllers, such as Pepcid AC or Tagamet HB. {**Note:** Read the labels before taking. Check with your doctor, too. Adverse side effects are more likely and more severe in older persons who take some acid controllers, such as Tagamet HB.}

- If you take aspirin, ibuprofen, or naproxen, take them with food.

## Contact Doctor When:

- The hiatal hernia causes frequent night pains.

- You have used antacids for a long time with little relief or not gotten any relief using self-care.

# 64. Irritable Bowel Syndrome

Irritable bowel syndrome (IBS) is a common disorder of the bowels. Also known as "spastic colon," it is marked by bouts of irregular bowel habits and abdominal pain that are not due to any other bowel disease.

IBS does not cause inflammation of the colon (colitis) or permanent harm to the bowels. It does not lead to bleeding of the colon or to cancer.

## Prevention

There is no known way to prevent IBS. Once you have it, though, you may be able to prevent future bouts and keep the condition under control with self-care.

## Signs & Symptoms

- Gas, bloating, cramps or pain in the abdomen

*Irritable Bowel Syndrome, Continued*

- Changes in bowel habits:
  - Constipation, diarrhea or both
  - Crampy urge, but not being able to move the bowels
  - Mucus in the stool

## Causes & Care

The actual cause is not known, but something disturbs the normal movement of the bowels. The person with IBS has a sensitive colon. This makes the colon respond strongly to stress, anxiety, smoking, eating certain foods, and alcohol and caffeine.

The goal of treatment is to reduce stress and relieve symptoms. Self-care helps in most cases. When self-care is not enough, your doctor may prescribe medicines to reduce spasms of the colon and to help with emotional distress.

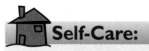 **Self-Care:**

- Keep a log of when symptoms occur. Note the things that preceded them. Avoid these "triggers."
- Manage stress. See "Managing Stress Checklist" on page 21 and "Self-Care" in "Stress" on page 323.

- Avoid foods that bring on symptoms for you. Common triggers are:
  - Eating large meals. Eat 5 to 6 small meals a day, instead.
  - Fats: butter and oils, deep fried foods; fats in meats, etc.
  - Beans, cabbage and broccoli
  - Chocolate, spicy foods, and the artificial sweetener, sorbitol.
  - Dairy products with milk sugar (lactose). Yogurts with live cultures of lactobacillus acidophilus may not cause symptoms. {**Note:** Make sure you get enough calcium in your diet from other sources, like tofu, and from calcium supplements, if needed.}

- Eat a high fiber diet. Good sources of fiber are whole grain breads and cereals, bran, fruits, and vegetables. Beans are a good source, if they do not cause IBS symptoms for you. Add oat bran to your foods and/or take fiber supplements, if needed. Talk to your doctor about which over-the-counter products to use . Too much fiber can make IBS symptoms worse or cause other problems. {**Note:** Add fiber and fiber supplements slowly. Too much, too soon, can worsen symptoms.}

*Continued on Next Page*

## *Irritable Bowel Syndrome, Continued*

### *Self-Care, Continued*

- For diarrhea, see "Self-Care" in "Diarrhea" on page 157.
- For constipation, see "Self-Care" in "Constipation" on page 156.
- Avoid alcohol and caffeine.
- Drink plenty of water.
- Get adequate rest.
- Exercise on a regular basis. This helps to reduce stress. It also helps to keep bowel movements regular.
- Don't smoke. If you smoke, quit.
- For pain:
  - Take an over-the-counter pain reliever. (See "Pain relievers" in "Your Home Pharmacy" on page 43.)
  - Put a hot water bottle or heating pad (set on low) on your abdomen.
  - Use relaxation therapy.

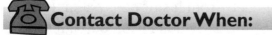

### Contact Doctor When:

- You have any of these problems:
  - Blood or excessive mucus in your stools

- Black stools that look like tar or maroon-colored stools
- A fever with cramps or pain in the abdomen or with diarrhea
- Weight loss
- You have been diagnosed with IBS and your symptoms have changed a lot or are getting worse.

### ♥ Get Immediate Care When:

You have very severe abdominal pain.

# 65. Kidney Stones

Kidney stones are hard masses of mineral deposits formed in the kidney(s). They are usually made of calcium oxalate or calcium phosphate. Less often, they are made of uric acid. The stones can be found in the kidney itself, in the duct (ureter) that carries urine from the kidney to the bladder, and in the bladder.

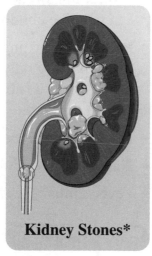

**Kidney Stones***

**II. Abdominal & Urinary Problems**

*Kidney Stones, Continued*

Kidney stones can be as small as a tiny pebble or an inch or more in diameter. They are more common in men.

## Signs & Symptoms

Some kidney stones cause no symptoms. Small ones can be passed, without pain, when you urinate. When symptoms occur, they include:

- Crampy pain (often very severe) that comes and goes. The pain starts in the lower back, travels down the side of the abdomen, and into the groin area. {**Note:** For women, the crampy pain can feel like childbirth pains.}

- Problems urinating, the need to urinate often; passing only small amounts of urine; or not be able to urinate except in certain positions

- Bloody, cloudy, or darkened urine

- Nausea and vomiting

- Fever, chills

## Causes, Risk Factors & Care

Causes and risk factors include:

- Too much calcium in the urine. This happens when the intestines absorb excess calcium.

- Too much calcium in the blood. This can result from vitamin D toxicity or an overactive parathyroid gland.

- High levels of uric acid in the blood. (See "Gout" on page 252.)

- A diet high in oxalic acid. Oxalic acid is found in spinach, leafy vegetables, rhubarb, and coffee.

- Repeated urinary tract infections

- Mild dehydration that persists

- Family traits

- Where you live in the U.S. Areas of the southeast have the highest rates.

In some cases, the cause is not known.

Treatment varies. If the stone is small and can be passed in the urine, treatment may be just drinking plenty of fluids. Save any stones you pass so your doctor can have them analyzed. For kidney stones too large to be passed, lithotripsy is used in most cases. With this, shock waves are directed to the areas where the stone is located. The shock waves break the stone into fragments. After treatment, the person drinks a lot of water to flush the stone fragments from his or her system. Lithotripsy is usually done in an outpatient setting. Lithotripsy causes little or no pain and costs less than invasive surgery.

*II. Abdominal & Urinary Problems*

*Kidney Stones, Continued*

### 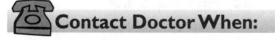 Self-Care/Prevention:

- Drink plenty of fluids. Drink at least 8, 8-ounce glasses of water a day.
- Eat a well-balanced diet. Vary your food choices.

Kidney stones can and do recur. If you're prone to getting stones:

- Follow your doctor's dietary advice. If you tend to form calcium stones, he or she will probably advise you not to take calcium in excess. If you form uric acid stones, your doctor may advise that you eat less foods with oxalic acid (spinach, leafy vegetables, etc.). You may also be told to eat less protein and to take sodium bicarbonate.
- Take medicines as prescribed.

### Contact Doctor When:

You have abdominal pain with these problems:

- The pain started in the side before it moved to the abdomen or groin.
- Blocked, painful, or frequent urination (but you only pass small amounts of urine)
- Bloody, cloudy, or dark urine
- Chills and/or fever
- Nausea and vomiting

## 66. Peptic Ulcers

An ulcer is a sore or break in one of the body's protective tissue layers. Ulcers located in the stomach (gastric ulcers) and ulcers in the first section of the small bowel (duodenal ulcers) are known as "peptic ulcers".

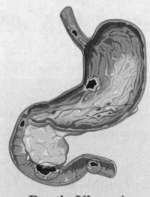

**Peptic Ulcers***

### Signs & Symptoms

Peptic ulcers do not always cause symptoms. When they do, symptoms include:

- A gnawing or burning pain in the abdomen between the breastbone and navel. This is the most common symptom. The pain with a peptic ulcer often occurs between meals and in the early hours of the morning. The pain may last from a few minutes to a few hours and may be relieved with eating or antacids.
- Appetite and weight loss

## Peptic Ulcers, Continued

- Nausea or vomiting dark, red blood or material that looks like coffee grounds

- Paleness and weakness, if anemia is present

- Bloody, black, or tarry stools

## Causes, Risk Factors & Care

In the past, it was thought that peptic ulcers were caused by stress, anxiety, and eating too many spicy or acidic foods. Today, the causes of peptic ulcers are known to be 2 things:

- An infection with bacteria called *Heliobacter pylori (H. pylori)*. About 80% of peptic ulcers result from this.

- About 20% of peptic ulcers may result from the repeated use of aspirin and other nonsteroidal anti-inflammatory drugs (NSAIDs). Examples of over-the-counter NSAIDs are ibuprofen, keto-profen, and naproxen sodium. Examples of prescribed NSAIDs are Anaprox, Feldene, and Relafen.

Family history, smoking, caffeine, and making excess digestive acids also play a role in peptic ulcers. So does stress, especially some types of physical stress, such as severe burns and major surgery.

After diagnosing a peptic ulcer, your doctor may prescribe:

- An antibiotic and a medicine that blocks acid if *H. pylori* is present

- Medicine to decrease or stop the stomach's acid production

- Over-the-counter antacids, acid controllers, or reducers

- Surgery

### Self-Care:

Peptic ulcers need medical care. These self-care measures help an ulcer heal:

- Eat healthy foods. Include foods rich in fiber, such as whole grain breads and cereals, fruits and vegetables, and dried beans and peas. In the past, persons with peptic ulcers were advised to eat bland food, drink a lot of milk, and eat many smaller meals a day. These measures may not help.

- Avoid things that stimulate excess stomach acid. These include: Coffee, regular and decaffeinated; tea; soft drinks with caffeine; and fruit juices high in acid, such as tomato juice.

- Avoid any foods that bother you.

*Continued on Next Page*

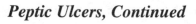

*11. Abdominal & Urinary Problems*

### Peptic Ulcers, Continued

#### Self-Care, Continued

- Limit or avoid alcohol.

- Don't use aspirin and other NSAIDs. These irritate the stomach lining. Don't stop taking NSAIDs your doctor has prescribed, though. Check with him or her first.

- Try over-the-counter antacids or acid controllers (with your doctor's okay). Use them on a short-term basis. Don't try to self-medicate an ulcer. You may soothe the symptoms without treating the problem.

- Don't smoke. If you smoke, quit.

- Lower stress in your life. Stress doesn't cause ulcers, but for some people, it may trigger ulcer flare-ups.

- Take medications as prescribed.

#### ☎ Contact Doctor When:

- You have bloody, black, or tarry stools and/or you are very, very tired, pale and weak. These can occur with a bleeding ulcer.

- No relief comes with self-care.

- The pain continues despite treatment.

- Bothersome side effects occur from prescribed or over-the-counter medicines.

- Symptoms return. The *H. pylori* bacteria may not be totally gone. A second course of medication therapy may be needed.

#### ♥ Get Immediate Care When:

- You have sudden, severe abdominal pain. It may be in the upper left stomach area below the ribs or below the ribs on the right side.

- You vomit bright red blood or material that looks like coffee grounds.

## 67. Rectal Problems

The rectum is the lowest part of the large bowel. The opening of the rectum is the anus. It is from here that bowel movements are passed.

### Signs & Symptoms

Rectal problems include rectal pain, bleeding, itching, and redness, swelling, or a rash.

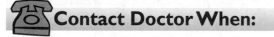

*Rectal Problems, Continued*

## Causes & Care

Common causes of rectal pain and/or bleeding include constipation, straining to have bowel movements, and hemorrhoids.

Other causes include anal fissures (splits or tears in the skin around the anus); polyps or small growths; and injury due to anal intercourse or the insertion of a foreign object. {**Note:** Although the most common causes of rectal bleeding are not serious, it is hard to tell them from polyps or cancer without a medical evaluation. To rule out colon cancer, if you have any sign of rectal bleeding, including blood on toilet paper, you should see a doctor, regardless of your age or family history.}

An intestinal obstruction and colon and rectal cancers (see page 153) also cause rectal pain and/or bleeding.

The most common cause of rectal itching in older persons is dry skin. Other causes of rectal itching include hemorrhoids; psoriasis (a chronic skin disease in which itchy, scaly red patches form on a part of the body); and products that irritate or cause a skin allergy in the rectal area. Examples are over-the-counter anesthetic ointments that end in "caine," such as benzocaine.

Often there is no clear cause. Persons with diabetes and liver disease are more prone to rectal itching. Also, some items, such as coffee, cola, and beer can lead to anal itching.

In most cases, rectal pain and/or bleeding is due to straining to have a bowel movement and/or hemorrhoids. (See "Constipation" on page 155 and "Hemorrhoids" on page 168.)

When rectal bleeding occurs, the color of the blood gives clues to the cause. A light amount of bright, red blood that appears on toilet paper or on the surface of the stool is usually, but not always, due to hemorrhoids. Burgundy, black, or tarry looking stool can signal bleeding from higher in the digestive tract. This needs medical diagnosis and treatment.

### Self-Care:

**For Rectal Pain:**

- Take warm baths. Use a warm water sitz bath for 15 minutes 2 to 3 times a day. A sitz bath is a shallow, warm water bath that fits over the toilet. You can get a sitz bath basin from medical supply and some drug stores.

*Continued on Next Page*

To Learn More, See Back Cover

*Rectal Problems, Continued*

*Self-Care, Continued*

- Put towels, soaked in warm water, or a cold compress to the painful area.

- Follow self-care, on page 156, to prevent constipation.

- Don't strain to have a bowel movement.

- Keep the rectal area clean. Use an over-the-counter wipe, such as Tucks, after using toilet paper.

- Take an over-the-counter pain medicine. (See "Pain relievers" in "Your Home Pharmacy" on page 43.)

- Use soft, plain, unscented, two-ply toilet paper. Use wet, not dry, toilet paper.

- Don't sit for long periods of time. When you do sit, raise your legs, when you can.

**For Rectal Bleeding:**

- Do not do heavy lifting.

- Stop taking anti-inflammatory medicines and/or aspirin, unless prescribed and monitored by your doctor.

- Don't strain to have a bowel movement.

**For Rectal Itching:**

- Practice good hygiene. Clean the rectal area daily.

- Use an over-the-counter ointment, such as one with zinc oxide or one for hemorrhoids, such as Preparation H. Follow package directions.

- Wear loose-fitting clothing and undergarments.

- Take a warm bath or sitz bath. Then dry the rectal area well. Use talcum powder, as needed.

- Take tub baths with a colloidal oatmeal product, such as Aveeno.

- Lose weight, if overweight. If you are diabetic, follow measures to keep you blood sugar under control.

See also "Self-Care" in "Constipation" on page 156, "Diarrhea" on page 157, and "Hemorrhoids" on page 169.

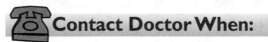

**Contact Doctor When:**

- You have symptoms of a thrombosed hemorrhoid:

  • A purple-colored hemorrhoid that bleeds heavily

  • Severe and constant pain with a sudden onset

*Rectal Problems, Continued*

■ Any of these problems occur with rectal bleeding:

- The bleeding is heavy or dark maroon or black in color.

- Bright red blood is present after an injury, intercourse, or having something inserted into the rectum.

- The rectal bleeding occurred after taking a new medicine or returning from a foreign country or between bowel movements.

■ You have any of these problems with rectal pain:

- The pain is severe or lasts longer than 1 week.

- Anal spasms after a bowel movement

- Diarrhea or mucus discharge

- Swelling or itching in the rectal area

■ You have rectal problems with any of these conditions:

- The problem came on or got worse after surgery.

- Diabetes or a heart condition

- Exposure to a sexually transmitted disease

- Rectal bleeding in a person with a family history of stomach, colon, or rectal cancer

### ♥ Get Immediate Care When:

■ You have bright red blood in the stools (not just blood on toilet paper).

■ You have maroon-colored or black, tarlike stools with any of these problems:

- Severe pain, cramps, and swelling in the abdomen

- Nausea and vomiting

- Weakness or dizziness

- Shortness of breath

■ Bright red blood from the rectum or in the stools occurs in a person with any of these conditions:

- Cirrhosis

- A bleeding disorder

- The person takes a blood-thinning medicine.

■ A foreign object is not able to be removed from the rectum.

■ Rape or sexual abuse has occurred.

# 68. Urinary Incontinence

If you have urinary incontinence, you suffer from a loss of bladder control or your body fails to store urine properly. As a result, you can't keep from passing urine, even though you try to hold it in.

Urinary incontinence is not a normal part of aging. It often affects older persons because the sphincter muscles that open the bladder into the urethra (the tube through which urine is passed) become less efficient with aging.

## Signs, Symptoms, & Causes

Two kinds of urinary incontinence are:

### Acute Incontinence

This form is generally a symptom of a new illness or condition, such as a bladder infection, diabetes (new or out-of-control), inflammation of the prostate, urethra, or vagina, or side effect of some medicines, such as water pills.

Acute urinary incontinence comes on suddenly. It is often easily reversed when the condition that caused it is treated.

### Persistent incontinence

This form comes on gradually over time. It lingers or remains, even after other conditions or illnesses have been treated. There are many types of persistent incontinence. The first 3 types, below, account for 80% of cases.

- Stress Incontinence. Urine leaks out when there is a sudden rise in pressure in the abdomen. This usually happens with coughing, sneezing, laughing, lifting, jumping, running, or straining to have a bowel movement. Stress incontinence is more common in women than in men.

- Urge Incontinence. This is an inability to control the bladder when the urge to urinate is so strong and comes on suddenly, that urine is released before the person can get to the toilet. It can be caused by an enlarged prostate gland, a spinal cord injury, or an illness, such as Parkinson's disease.

- Mixed Incontinence. This type has elements of both stress and urge incontinence.

- Overflow Incontinence. This is the constant dribbling of urine because the bladder overfills. This may be due to an enlarged prostate, diabetes, or multiple sclerosis.

11. Abdominal & Urinary Problems

***Urinary Incontinence, Continued***

- Functional Incontinence. With this type, a person has trouble getting to the bathroom fast enough, even though he or she has bladder control. This can happen in a person who is physically challenged.

- Total Incontinence. This is a rare type with complete loss of bladder control Urine leakage can be continual.

## Care

You might feel embarrassed if you have urinary incontinence, but let your doctor know about it. It may be a symptom of a disorder that could lead to more trouble if not treated. In most cases, the problem is curable and treatable.

Treatment will depend on the type and cause.

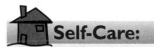

### Self-Care:

- Keep a diary of how often and how much you urinate in a 24 hour period.

- Avoid caffeine. Limit or avoid fluids 2 to 3 hours before bedtime.

- Limit carbonated drinks, alcohol, citrus juices, greasy and spicy foods, and items that have artificial sweeteners. These can irritate the bladder.

- Go to the bathroom often, even if you don't feel the urge. When you urinate, empty your bladder as much as you can. Relax for a minute or 2 and then try to go again. Keep a diary of when you have episodes of incontinence. If you find that you have accidents every 3 hours, empty your bladder every 2 hours. Use an alarm clock or wristwatch with an alarm to remind you.

- Wear clothes you can pull down easily when you use the bathroom. Wear elastic-waist bottoms and items with velcro closures or snaps instead of buttons and zippers.

- Wear absorbent pads or briefs, if needed.

- Empty your bladder before you leave the house, take a nap, or go to bed.

- Keep the pathway to your bathroom free of clutter and well lit. Leave the bathroom door open until you use it. Have a night light on in your bathroom when it is dark.

- Use an elevated toilet seat and grab bars if these will make it easier for you to get on and off the toilet.

- Keep a bedpan, plastic urinal (for men), or portable commode chair near your bed.

*Continued on Next Page*

## *Urinary Incontinence, Continued*

### *Self-Care, Continued*

- Ask your doctor if your type of incontinence could be managed by using self-catheters. These help to empty your bladder completely. You need a prescription for self-catheters.

### Kegel Exercises

Do pelvic floor exercises (Kegel exercises). These can help treat or cure stress incontinence. Even elderly women who have leaked urine for years can benefit greatly from these exercises. Here's how to do them:

- First, start to urinate, then hold back and try to stop. If you can slow the stream of urine, even a little, you are using the right muscles. You should feel muscles squeezing around the urethra (the tube through which urine is passed) and the anus (the opening though which stool is passed).

- Next, relax your body, close your eyes, and just imagine that you are going to urinate and then hold back from doing so. You should feel the muscles squeeze like you did in the step before this one.

- Squeeze the muscles for 3 seconds and then relax them for 3 seconds. When you squeeze and relax, count slowly. Start out doing this 3 times a day. Gradually work up to 3 sets of 10 contractions, holding each one for 10 seconds at a time. You can do them in lying, sitting, and/or standing positions.

- When you do these exercises, do not tense the muscles in your belly or buttocks. Do not hold your breath, clench your fists or teeth, or make a face.

- Squeeze your pelvic floor muscles right before and during whatever it is (coughing, sneezing, jumping, etc.) that causes you to lose urine. Relax the muscles once the activity is over.

- Women can also use pelvic weights prescribed by their doctor. A women inserts a weighted cone into the vagina and squeezes the correct muscles to keep the weight from falling out.

It may take several months to benefit from pelvic floor exercises and they should be done daily.

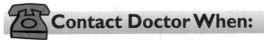

## Contact Doctor When:

- The loss of bladder control is ongoing after surgery or an injury.

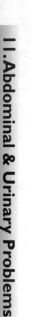

### Urinary Incontinence, Continued

- With loss of bladder control, you have signs and symptoms of a urinary tract infection (see page 187).

- The loss of bladder control occurs in a person with diabetes or with symptoms of diabetes (see page 276).

- With loss of bladder control, you are male, and you have symptoms of prostate problems (see page 331).

- You leak urine when you cough, run, sneeze, laugh, or lift heavy objects.

- You have loss of bladder control after you take a new medicine or change the dose of a medicine you take.

### ♥ Get Immediate Care When:

- Loss of bladder control occurs after an injury to your spine or back.

- Loss of bladder control occurs with signs and symptoms of a stroke. See "Stroke Warning Signs" on page 229.

- Loss of bladder control occurs with signs of an acute kidney infection:

  - Change in mental status. This can be the first sign in persons over age 70.

  - Back pain (sometimes severe) in one or both sides of your back

- Fever and shaking chills (maybe)

- Nausea and vomiting

## For Information Contact:

National Association for Continence
1-800-BLADDER (252-3337)
www.nafc.org

American Foundation for Urologic Disease
1-410-468-1800
www.afud.org

# 69. Urinary Tract Infection (UTIs)

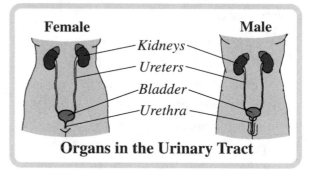

**Organs in the Urinary Tract**

Urinary tract infections are ones that occur in any organs that make up the urinary tract. The kidneys filter waste products from the blood and make urine. Ureters connect the kidney to the bladder, which holds urine until it is passed through the urethra.

*Urinary Tract Infection (UTIs), Continued*

## Prevention

- Drink plenty of fluids to flush bacteria out of your system. Drink fruit juices, especially one made from unsweetened cranberry juice concentrate.

- Empty your bladder as soon as you feel the urge.

- Drink a glass of water before you have sex. Go to the bathroom as soon as you can after sex.

- If you use a lubricant when you have sex, use a water-soluble one, such as K-Y Jelly.

- Wear cotton underwear. Bacteria like a warm, moist, wet place to grow. Cotton helps keep you cool and dry.

- If you're prone to UTIs, don't take bubble baths. Take showers instead.

- Don't wear tight-fitting jeans, slacks, and undergarments.

- If you're a woman, you should wipe from front to back after using the toilet to keep bacteria away from the opening of the urethra.

- If you need to use a catheter to draw your own urine, make sure to wash your hands and clean the area around the urethra. Wash the catheter in soapy water after each use or use disposable ones. If you have a catheter that is kept in place, follow the instructions for proper use and cleaning.

## Signs & Symptoms

- A strong need to urinate

- Urinating more often than usual

- A sharp pain or burning sensation in the urethra when you pass urine

- Bloody or cloudy urine

- The feeling that the bladder is still full after you pass urine

- Pain in the abdomen, back, or sides

- A change in mental status, especially in persons over age 70.

Sometimes there are no symptoms with a UTI.

## Causes, Risk Factors & Care

UTIs are caused by bacteria that infect any part of the urinary tract. The bladder is the most common site.

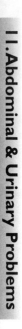

*Urinary Tract Infection (UTIs), Continued*

Things that increase the risk of UTIs include any obstruction in the flow of urine, like a kidney stone or an enlarged prostate gland; having a history of urinary tract infections, urinary tract defects, and diabetes; having a urinary catheter to empty the bladder.

Treatment for a UTI includes an antibiotic to treat the specific infection and pain relievers, if needed.

## Self-Care:

- Avoid alcohol, spicy foods, and caffeine.
- Drink at least 8 glasses of water and other liquids a day.
- Drink juice made from unsweetened cranberry juice concentrate. Take cranberry tablets or the herb *uva-ursi*. Look for these at health food stores.
- Get plenty of rest.
- Check for fever twice a day. Take your temperature in the morning and in the afternoon or evening.

- Take an over-the-counter medicine for pain. (See "Pain relievers" in "Your Home Pharmacy" on page 43). Or take an over-the-counter medicine, such as Uristat, which relieves pain and spasms that come with a bladder infection. {**Note:** Uristat helps with symptoms, but doesn't get rid of the infection. If you take Uristat, you should see your doctor to diagnose and treat the problem.}
- Go to the bathroom as soon as you feel the urge. Empty your bladder completely. If you have a condition that might keep you from doing this, such as multiple sclerosis, ask your doctor about using self-catheters.
- Empty your bladder as soon as you can after sex.

## Contact Doctor When:

- You have any signs or symptoms of a urinary tract infection listed on page 187.
- You have had symptoms for more than 3 days, without getting better.
- Medicine the doctor prescribed gave you side effects, such as a skin rash, or made you sick.
- You get UTIs a lot.

*Urinary Tract Infection (UTIs), Continued*

### Get Immediate Care When:

- You have a change in mental status, such as confusion.

- You have signs of a kidney infection: Vomiting and nausea, fever and shaking chills, and pain in one or both sides of your back.

## 70. Vomiting & Nausea

### Signs & Symptoms

Vomiting is when you throw up what is in your stomach. Nausea is when you feel like you're going to throw up.

### Causes & Care

Common causes are: Viruses in the intestines; diarrhea; some medicines; spoiled food; and eating or drinking too much.

Medical conditions that cause vomiting include:

- **Labrynthitis**. This is inflammation of an area in the ear that usually results from an upper respiratory infection.

- Vertigo (see page 222)

- Migraine headaches

- Acute glaucoma (see page 68)

- Stomach ulcers. (See "Peptic Ulcers" on page 177.)

- Intestinal obstruction

- Hepatitis (see page 290)

- Meningitis. This is inflammation of membranes that cover the brain and spinal cord.

- Heart attack (see page 201)

Self-care treats most cases of nausea and vomiting from common causes. Treatment for a medical condition treats the nausea or vomiting that comes with that condition.

### Self-Care:

**For Vomiting:**

- Don't eat solid foods. Don't drink milk.

- Drink clear liquids at room temperature (not too cold or too hot). Take small sips. Drink only 1 to 2 ounces at a time. Drink water, sport drinks, such as Gatorade, diluted fruit juices, flat cola and ginger ale, etc. Stir any carbonated beverages to get all the bubbles out before sipping them. Suck on ice chips if nothing else will stay down.

*Continued on Next Page*

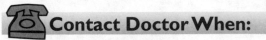

**11. Abdominal & Urinary Problems**

*Vomiting & Nausea, Continued*

### Self-Care, Continued

- Gradually return to a regular diet, but wait 8 hours from the last time you vomited. Eat foods as tolerated. Avoid greasy or fatty foods.

- Take an over-the-counter medicine, like Emetrol, as directed.

- Don't smoke, drink alcohol, or take aspirin.

{**Note:** Call your doctor if you don't get better or if the vomiting comes back.}

### Nausea Without Vomiting:

- Drink clear liquids. Eat small amounts of dry foods, such as soda crackers, if tolerated.

- Avoid things that irritate the stomach, such as alcohol and aspirin.

- For motion sickness, use an over-the-counter antinausea medicine, such as Dramamine, as directed.

## Contact Doctor When:

- You have stomach pain that lasts for more than 2 hours, interferes with your activities, and keeps hurting even after you vomit.

- With vomiting, you have a fever or chronic medical condition, such as diabetes, cancer, HIV infection, etc. and self-care measures do not control the vomiting.

- With nausea and/or vomiting, you have any of these problems:

  - The whites of your eyes or your skin look yellow.

  - Ear pain or a feeling of fullness in your ear

- With vomiting or nausea, you have signs and symptoms of a urinary tract infection (see page 187).

- The vomiting has lasted more than 24 hours without getting better using self-care.

- You are throwing up medicine that is necessary for you to take, such as one for high blood pressure.

To Learn More, See Back Cover

*Vomiting & Nausea, Continued*

♥ **Get Immediate Care When:**

- Nausea and/or vomiting occurs with signs of a heart attack. (See "Heart Attack Warning Signs" on page 202.)

- You vomit bright red blood or material that looks like coffee grounds.

- You vomit in an unusually violent way and/or the vomiting is continuous and hard to manage.

- You vomit and have any of these problems:

  - Stiff neck, fever, severe headache, <u>and</u> drowsiness

  - Severe pain in and around one eye, blurred vision, headache, and you see rainbow-colored halos around lights

  - A blind spot, a loss of part of your visual field, or you see sparkling lights

  - A head or abdominal injury that happened a short time ago

  - Fever and shaking chills and pain in one or both sides of your back

  - Mental confusion

- You vomit and have signs of dehydration (see page 391).

Heart disease is America's number 1 cause of death. Many people face heart problems because of their past and present lifestyle choices.

## 71. Angina

Angina is chest pain or discomfort. It occurs when the heart muscle does not get as much blood and oxygen as it needs for a given level of work.

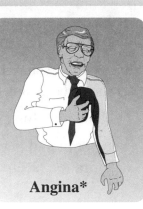

**Angina***

## Signs & Symptoms

- Squeezing pressure, heaviness, or mild ache in the chest (usually behind the breastbone)

- Aching in a tooth with or without squeezing pressure in the chest

- Aching into the neck muscles, jaw, one or both arms, or back

- A feeling of gas in the upper abdomen and lower chest

- A feeling that you're choking or shortness of breath

- Paleness and sweating

- Nausea and vomiting

Many people who experience angina for the first time fear they're having a heart attack. A heart attack damages or injures the heart muscle. Angina does not. Pain from angina is a warning sign that heart attack can occur, though.

## Causes, Risk Factors & Care

Angina is caused by blocked or narrowed blood vessels that supply blood to the heart.

Episodes of angina are often brought on by anger, excitement, or emotional shock. Exertion or heavy

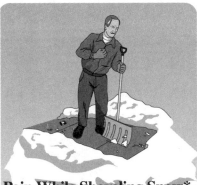

**Pain While Shoveling Snow***

physical work, hurrying up the stairs, or walking rapidly uphill can also bring on an angina episode.

If you have angina, your doctor or a cardiologist should follow you closely. He or she may prescribe:

- Medications, such as nitroglycerin; beta-blockers; and a low-dose daily aspirin

To Learn More, See Back Cover

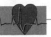

*Angina, Continued*

- Daily physical exercise specific for you
- Surgery, such as angioplasty or bypass surgery

## Self-Care:

Medical care is needed to treat angina. If you have angina, these self-care measures can be part of your treatment plan.

- Don't smoke. If you smoke, quit.
- Follow a low-saturated fat, low cholesterol diet.
- Eat 5 to 6 small meals instead of 3 large meals a day.
- Maintain a healthy weight. If you are overweight, lose weight
- After you eat, rest or do a quiet activity.
- Minimize exposure to cold, windy weather.
- Take medication(s), as prescribed.
- Avoid sudden physical exertion, such as running to catch a bus.
- Avoid anger whenever you can.
- Manage stress.

## Contact Doctor When:

- You have been diagnosed with angina and there is a change in your angina symptoms. You may, for example, start to feel symptoms at rest.
- You have minor chest pain that is not due to an injury or strain; does not let up; and/or is not relieved by rest.

## Get Immediate Care When:

- You have symptoms of a heart attack. (See "Heart Attack Warning Signs" on page 202.)
- You have been diagnosed with angina and your chest pain does not respond to your prescribed medicine or the pain does not go away in 10 to 15 minutes.

**12. Heart & Circulation Problems**

# 72. Chest Pain

**Chest Pain Chart**

| Signs & Symptoms | What It Could Be | What to Do |
|---|---|---|
| Feeling of pressure, tightness, squeezing, or heaviness in the chest that lasts more than a few minutes or goes away and comes back. The pain may spread to the arm, neck, jaw, or teeth. <br><br> Chest discomfort with one or more of these problems: <br> ▪ Shortness of breath or trouble breathing <br> ▪ Fast or uneven heartbeat <br> ▪ Bluish lips, skin, or fingernails <br> ▪ Sweating; pale or clammy skin <br> ▪ Lightheadedness, dizziness, fainting, or sense of doom <br> ▪ Nausea and/or vomiting <br> ▪ Persistent cough with pink, blood-tinged mucus and/or swelling in the lower legs or ankles. {**Note:** Women may show these signs of a heart attack more often than men.} | Heart Attack | Get immediate care. (Call 911 or go to the emergency department of a hospital). <br><br> {**Note:** Before emergency care, take a regular aspirin unless you are allergic to aspirin or take a blood-thinning medicine.} |
| Severe chest pain with extreme pain felt across the upper back (not just on one side) that came on within 15 minutes for no apparent reason, such as an injury or back strain. The pain can spread to the abdomen. Dizziness and fainting. | Dissecting aortic aneurysm. This is a tear in the main artery from the heart. | Get immediate care. (Call 911 or go to the emergency department of a hospital. Do not take aspirin). |

To Learn More, See Back Cover

## Chest Pain, Continued

| Chest Pain Chart, Continued | | |
|---|---|---|
| **Signs & Symptoms** | **What It Could Be** | **What to Do** |
| Chest pain that gets worse when taking deep breaths and is present with any of these conditions:<br>■ Sudden shortness of breath and severe problems breathing<br>■ Rapid heartbeat<br>■ Cough with bloody sputum<br>■ Sudden onset of chest pain with calf pain<br>■ Recent surgery or illness with prolonged bed rest | Blood clot(s) to the lungs | Get immediate care. (Call 911 or go to the emergency department of a hospital.)<br>See "Phlebitis & Thrombosis" topic on page 207. |
| Sudden and sharp chest pain or tightness with breathing. Increasing shortness of breath. | Collapsed lung. Could result from a recent chest injury or from asthma or chronic bronchitis. | Get immediate care. (Call 911 or go to the emergency department of a hospital.) |
| Squeezing, pressure, or pain (often dull) in the chest. The pain may spread to the arm, neck, jaw, or back. Symptoms come on or are made worse by stress or physical activity and ease with rest. | Angina | See "Angina" on page 192. |
| The pain is on only one side of the chest and is not affected by breathing. A burning feeling and a skin rash are at the site of the chest pain. | Shingles | See "Shingles" on page 134. |

## Chest Pain, Continued

| Chest Pain Chart, Continued | | |
| --- | --- | --- |
| **Signs & Symptoms** | **What It Could Be** | **What to Do** |
| Chest pain with shortness of breath; chronic fatigue; cough with phlegm or blood; night sweats; appetite and weight loss; and low grade fever. | **Tuberculosis (TB).** This is a chronic lung infection with a certain bacteria. | Contact doctor. |
| Pain felt is a burning feeling in the chest or just above the stomach. The feeling comes and goes before, during, or after eating. It gets worse when you bend over or lie down. | Heartburn or hiatal hernia. {**Note:** This could also signal a heart attack.} | See "Heart Attack Warning Signs" on page 202, "Heartburn" on page 166, "Hiatal Hernia" on page 172, or "Peptic Ulcers" on page 177. |
| Chest pain that gets worse when taking deep breaths or when you touch the chest or ribs. | Muscle strain or rib injury | See "Sprains & Strains" on page 267. |
| Chest pain with fever and coughing up green, yellow, or gray mucus | Flu, pneumonia, bronchitis, or other upper respiratory infection | Contact doctor. See "Flu" on page 100 or "Pneumonia" on page 104, or "Bronchitis" on page 93. |
| Pain or tightening feeling in the chest with rapid pulse and/or breathing; feeling a "lump in the throat"; sweating; numbness or tingling of the hands, feet, or mouth, or it feels like you can't get enough air | Anxiety. {**Note:** This could also signal a heart attack.} | See "Heart Attack Warning Signs" on page 202. See "Anxiety" on page 306. |

 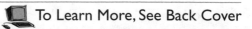

# 73. Congestive Heart Failure

The heart is the body's pump. When the heart can't pump well enough to meet the body's needs, it is called congestive heart failure (CHF). The heart itself doesn't fail, but "fails" to supply the body with enough blood and oxygen.

## Prevention

These causes of CHF can be prevented:

- Coronary artery disease
- High blood pressure
- Alcohol and drug abuse
- Some cases of heart valve damage. Rheumatic fever can be prevented if strep throat is treated.

## Signs & Symptoms

- Shortness of breath
- Feeling very tired or very weak
- Swelling of the lower legs, ankles, and feet. Shoes can suddenly feel tight.
- Rapid weight gain (up to 1 pound a day) over several days or weeks without eating too much.
- Dry cough or a cough with pink mucus

- A fast (sometimes irregular) heartbeat.
- Feeling anxious and/or restless
- A feeling of suffocation. It can be difficult to lie flat.

At first, symptoms come on with physical exertion. As CHF gets worse, symptoms occur even at rest.

## Causes & Care

Causes of CHF include:

- One or more heart attacks. This is the number 1 cause.
- Advanced coronary artery disease.
- Uncontrolled high blood pressure
- Pulmonary hypertension. This is high blood pressure in the lungs.
- Alcohol and drug abuse
- Pericarditis. This is a swelling of the lining that surrounds the heart.
- Heart valve damage. Rheumatic heart disease and rheumatic fever are 2 conditions that can result in this.
- Liver and kidney disease

Treatment for CHF depends on the cause. Most cases can be treated with success. Both medical care and self-care are needed.

12. Heart & Circulation Problems

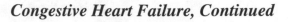

*12. Heart & Circulation Problems*

### Congestive Heart Failure, Continued

Medicines to treat CHF include:

- Vasodilators. These drugs open blood vessels to reduce the force the heart must pump against. Ones called ACE inhibitors can help persons with CHF live longer and feel better. Federal health guidelines recommend them as first-line therapy for CHF.

- Diuretics (water pills), such as spirono-lactone and furosemide. These drugs rid the body of extra fluids and salt.

- Digitalis. This strengthens the pumping action of the heart muscle.

### Self-Care:

Your doctor may advise you to:

- Weigh yourself and record your weight daily. Take this record to doctor visits.

- Limit your salt and fluid intakes. Follow your doctor's guidelines.

- Have 5 to 6 small meals a day instead of 3 larger meals.

- Stay as active as you can.

- Eat healthy foods and get regular exercise. Follow your doctor's plan.

- Limit alcoholic drinks to 1 a day, if at all. One drink = 5 oz. of wine; 12 oz. of beer; or $1^{1}/_{2}$ oz. of 80 proof hard liquor.

- Modify your daily activities as needed. Pace yourself. Do not place too heavy a demand on your heart.

- Alternate activity with rest. Sit up when you rest, if this makes breathing easier.

- Sleep on 2 or more pillows or raise the head of your bed 6 inches when you sleep.

- Don't smoke. If you smoke, quit.

- Lose weight if you are overweight.

### Contact Doctor When:

- You cough up pink or frothy mucus with mild shortness of breath.

- You have an unexplained weight gain of 3 to 5 pounds.

- You have CHF and have symptoms of a cold or flu or your CHF symptoms get worse.

- You have 1 or more signs and symptoms of CHF listed on page 197.

To Learn More, See Back Cover

*Congestive Heart Failure, Continued*

## ♥ Get Immediate Care When:

- You have heart attack symptoms. (See "Heart Attack Warning Signs" on page 202.)

- You have severe shortness of breath (you are too short of breath to say a few words) with or without wheezing (a high pitched whistling sound).

# 74. Coronary Artery Disease

The coronary arteries supply blood to the heart muscle. When they become narrowed or blocked (usually by fatty deposits and/or blood clots), this is coronary artery disease (CAD). Two conditions of CAD are angina (see page 192) and heart attacks (see page 201).

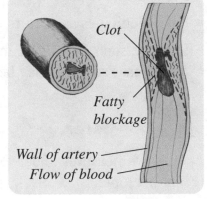

*Clot*

*Fatty blockage*

*Wall of artery*

*Flow of blood*

## Prevention

- Have your blood pressure checked regularly. Follow your doctor's advice to control it.

- Don't smoke. If you smoke, quit.

- Know the signs and symptoms of diabetes (see page 276). If you have diabetes, follow your doctor's advice.

- Maintain a normal body weight. Lose weight if you are overweight.

- Follow a diet low in saturated fats and cholesterol.

- Reduce your intake of salt and foods high in salt if you are "salt-sensitive." Salt-sensitive persons' blood pressure goes up if they eat too much salt.

- Get regular exercise. Follow your doctor's advice.

- Practice relaxation techniques.

- Take medicines as prescribed.

## Signs & Symptoms

In the early stages, CAD has no symptoms. When symptoms occur, they include:

- Irregular heartbeats, such as palpitations
- Shortness of breath
- Dizziness, lightheadedness, or fainting
- Angina symptoms (see page 192)
- Heart attack symptoms (see page 202)

*12. Heart & Circulation Problems*

*Coronary Artery Disease, Continued*

## Causes, Risk Factors & Care

Some factors make people more likely to suffer from heart disease. The more risk factors you have, the more you are at risk.

Risk Factors You Can't Change:

- A past heart attack or stroke
- Family history of heart disease:
  - You have a father or brother who had heart disease before age 55.
  - You have a mother or sister who had heart disease before age 65.
  - You have a family history of high blood cholesterol
- Being a male 45 years or older
- Being a female past menopause and not on estrogen replacement therapy (ERT)
- Race. African Americans have a higher risk than Caucasians.

Risk Factors You Can Control:

- High blood pressure
- High blood cholesterol
- Smoking
- Being overweight
- Lack of physical activity

- Having diabetes and high blood cholesterol
- Using cocaine or amphetamines
- Stress

High blood pressure, high blood cholesterol, and smoking are the 3 most important risk factors for heart disease. On the average, each one doubles your chance of having heart disease.

Treatment for CAD will depend on the diagnosis and severity of the disease.

- If you think you're having a heart attack, get to a hospital as soon as possible. If given within 4 hours, an injection that dissolves clots can reduce the risk of death and severity of damage to the heart muscle. Other emergency procedures can also prevent damage to the heart muscle.
- For angina, see page 192.
- Take medicines as prescribed.
- Surgery, such as balloon angioplasty and bypass surgery, may be needed.

### Self-Care:

- Follow measures under "Prevention" in this topic.
- Take medicines as prescribed.

*Continued on Next Page*

 To Learn More, See Back Cover

**12. Heart & Circulation Problems**

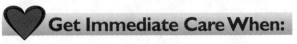

## Coronary Artery Disease, Continued

### Self-Care, Continued

- Ask your doctor about taking vitamins C, E, folic acid and other B vitamins.

- If you drink alcohol, do so in moderation. Too much alcohol can raise the risk for high blood pressure, heart disease, stroke, and other health problems. Moderate drinking, though, is associated with a lower risk of coronary heart disease in some persons. Moderation means no more than 1 drink a day. One drink = 4 oz. of wine; 12 oz. of beer; or $1\frac{1}{2}$ oz. of 80 proof liquor.

- Limit caffeine

### ☎ Contact Doctor When:

- You have been diagnosed with angina and have a change in your angina symptoms. You may, for example, start to feel symptoms at rest.

- You have minor chest pain that is not due to an injury or strain, does not let up, and/or is not relieved by rest.

- You need help to quit smoking and/or to lose excess weight.

### ♥ Get Immediate Care When:

You have heart attack symptoms. (See "Heart Attack Warning Signs" box on page 202.)

### For Information Contact:

The American Heart Association
1-800-242-8721
www.americanheart.org

National Heart, Lung, and Blood Institute
1-800-251-1222
www.nhlbi.nih.gov

## 75. Heart Attack

A heart attack happens when the heart does not get enough blood supply for a period of time. Part or all of the heart muscle dies.

### Prevention

- Follow prevention measures in "Coronary Artery Disease" on page 199.

- Don't use amphetamines and/or cocaine.

- Don't shovel snow or carry heavy objects, especially if you are not physically fit.

12. Heart & Circulation Problems

*Heart Attack, Continued*

## Signs & Symptoms

A heart attack may be painful or "silent."

| Heart Attack Warning Signs | |
|---|---|
| ■ Chest pain. This may spread to the arm, neck, or jaw.<br><br>■ A feeling of tightness, burning, squeezing, fullness, or heaviness in the chest. This lasts more than a few minutes or goes away and comes back.<br><br>■ Chest discomfort with one or more of these problems:<br><br>• Shortness of breath or trouble breathing<br><br>• Fast or uneven heartbeat or pulse<br><br>• Bluish lips, skin, or fingernails<br><br>• Sweating; pale, gray-colored, or clammy skin<br><br>• Lightheadedness, fainting, or sense of doom<br><br>• Nausea, and/or vomiting | ■ Chest pain in a person with a heart condition that does not respond to their prescribed medicine<br><br>In women, common heart attack warning signs are:<br><br>■ Heavy fullness or pressure-like chest pain between the breasts and spreading to the left arm, shoulder, or throat<br><br>■ An uneasy feeling in the chest with any problem listed in the left column of this chart or any of these problems:<br><br>• Persistent cough, especially with pink, blood-tinged mucus<br><br>• Swelling in the lower legs or ankles<br><br>• Fatigue<br><br>• Fluttering or rapid heartbeats<br><br>(These signs can occur in men, too.) |

## Causes, Risk Factors & Care

■ The most common cause is 1 or more blood clots that block a coronary artery. Often, a blood clot forms in the coronary artery already narrowed by plaque.

■ Having already had a heart attack increases the risk for another one.

■ Cocaine or amphetamine abuse can cause a sudden heart attack, even in persons with no signs of heart disease.

To Learn More, See Back Cover

### *Heart Attack, Continued*

- Spasms of the large coronary artery. This can be triggered by: Heavy physical exertion, such as shoveling snow; exposure to cold; severe emotional stress; and having a heavy meal.

These triggers are more likely to affect persons who are sedentary.

## ♥ Get Immediate Care When:

- You have heart attack symptoms. (See "Heart Attack Warning Signs" on page 202.) Shout for help. Call 911!

### First Aid for a Heart Attack Before Emergency Care:

- If there is no breathing and no pulse, do CPR (see page 381).

- Ask the victim if he or she uses heart medicine (nitroglycerin). If yes, ask where it is, find it, and place the nitroglycerin tablet under the tongue. Give as many as 3 tablets in 10 minutes.

- Give the victim a regular aspirin to chew on, if able, at the onset of symptoms.

- Loosen any clothing around the victim's neck, chest, and waist.

- Don't let the victim lie down, especially if he or she has breathing problems. A half-sitting position is better – with the legs up and bent at the knees. Put a pillow or rolled towel under the knees. Support the back.

- Reassure the victim that you have called for help and will stay with him or her until help arrives.

After a heart attack, follow your doctor's treatment plan.

- Chest pain does not respond to prescribed medicine or go away in 10 to 15 minutes, if you have angina.

# 76. High Blood Pressure

High blood pressure (HBP) happens when your blood moves through your arteries at a higher pressure than normal. The heart is actually straining to pump blood through the arteries.

Blood pressure is normally measured with a blood pressure cuff placed on the arm.

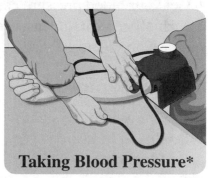

**Taking Blood Pressure***

## High Blood Pressure, Continued

The first (higher) number measures the maximum pressure exerted against the artery walls while the heart is beating (systolic pressure). The second (lower) number measures the pressure between heartbeats, when the heart is resting (diastolic pressure). The results are then recorded as systolic/diastolic pressure (120/80 mmHg, for example). Blood pressure is high if readings are consistently 140 or higher for first number and/or 90 or higher for second number.

## Prevention

- Get to and/or stay at a healthy weight.
- Don't smoke. If you smoke, quit.
- Limit alcohol to 1 drink or less a day.
- Exercise regularly.
- Learn to handle stress.
- Get your blood pressure checked at each office visit, at least every 2 years, or as your doctor advises.

## Signs & Symptoms

There are usually no signs or symptoms. When blood pressure is very, very high, these symptoms may occur:

- Headache
- Nosebleeds
- Palpitations
- Dizziness
- Numbness or tingling in the hands or feet
- Confusion

## Causes, Risk Factors & Care

There is no known cause for 90% of HBP. When this is the case, it is called primary hypertension. About 10% of persons with HBP get it from another medical disorder or as a side effect of some medicines. This is called secondary hypertension.

Risk factors for primary hypertension:

- Family history of HBP
- Aging. More than half of older adults have HBP.
- Smoking cigarettes
- Race. Black persons are twice as likely to have HBP as are white persons.
- Gender. Men are more likely to have HBP than women.
- Sedentary lifestyle; obesity
- Emotional distress
- High-sodium diet in some persons

If left untreated, HBP can lead to stroke, heart, kidney, and eye problems.

To Learn More, See Back Cover

*High Blood Pressure, Continued*

High blood pressure is one of the easiest health problems to control.

### For Primary Hypertension:

When self-care is not enough, your doctor will prescribe one or more medicines.

### For Secondary Hypertension:

The root cause needs to be found. Once the cause is found and treated, blood pressure usually goes back to normal.

## Self-Care:

- Follow prevention tips in this topic.

- Limit salt and foods high in salt. (This is helpful for many people). Use salt substitutes only if your doctor says it's okay.

- Reduce fat and cholesterol. Get good sources of calcium and potassium. Don't eat black licorice. It can lower potassium. Limit caffeine

- Take medicine as prescribed. Tell your doctor if you have any side effects, such as dizziness, faintness, or a dry cough in the absence of a cold. Don't stop taking your pre-scribed medicine unless your doctor tells you to.

- Talk to your physician or pharmacist before you take antihistamines and decongestants. An ingredient in some of these can raise your blood pressure.

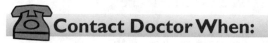

## Contact Doctor When:

- You have signs of very, very high blood pressure listed under "Signs & Symptoms" on page 204.

- You take medicine for high blood pressure and have side effects, such as dizziness.

- You need office visit checks of your blood pressure.

## Get Immediate Care When:

- You have heart attack symptoms. (See "Heart Attack Warning Signs" on page 202.)

- You have stroke symptoms. (See "Stroke Warning Signs" on page 229.)

## For Information Contact:

The American Heart Association
1-800-242-8721
www.americanheart.org

National Heart Lung and Blood Institute
1-800-251-1222
www.nhlbi.nih.gov

12. Heart & Circulation Problems

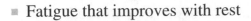

# 77. Peripheral Vascular Disease

Peripheral vascular disease occurs when arteries to the limbs become too narrow to supply enough oxygen to the tissues. Blood flow is reduced. This is most common in the legs and much less common in the arms. Peripheral vascular disease often occurs with coronary artery disease (see page 199).

## Prevention

- Don't smoke. If you smoke, quit.
- Get regular exercise.
- Get to and/or stay at a healthy weight.
- Follow a diet low in saturated fat and cholesterol.

## Signs & Symptoms

- Muscle pain in one or both legs when walking, especially when walking fast or uphill. The pain lessens or goes away with rest. Pain can be in the calves (most often) or thighs. Much less often, it can also be in the arms, fingers, lower back, buttocks, or the foot arches.

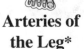

**Arteries of the Leg***

- Fatigue that improves with rest
- Impotence in men (sometimes)

With severe disease symptoms are:

- Muscle pain at rest, especially at night
- Cold or numb feet
- Weak or no pulse in the affected limb
- Pale, bluish-colored toes
- Open sores on the lower leg, toes, or ankles
- Shiny and hairless skin on affected areas

## Causes, Risk Factors & Care

- Smoking
- Diabetes, especially in women {**Note:** If you have diabetes and smoke cigarettes, you are very prone to peripheral vascular disease. If you have diabetes, YOU MUST NOT SMOKE.}
- Fatty buildup (plaque) in the arteries
- High cholesterol
- High blood pressure
- Being elderly
- Taking some medications, such as beta-blockers, to lower high blood pressure {**Note:** Don't stop taking any prescribed medicines on your own. Consult with your doctor.}

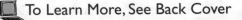 To Learn More, See Back Cover

12. Heart & Circulation Problems

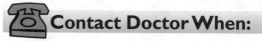

*Peripheral Vascular Disease, Continued*

Treatment for peripheral vascular disease includes:

- A graduated exercise program, such as walking.

- Medicines, such as ones to lower cholesterol and/or high blood pressure and to improve blood flow

- Surgery, if needed, such as balloon angioplasty or bypass surgery

## Self-Care:

- Follow measures under "Prevention" in this topic.

- Follow a graduated walking program as advised by your doctor.

- Take good care of your feet:
  - Check the feet daily.
  - Don't walk barefoot.
  - Wear comfortable, roomy shoes. Avoid sandals and high heels.
  - Cut toenails straight across. Do not cut nails close to the skin.
  - Use an antifungal foot powder to avoid athlete's foot.

- Take medicines as prescribed.

## Contact Doctor When:

- You have any pain, redness, or a leg or foot wound and you have a history of diabetes or peripheral vascular disease.

- The pain, redness, and swelling extend up the ankle to the leg.

- The skin of your foot has turned grayish to black in color.

- Repeated muscle pain occurs in a leg when you walk and it goes away with rest.

- Leg pain occurs when you are at rest.

## Get Immediate Care When:

You have all of these problems:

- Sudden onset of pain

- Rapid skin color changes: white, red, blue, grayish, or black

- You cannot feel sensation in your foot for the first time.

# 78. Phlebitis & Thrombosis

Phlebitis is inflammation in a vein. Thrombosis is when a blood clot forms. When both of these occur together, it is called thrombophlebitis.

**12. Heart & Circulation Problems**

*Phlebitis & Thrombosis, Continued*

## Prevention

- Avoid sitting or standing for long periods without moving around.

- Inform your doctor if you have a history of varicose veins, superficial phlebitis (SP), or deep-vein thrombosis (DVT) and take estrogen.

- Don't sit with your legs crossed. Don't wear tight garments below the waist, such as knee-high hosiery. These restrict blood flow.

- On trips, drink a lot of fluids (no alcohol) and move about at least every hour. Exercise the legs, while sitting.

- If you're confined to a bed or a chair, stretch often. Push with the feet, pretending you're pressing on a gas pedal and then release it. Do this with one foot, then the other.

- Avoid tobacco.

## Signs & Symptoms

- Superficial phlebitis (SP) occurs just under the skin's surface. The affected area is swollen and feels warm and tender. At times, a hard ropy vein is felt. This type seldom showers clots into the bloodstream.

- Deep-vein thrombosis (DVT) occurs within a muscle mass (commonly the leg). It is apt to release showers of clots (emboli) that often go to the lung (pulmonary emboli). The symptoms may resemble those of SP; the limb may swell and/or the muscle involved may ache. Often, DVT symptoms are silent and can't be seen. In silent DVT, the first symptoms may be from a blood clot to the lung. These include sudden shortness of breath and severe problems breathing; sudden chest pain; and/or collapse.

## Cause, Risk Factors & Care

Phlebitis is usually caused by infection, injury, or poor blood flow in a vein. It is common in women over age 50.

Conditions that can lead to SP and/or DVT include:

- Inactivity. This could result from prolonged bed rest, a sedentary job, or a long trip, especially in a cramped space, such as sitting in the economy class section of a plane.

- Varicose veins

- Being overweight, in poor physical condition, or older in age

- Estrogen therapy

- Trauma to an arm or leg. Examples are a fall or injury to the vein, such as from injections or IV needles.

To Learn More, See Back Cover

12. Heart & Circulation Problems

*Phlebitis & Thrombosis, Continued*

- Heart failure or heart attack
- Some cancers

A doctor needs to diagnose SP with or without DVT or DVT alone. Treatment for SP alone includes resting the affected limb, warm compresses, and pain relievers.

Treatment for DVT includes blood thinning medicine, possible hospitalization, and surgery if a blood clot to the lung has occurred.

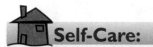 **Self-Care:**

It is best to let your doctor diagnose if you have phlebitis or thrombosis. If SP is diagnosed, you may be told to follow these self-care measures:

- Wear elastic support stockings as prescribed by your doctor.
- Rest the affected limb as advised. Elevate it when you rest.
- Apply moist, warm compresses to the area of pain.
- Take an over-the-counter medicine for pain and inflammation. (See "Pain relievers" in "Your Home Pharmacy" on page 43. ) Take the one your doctor advises.

- Don't massage or rub the limb.
- Don't sit or stand for long periods of time. When you sit, elevate the limb. Continue with your regular activities, though, as much as you can.
- Follow "Prevention" measures in this topic.

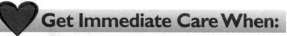 **Contact Doctor When:**

You have 1 or more of these problems:

- Redness, pain, and a burning feeling in the leg
- Swelling and the feeling of a cordlike vein beneath the skin along the length of the vein

**Get Immediate Care When:**

- You have symptoms of a blood clot to the lung:
  - Sudden onset of chest pain with calf pain
  - Sudden shortness of breath and severe problems breathing
  - Rapid heartbeat
  - Cough with bloody sputum (sometimes)

**_Phlebitis & Thrombosis, Continued_**

- Chest pain in a person who has had a recent operation or illness that has kept them in bed

■ You have symptoms of deep-vein thrombosis (DVT):

- Swelling and warmth in the leg
- Pain in the ankle, calf, or thigh that does not go away with rest
- The affected skin area is red and tender

# 79. Varicose Veins

Varicose veins may occur in almost any part of the body. They are most often seen in the back of the calf or on the inside of the leg between the groin and the ankle. Hemorrhoids (veins around the anus) can also become varicose.

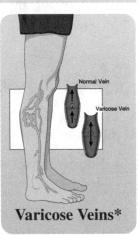

**Varicose Veins\***

## Signs & Symptoms

■ Swollen and twisted veins that look blue and are close to the surface of the skin.

■ Veins bulge and feel heavy.

■ The legs and feet can swell.

■ The skin can itch.

## Causes, Risk Factors & Care

■ Obesity

■ Hormonal changes at menopause

■ Activities or hobbies that require standing or lifting heavy objects for long periods of time

■ A family history of varicose veins

■ Past vein diseases such as thrombophlebitis

■ Often wearing clothing that is tight around the upper thighs

■ Body positions that restrict lower leg blood flow for long periods of time. One example is sitting on an airplane, especially in the economy class section on a long flight.

Medical treatment is not required for most varicose veins unless problems result. If so, treatment includes:

■ Surgery to remove the vein or part of the vein

■ Sclerotherapy, which uses a chemical injection into the vein, causing it to close up

■ Laser therapy, which causes the vein to fade away

12. Heart & Circulation Problems

## Varicose Veins, *Continued*

### Self-Care:

- Don't cross your legs when sitting.

- Exercise regularly. Walk. It improves leg and vein strength.

- Keep your weight down.

- Don't stand for long periods of time. If you must, shift your weight from one leg to the other every few minutes or wiggle your toes.

- Don't wear tight clothing or undergarments that constrict your waist, groin, or legs.

- Eat high-fiber foods, like bran cereals, whole grain breads, and fresh fruits and vegetables. Drink at least 8 glasses of water a day.

- To prevent swelling, limit your salt intake.

- Exercise your legs. From a sitting position, rotate your feet at the ankles. Turn them clockwise, then counterclockwise, using a circular motion. Next, extend your legs forward and point your toes to the ceiling, then to the floor. Then, lift your feet off the floor and gently bend your legs back and forth at the knees.

- Elevate your legs when resting.

- Get up and move about every 35 to 45 minutes when traveling by air or even when sitting for hours. Opt for an aisle seat in theaters, etc. Stop and take short walks at least every 45 minutes when taking long car rides.

- Wear elastic support socks that go up to the knee, but do not cover the knee. The top of these socks must not be tight.

### Contact Doctor When:

- A varicose vein looks like it has broken open and is bleeding a lot under the skin. {**Note:** Apply direct pressure on the skin area over the varicose vein.}

- A varicose vein has become swollen, red, very tender, or warm to the touch.

- You have varicose veins with a rash or sores on the leg or near the ankle; or the varicose vein(s) have caused circulation problems in the feet.

12. Heart & Circulation Problems

## 80. How Aging Affects Memory

Many people are afraid that growing old means losing the ability to think, reason, or remember. They worry when they feel confused or forgetful that these feelings are the first signs of being "senile."

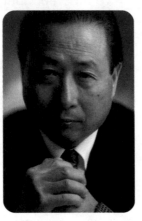

Some short-term memory loss does come with aging. You may, for example, forget where you put your keys or not remember the name of a person you just met. This is normal. Memory lapses that interfere with your normal activities, though, are not a normal part of aging. Nor is confusion.

People who have changes in personality, behavior, or skills may have a brain or nervous system condition. These problems could also be a side effect of certain medicines, too much alcohol, or depression, to name a few causes. There are many more. This chapter gives information on common brain and nervous conditions in older persons. It can help you decide when to get medical care for yourself or for someone else.

## 81. Alzheimer's Disease

Alzheimer's disease (AD) afflicts nearly 4 million Americans. It strikes over 45 percent of the population over age 85 and about 5 to 10 percent of those over age 65. In rare instances, AD comes earlier than age 65. It is the 4th leading cause of death in older adults.

AD is the most common cause of dementia in older persons. It affects the parts of the brain that control memory, thought, and language.

### Prevention

There is no known prevention. Some studies suggest the following may lower the risk of AD and delay the onset of AD symptoms:

- For women, estrogen replacement taken during and after menopause

- Taking nonsteroidal anti-inflammatory drugs (NSAIDs) other than aspirin. Examples are ibuprofen, naproxen sodium, and indomethacin.

- Taking the drug selegiline (used to treat Parkinson's disease) and taking vitamin E. These act as anti-oxidants.

*Alzheimer's Disease, Continued*

## Signs & Symptoms

Alzheimer's disease has a gradual onset. The signs and symptoms progress in stages. How quickly they occur varies from person to person. The time span of the disease varies from 3 to 20 years. It averages 8 years from the time symptoms start.

### Stage One

- Forgetfulness. Short-term memory loss.
- Disorientation of time and place
- Increasing inability to do routine tasks
- Impairment in judgement
- Lessening of initiative
- Lack of spontaneity
- Depression and fear

{**Note:** As soon as symptoms develop, the person's ability to drive should be carefully monitored. Seek professional help to determine this.}

### Stage Two

- Increasing forgetfulness. Short and long-term memory loss.
- Increasing disorientation
- Wandering

- Restlessness and agitation, especially at night
- Repetitive actions
- Muscle twitching and/or convulsions may develop

### Stage Three

- Disorientation
- Inability to recognize either themselves or other people
- Speech impairment (may not be able to speak at all)
- A need to put everything into the mouth
- A need to touch everything in sight

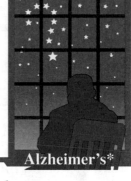

Alzheimer's*

- Becoming emaciated
- Complete loss of control of all body functions

{**Note:** The stages very often overlap.}

## Causes, Risk Factors & Care

No one knows what causes Alzheimer's disease. It is probably not caused by any one factor. Studies suggest these possible causes:

- A virus

**13. Brain & Nervous System Conditions**

*Alzheimer's Disease, Continued*

- Lower levels of certain brain chemicals (acetylcholine and somatostatin)

- Family traits. Having certain genes increases the risk.

- Lower education level increases the risk.

- Having Down Syndrome increases the risk.

Whatever the cause, the end result is the death of brain cells that control the way the brain receives and processes information.

{**Note:** There are many diseases or other problems that can cause symptoms of Alzheimer's disease. See "Dementias" on page 220. Many of these problems can be treated. It is very important to have the person evaluated for other problems.}

If someone shows signs of Alzheimer's disease, see that they get medical care to confirm (or rule out) the diagnosis.

There is no known cure for Alzheimer's disease. Good planning, medical care, and social management are needed. These help both the victim and caregivers cope with the symptoms and maintain the quality of life for as long as possible. An advance directive should be drafted in the early stages to allow for the person's wishes. (See "Advance Directives" on page 33.) It is especially helpful to put structure in the life of someone who is in the early stages of AD. See "Self-Care" in this topic.

Prescription medicines, such as tacrine, (Cognex), and donepezil (Aricept) may help some persons in early and middle stages of AD. Sometimes medicines to treat depression, paranoia, and agitation, etc. can minimize symptoms. They may not, though, improve memory.

Many persons with AD eventually need 24-hour care. Caregivers of Alzheimer's victims should also be given "care". (See "Caregivers Guide" on page 54.)

### Self-Care:

- Post safety reminders, like "Turn off the stove" at appropriate places.

- See that the person with AD eats well-balanced meals, goes for walks with family members, and continues to be as active as possible.

- Maintain daily routines.

- Post reminders on a large calendar that can be easily seen.

*Continued on Next Page*

13. Brain & Nervous System Conditions

*Alzheimer's Disease, Continued*

*Self-Care, Continued*

- Make "to do" lists of daily tasks for the person with AD. Ask him or her to check them off as they are done.

- Put things in their proper places after use. This helps the person with AD find things as needed.

### Contact Doctor When:

- The person needs a consult, medical history, and tests to rule out or confirm Alzheimer's disease.

- The person has an increase in memory lapses or any other symptom listed in "Stage One" under "Signs & Symptoms" on page 213.

- Help is needed to care for a person with Alzheimer's disease or if his or her symptoms worsen.

- The caretaker of the person with Alzheimer's needs guidance.

### Get Immediate Care When:

The person has sudden confusion, disorientation, loss of reasoning or ability to communicate.

## For Information Contact:

Alzheimer's Disease Education and Referral (ADEAR) Center
1-800-438-4380.
www.alzheimers.org/adear

Alzheimer's Association
1-800-272-3900
www.alz.org

# 82. Bell's Palsy

With Bell's palsy, a nerve that runs between the ear and the jaw becomes inflamed. This paralyzes the muscles on one side of the face. Bell's palsy occurs in about 1 in 2,000 people each year. It can occur at any age. In older persons, it is especially important to distinguish Bell's palsy from a stroke.

## Signs & Symptoms

The onset of signs and symptoms is usually sudden. You may have pain or tingling on one side of your face 1 or 2 days before signs and symptoms occur. Often, symptoms will be noticed when you wake up.

- These problems occur on one side of your face:

  - It droops or sags, has no expression, or looks flat.

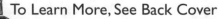

*Bell's Palsy, Continued*

- The muscles are weak or paralyzed.

- You can't smile or frown or if you can, these look distorted. You drool.

- Pain. The area behind the ear on that side of your face can hurt, too.

■ These problems occur with your eye:

- Your eyelid droops.

- You can't close your eye.

- Your eye tears.

■ Other problems can occur:

- You have changes in taste.

- You are more sensitive to noise.

## Causes, Risk Factors & Care

The cause is not known. These factors may cause the facial nerve to swell:

■ A virus, such as shingles (see page 134).

■ A physical blow that damages the facial nerve

■ Decrease in blood flow and pressure on the facial nerve. This could be due to circulation problems.

■ Family traits

Most of the time, Bell's palsy goes away on its own. If you have symptoms, though, you should see your doctor. He or she can make the diagnosis and rule out other conditions, such as a stroke. The time it takes to recover varies and depends on the extent of nerve damage and how severe the paralysis is.
Even 80% to 90% of persons with severe facial paralysis have a complete recovery. Symptoms start to go away in 2 to 3 weeks. It could take months for them to be all gone.

Self-care can help with the discomfort. For severe cases, a doctor may prescribe:

■ Nerve conduction tests of the facial nerves

■ Physical and/or speech therapy

■ Corticosteroid medicine to reduce swelling of the affected nerve

■ Eye drops to comfort and protect the affected eye

■ Electric stimulation to the affected muscle

■ Surgery, on occasion, to reduce pressure on the facial nerve

■ Plastic surgery may be done in rare cases, if the face remains paralyzed.

To Learn More, See Back Cover

*Bell's Palsy, Continued*

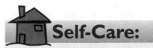 **Self-Care:**

Try to be patient. Bell's palsy is a cause for distress, but is not dangerous. The goal of self-care is to ease symptoms and to prevent damage to the eye.

**For Pain:**

- Take an over-the-counter medicine for pain. (See "Pain relievers" in "Your Home Pharmacy" on page 43.)
- Cover or close your eye. Apply a heating pad (set on low) to the painful area. Do this for 15 minutes at a time, 2 times a day.
- Soak a washcloth in hot water. Wring it out. Close your eye and place it over the eye for 15 minutes.

**If You Cannot Close Your Eye:**

- Wear wraparound goggles during the day to protect your eyes from dust, dirt, and dryness. Wear an eye patch at night to help hold the eyelid shut.
- Exercise the affected facial muscles as advised by your doctor or physical therapist. Do a facial massage for 15 to 20 minutes a day. With an oil or a cream, massage the muscles of your forehead, cheek, lips, and eye area.

- Use over-the-counter artificial tears as advised by your doctor.
- Keep up with your normal activities.
- Eat soft foods, if you need to.

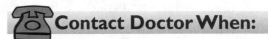 **Contact Doctor When:**

- You have any of these problems after a diagnosis of Bell's palsy:
  - Symptoms get worse.
  - The numbness or weakness appear to be spreading or affect an area or body part not affected before.
  - Your eye gets very red or irritated.
  - Fever.
  - Severe pain
  - Swelling or a lump in front of the ear
- You have no improvement in symptoms 3 weeks after you have been diagnosed with Bell's palsy.

**Get Immediate Care When:**

You have signs of a stroke. (See "Stroke Warning Signs" on page 229.)

{**Note:** Immediate care is advised because the initial symptoms of Bell's palsy are so like ones of a stroke. This is especially true for older persons.}

**13. Brain & Nervous System Conditions**

**The "Exam to Assess Mental Status, below, can help detect cognitive problems, such as seen in dementias (see page 220).**

## Exam to Assess Mental Status

A number of tests can assess mental status. A common one used is called "Mini-Mental State Examination". It was written by M.S. Folstein, S.E. Folstein, and P.R. McHugh in 1975. The questions that follow are adapted from this examination. They were taken from "Working With Your Older Patient: A Clinician's Handbook" by B. Gaskel, Bethesda, MD: National Institute on Aging, National Institutes of Health, 1994.

| Questions and Tasks | Score |
|---|---|
| **1.** These questions test for orientation to time and place. Give 1 point for each correct answer. | |
| ▪ What year is it? | _____ out of 1 |
| ▪ What season is it? | _____ out of 1 |
| ▪ What is today's date? | _____ out of 1 |
| ▪ What day is it? | _____ out of 1 |
| ▪ What month is it? | _____ out of 1 |
| ▪ What state are you in? | _____ out of 1 |
| ▪ What country are you in? | _____ out of 1 |
| ▪ What city or town are you in? | _____ out of 1 |
| ▪ What place (home, building, etc.) are you in? | _____ out of 1 |
| ▪ What room are you in or what floor are you on in this place? | _____ out of 1 |
| **2.** This part tests instant recall. (These things will be asked to be recalled later.) Give 1 point for each object named.<br>▪ Name 3 objects (e.g. apple, table, dime.) Take 1 second to name each object. Have the person repeat the 3 objects named. | _____ out of 3 |
| **3.** This part of the exam tests for attention and calculation skills. Give 1 point for each correct answer.<br>▪ Count backwards from the number 100 by 7s. Do this for 5 numbers. (The answers are 93, 86, 79, 72, and 65.)<br>▪ Another option is to spell the word WORLD backwards. (The answer is D L R O W.) | _____ out of 5 |

| Questions and Tasks | Score |
|---|---|
| **4.** This part tests for recall. Give 1 point for each object named.<br>   ■ Ask for the 3 objects stated in step 2 (i.e., apple, table, dime). | _____ out of 3 |
| **5.** This part tests for language skills.  Give 1 point for each correct answer. | |
|    ■ Point to a pencil or pen. Ask the person to name it. | _____ out of 1 |
|    ■ Point to a wristwatch or clock. Ask the person to name it. | _____ out of 1 |
|    ■ Ask the person to repeat this phrase "No ifs, ands, or buts". | _____ out of 1 |
|    ■ Ask the person to do these 3 things: Give 1 point for each step done correctly. | |
|       • Take a piece of paper in your right hand. | _____ out of 1 |
|       • Fold the paper in half. | _____ out of 1 |
|       • Put the paper on the floor. | _____ out of 1 |
|    ■ Write CLOSE YOUR EYES in large letters on a piece of paper. Ask the person to read the phrase and to do what it says. Give 1 point for following the command. | _____ out of 1 |
|    ■ Give the person a pen or pencil and a piece of paper. Tell him or her to write a sentence with a subject and an object. It's okay if words are not spelled correctly. Give 1 point for writing a sentence. | _____ out of 1 |
|    ■ Give this design on a piece of paper to the person. Tell the person to copy it on the same piece of paper. Give 1 point if the person copies the design correctly. | _____ out of 1 |
| **Total** | _____ out of 30 |

In general, a score of 24 or less for persons with 12 or more years of schooling and 20 or less for persons with 4 or fewer years of schooling may mean a cognitive problem. Check, though, with a health care provider. A more complete assessment may need to be done to check for mental status.

**13. Brain & Nervous System Conditions**

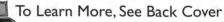

# 83. Dementias

Dementias are brain diseases. They result in a decline of all areas of mental ability. This includes learning, memory, problem solving, behaviors, and language.

## Signs & Symptoms

Symptoms of most forms of dementia usually appear slowly over time. However, with a certain form, multi-infarct dementia, the onset of symptoms can be sudden. Symptoms of dementia include:

- Poor memory of recent events, etc.

- Making up stories to explain memory loss

- Getting lost in familiar settings

- Not being able to finish tasks

- Decreased energy

- Social withdrawal or depression

- General confusion

- Behaviors that are paranoid, anxious, irritating, childlike, or rigid

- No interest in personal hygiene, grooming, or dressing oneself

- Unclear speech

## Causes & Care

There are 2 types of dementias.

### Primary or True Dementias

The origin of the dementia is in the brain itself. Examples of this type are:

- Alzheimer's disease (see page 212). This is the most common type of dementia.

- Multi-infarct dementia. This is due to blocked blood vessels in the brain. Often the cause is a stroke.

- Parkinson's disease (see page 226)

- Pick's disease. This is like Alzheimer's disease, but has different changes in the brain.

- Huntington's disease. This is an inherited disease. Dementia symptoms usually start in middle age. Facial tics and other uncontrolled movements also occur.

- Creutzfeldt-Jacob disease. This is caused by a virus that lies dormant in the body for years. When the virus is activated, the dementia progresses quickly.

- Multiple sclerosis. With this, scar tissue in the brain can prevent the normal travel of nerve impulses used for mental function. Dementia with multiple sclerosis is rare, though, and may occur with the end stage of this disease.

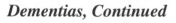

## Dementias, Continued

### Secondary Dementias

The dementia results from other conditions, such as:

- Depression (see page 312)
- Alcohol problems (see page 303)
- Reactions to certain medicines
- Poor nutrition. This includes a vitamin $B_{12}$ deficiency.
- Hypothyroidism (see page 301)
- Dehydration (see page 391)
- Head injuries (see page 403)
- Infections, such as HIV which causes AIDS (see page 294) or syphilis (see page 365)
- Brain tumors

Dementias need medical diagnosis and treatment. When another condition, such as depression or vitamin $B_{12}$ deficiency is the cause and is treated with success, the dementia can be cured. For others, such as Alzheimer's Disease, there is no cure. The goal of treatment is to treat symptoms and provide safety and comfort.

## Self-Care:

The person with dementia needs to:

- Follow a simple daily routine
- Limit activities
- Wear an ID tag
- Be kept in a safe environment
- Have labels put on objects
- Be given written notes for tasks
- Eat a well balanced diet and drink plenty of fluids
- Have regular sensory stimulation, like touching, exercising, etc.

Caretakers should:

- Assume a non-combative approach to difficult behaviors. Steer the person into another activity.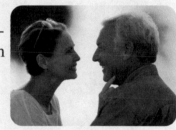

- Give medicines as advised by the person's doctor; report and review medicines with the doctor and/or pharmacist.

- Get home care, respite care, hospital, or nursing home care, if needed.

13. Brain & Nervous System Conditions

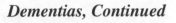

*Dementias, Continued*

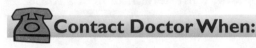

## Contact Doctor When:

- You are unable to care for someone with dementia or he or she is too agitated or hostile to control.

- A medical evaluation is needed for a person with symptoms of dementia. See "Signs & Symptoms" in this topic. See also "Exam to Assess Mental Status" on page 218.

## Get Immediate Care When:

Signs and symptoms of a stroke are present. (See "Stroke Warning Signs" on page 229.)

### Delirium

Delirium is mental confusion, behavior changes, etc. that develop in a matter of hours to a day or so. Delirium is a symptom of another condition, such as:

- A high fever

- Pneumonia or other infection

- Diabetes

- Substance abuse or withdrawal

- Misuse or withdrawal of certain medicines

Immediate medical care is needed for delirium so the cause can be found and treated.

# 84. Dizziness & Vertigo

Dizziness is feeling lightheaded. It is a symptom of another condition. Vertigo is a spinning feeling. It affects the inner ear, the brain's gravity-and-motion detector.

| Dizziness Chart | | |
| --- | --- | --- |
| **Signs & Symptoms** | **What It Could Be** | **What to Do** |
| Sudden dizziness with:<br>- Hot, dry, red skin<br>- High fever. No sweating.<br>- Pulse that is rapid and then gets weak<br>- Exposure to very, very hot conditions | Heat stroke | Get immediate care. Follow "Immediate Care" guideleines on page 407. |

 To Learn More, See Back Cover

**13. Brain & Nervous System Conditions**

## Dizziness & Vertigo, Continued

### Dizziness Chart, Continued

| Signs & Symptoms | What It Could Be | What to Do |
|---|---|---|
| Dizziness with "Stroke Warning Signs" (see page 229) | Stroke or transient ischemic attack (TIA) | Follow "Immediate Care" guideline on page 230. |
| Dizziness with "Heart Attack Warning Signs" (see page 202) | Heart Attack | Follow "Immediate Care" guidelines on page 203. |
| Dizziness with a heart rate greater than 130 beats per minute or less than 50 beats per minute or an irregular heart rhythm | Irregular heartbeat | Get immediate care. |
| Dizziness with signs and symptoms of dehydration (see page 391) | Dehydration | Get immediate care. |
| Dizziness with:<br>▪ Abdominal pain and swelling that get worse<br>▪ Inability to pass stool or gas<br>▪ Vomiting | Intestinal obstruction | Get immediate care. |
| Dizziness and fainting. Severe chest pain with extreme pain felt across the upper back (not just on one side) that came on within 15 minutes for no apparent reason, such as an injury or back strain. The pain can spread to the abdomen. | Dissecting aortic aneurysm. This is a tear in the main artery from the heart. | Get immediate care. (Do not take aspirin.) |
| Dizziness with ear pain, ringing in the ear, pus or other ear discharge, fever | Ear infection | Contact doctor. See "Earaches" on page 74. |

*Dizziness Chart Continued on Next Page*

13. Brain & Nervous System Conditions

*Dizziness & Vertigo, Continued*

| Dizziness Chart, Continued | | |
| --- | --- | --- |
| **Signs & Symptoms** | **What It Could Be** | **What to Do** |
| Dizziness with:<br>■ True spinning sensation<br>■ Loss of balance<br>■ Nausea and vomiting<br>■ Ringing in the ears<br>■ Jerky movements of the eye | **Labrynthitis**. This is an inflammation in the ear that usually results from an upper respiratory infection. | Contact doctor. |
| Dizziness with hunger, sweating, trembling, anxiety, and confusion | Low blood sugar. This can occur in persons taking insulin or oral pills for diabetes and/ or after not eating for 4 or more hours. | Use self-care. (See "Self-Care" in "Diabetes" on page 278 and "Self-Care/ First Aid for a Low Blood Sugar Reaction" on page 398.) |
| Dizziness when getting up too quickly from a seated or lying position | Temporary drop in blood pressure (orthostatic hypotension). This could be a side effect of taking medicines, such as ones for high blood pressure and depression. | Use self-care. (See "Self-Care for Orthostatic Hypotension" on page 225.) |

**Other Causes of Dizziness:**

■ Alcohol

■ New medications, antibiotics, or high doses of aspirin

■ A change in altitude or motion sickness

■ Sudden movement, such as with turning the head quickly

■ Seeing fast moving objects

Treatment for dizziness depends on the cause.

13. Brain & Nervous System Conditions

*Dizziness & Vertigo, Continued*

# Vertigo

## Signs & Symptoms

- Wooziness
- Sense that the room is spinning
- Nausea
- Blurred vision
- Floating, rocking, and/or rolling feeling
- Sense of walking on an uneven surface
- Loss of balance

## Causes, Risk Factors & Care

Vertigo is caused by a problem with the inner ear. Causes of vertigo are:

- **Benign Positional Vertigo (BPV)**. This is the most common type. It may happen when you turn over in bed, get up, sit down, bend over, or just tilt your head. The sensations start within seconds of changing positions and last less than a minute. As bothersome as BPV is, it rarely signals more serious disease. Risk factors for BPV are aging, viral infections, and a prior head injury.

- **Ménière's disease**. This condition may be due to spasms of blood vessels in the inner ear, fluid retention in the inner ear, or allergic reactions. Meniere's disease is linked with a decrease in hearing and tinnitus. It sometimes leads to permanent hearing loss.

- **Multiple sclerosis**. With this, the covering that protects nerves (myelin) is destroyed. Over time, scar tissue (sclerosis) forms where the myelin used to be in the brain and spinal cord. Scar tissue or inflammation in the brain may cause vertigo symptoms.

After proper diagnosis, most cases of vertigo are easily treated in the doctor's office or at home with self-care.

While attacks of Meniere's disease can continue for many years, some symptoms can be controlled by antinausea medicines, tranquilizers, antihistamines, and/or diuretics (water pills).

### Self-Care:

**For Orthostatic Hypotension:**

- Don't jump out of bed. Go from a lying position to a sitting position slowly. Sit on the edge of the bed a few minutes. Stand up slowly.

*Continued on Next Page*

**13. Brain & Nervous System Conditions**

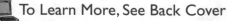

*Dizziness & Vertigo, Continued*

### Self-Care, Continued

- From a sitting position, stand up slowly. Hold onto the arms of the chair or the head of the bed for support.

- If you feel lightheaded, sit back down for a few minutes. Take a few deep breaths. Get up again, slowly.

### For Benign Positional Vertigo (BPV):

- Sit on the side of the bed and lean to your right, resting the right ear on the bed. This might make you dizzy and nauseous at first.

- Wait 20 seconds until the dizziness stops and sit up straight.

- Wait another 20 seconds and repeat steps 1 and 2 on your left side.

- Do this exercise 10 to 15 times, 3 times a day.

### For Meniere's Disease:

- Lie still in bed until the dizziness and nausea are gone.

- Walk with assistance.

- Don't change positions too fast.

- Do not drive, climb ladders, or work around dangerous machinery.

- Decrease the amount of salt and fluids in your diet.

- Avoid bright lights. Do not read when you have a spinning feeling.

- Resume your normal activities when symptoms go away.

- Avoid alcohol, caffeine, and tobacco.

# 85. Parkinson's Disease

Parkinson's disease is a nervous system disorder. It causes tremors (involuntary shaking in the limbs and head), a shuffling gait, and a gradual, progressive stiffness of muscles. Parkinson's disease is found equally in men and women of all races and ethnic groups. It most often strikes people over the age of 50. The average age of onset is 60 years.

## Signs & Symptoms

Early symptoms can be subtle. They occur gradually and include:

- Feeling a little shaky. A person's handwriting can look spidery.

- Being tired. Speaking too softly.

- Losing track of a word or thought

- Having no facial expression

- Feeling irritable or depressed for no apparent reason

To Learn More, See Back Cover

## Parkinson's Disease, Continued

The 4 main symptoms are:

- Tremor. This usually starts in the head, but can start in a foot or in the jaw.

- Rigidity. The person has stiffness of the limbs and trunk.

- Slow movement and loss of automatic and spontaneous movement. The person may not be able to wash or dress quickly or easily.

- Impaired balance and coordination. This can lead to a stooped posture, a shuffling gait, and falls.

Other symptoms include:

- Problems in chewing and swallowing

- Having a hard time changing positions

- Depression and anxiety

- Speech changes. The person may speak too softly, in a monotone, slur or repeat words, or speak too fast.

- Bladder or bowel problems, such as constipation

- Skin that is too oily or too dry

- Sleep problems. These include restless sleep, daytime drowsiness, and having a harder time staying asleep at night.

- Dementia (in advanced stages)

## Causes, Risk Factors & Care

The exact cause of Parkinson's disease is not known. What is known, though, is that certain cells in the lower part of the brain can't produce dopamine, a substance nerves need for coordination of body movement.

{**Note:** Some medicines can bring on Parkinsonian symptoms. Examples are major tranquilizers and Reglan, a drug used for some digestive problems.}

Risk factors for Parkinson's disease are:

- Family traits

- Aging. For some persons, the neurons that produce dopamine wear away with aging.

- Rarely, recurring trauma to the head, such as occurs to boxers. Muhammad Ali suffers from this condition.

- Damage to nerve cells through a chemical process called oxidation

- Toxins in the environment

Parkinson's disease is not yet curable. Symptoms can be relieved or controlled, though. Treatment includes:

- Medicines, such as Sinemet and Selegiline

- Neurosurgery and direct electrical brain stimulation

- Physical therapy and/or speech therapy

13. Brain & Nervous System Conditions

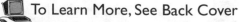

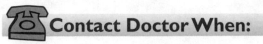

*Parkinson's Disease, Continued*

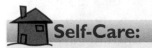

## Self-Care:

Medical treatment is needed for Parkinson's disease. These self-care measures are a part of overall care.

- Take care to maintain a safe home environment. Replace razor blades with electric shavers; use nonskid rugs and handrails to prevent falls, etc.

- Simplify tasks. Replace tie shoes with loafers. Wear clothing that can be pulled on or that has zippers or Velcro closures instead of buttons.

- Prevent constipation. (See "Self-Care" on page 156.)

- Remain as active as possible. Do the activities and exercises advised by your doctor and/or physical therapist.

- Take warm baths and have massages to help with rigid muscles.

- Eat healthy foods. If you take levodopa, limit the protein in your diet, if and as advised by your doctor. A high protein diet can make levodopa less effective.

## Contact Doctor When:

- You have one or more signs and symptoms of Parkinson's disease listed on page 226.

- You have side effects from medicines taken for Parkinson's disease or if new, unexpected symptoms occur during treatment.

## For Information Contact:

American Parkinson's Disease Association
1-800-223-2732
www.apdaparkinson.com

National Parkinson Foundation
1-800-327-4545
www.parkinson.org

# 86. Stroke

A stroke is also called a "brain attack." With a stroke, brain cells die because of a blood clot or rupture of a blood vessel in the brain. The end result is brain damage (and possible death).

Strokes are the 3rd leading cause of death in the United States. They are the leading cause of adult disability.

To Learn More, See Back Cover

**13. Brain & Nervous System Conditions**

*Stroke, Continued*

## Prevention

To reduce the risks of a stroke:

- Get your blood pressure checked at every office visit or at least every 2 years. Follow your doctor's advice to keep your blood pressure under control. Take medicines as prescribed.

- Get checked at your doctor's office for **atrial fibrillation**, a form of irregular beating of the heart. Although in itself, it is not terribly serious, it can cause small blood clots to form that then go up to the brain and cause a stroke. These strokes can be greatly reduced by taking medication.

- Reduce blood levels of cholesterol to below 200 milligrams per deciliter.

- Get regular exercise.

- Get to and stay at a healthy weight.

- Don't smoke. If you smoke, quit.

- If you have diabetes, keep blood sugar levels under control.

- Use alcohol in moderation.

- Learn to manage stress.

- Ask your doctor about taking an aspirin every day or every other day.

- Ask your doctor to evaluate you for a surgical procedure that scrapes away fatty deposits in one or both of the main arteries in the neck.

- Take medicine(s) your doctor has prescribed to help prevent strokes.

## Signs & Symptoms

| Stroke Warning Signs |
|---|
| - Sudden numbness or weakness of the face, arm, or leg, especially on one side of the body |
| - Sudden confusion, trouble speaking or understanding |
| - Sudden trouble seeing in 1 or both eyes |
| - Sudden trouble walking, dizziness, loss of balance or coordination |
| - Sudden severe headache with no known cause |

{**Note:** Stroke symptoms can appear for a short time and then go away. This could be a sign of a **transient ischemic attack (TIA)**. A TIA is a temporary lack of blood supply to the brain. It is a warning that a stroke may follow. See your doctor right away if you have any TIA episodes.}

**13. Brain & Nervous System Conditions**

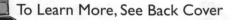

*Stroke, Continued*

## Causes, Risk Factors & Care

About 80% of strokes are caused by a blood clot in an artery in the neck or brain. The rest are caused by bleeding into or around the brain.

Risk factors for a stroke are:

- High blood pressure (see page 203)
- Cigarette smoking
- Heart disease. (See "Coronary Artery Disease" on page 199.)
- Diabetes (see page 276)
- Transient ischemic attack (TIA)
- Atrial fibrillation. This is an irregular beating of the heart.

A stroke needs emergency medical treatment without delay. For a stroke caused by a blood clot, it is important to get some medicines as soon as possible (ideally 1 to 2 hours) after the onset of symptoms to prevent further damage to the brain. After a stroke, rehabilitation by speech, physical, and occupational therapists is prescribed as needed.

## Self-Care:

Medical care, not self-care, is needed.

- Your role is to know the warning signs of a stroke, listed on page 229, and to get emergency medical care right away if any occur.
- After a stroke, a recovery program will be planned by your doctor. A caretaker's help is often needed.
- Follow measures listed in "Prevention" in this topic.

## Contact Doctor When:

You think you may have had a transient ischemic attack (TIA) in the past.

## Get Immediate Care When:

You have one or more stroke warning signs listed on page 229. Call 911 or your local rescue squad right away.

## For Information Contact:

National Stroke Association
1-800-787-6537
www.stroke.org

American Heart Association
1-800-553-6321
www.americanheart.org

To Learn More, See Back Cover

**13. Brain & Nervous System Conditions**

## 87. How Aging Affects the Bones & Muscles

As you age, you lose bone mass. Your bones become weaker and more porous. You may not feel these changes, but one sign of them is a gradual loss of height. This could come from osteoporosis (see page 259). It could also come from flattening of your feet and a shrinkage of cartilage, which cushions and lubricates the joints. Years of wear and tear on cartilage and joints can make your joints ache and make it harder to move them. (See "Osteoarthritis" on page 232.)

As you get older, you may lose muscle mass. This is not due to aging itself, but usually due to using your muscles less.

Keep your muscles healthy by doing stretching and strengthening and weight-bearing exercises. (See "Stay Active with Exercise" on page 12.)

This chapter gives common conditions that affect the bones, joints, and muscles. It tells you how to prevent problems and what to do if you have any of them.

## 88. Arthritis

Arthritis is joint inflammation. It causes pain and loss of movement. It can affect joints in any part of the body. There are over 100 different forms of arthritis. Half of all people aged 65 or older have arthritis. The most common type is osteoarthritis. It is also called degenerative joint disease. Two other common types in older persons are rheumatoid arthritis (RA) and gout. (For information on gout, see page 252.)

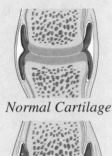

*Normal Cartilage*

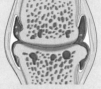

*Deteriorated Cartilage*
**Osteoarthritis***

### Prevention

You may not be able to keep from getting arthritis, but to keep your joints healthy:

- Get to and stay at a healthy weight.
- Exercise on a regular basis to keep the muscles around joints strong and to keep joint cartilage healthy. When you exercise:
  - Do low-impact exercises, like walking, not high impact ones, like jogging.

*Arthritis, Continued*

- • Do stretching exercises before aerobic activities.
- • Don't overdo it. If you feel pain, stop.
- ▪ Avoid activities that can injure your joints. (See "Use fall prevention measures" under "Self-Care" on page 262.)

## Signs & Symptoms

### For Osteoarthritis:

- ▪ Joint pain and stiffness, often in the hands, knees, ankles, and hips
- ▪ Early in the disease, pain occurs after activity. Rest brings relief. Later on, pain can occur with even minimal movement or while at rest.
- ▪ Swollen joints (sometimes)

### For Rheumatoid Arthritis:

- ▪ Morning stiffness that lasts longer than an hour
- ▪ Swelling in 3 or more joints
- ▪ Swelling of the same joints on both sides of the body, such as both knees or both wrists
- ▪ Joint tenderness, warmth, or redness

## Causes, Risk Factors & Care

### For Osteoarthritis:

- ▪ Wear and tear on joints
- ▪ Injuries and overuse of joint(s)
- ▪ Being overweight
- ▪ Family traits, especially when the hands and hips are affected

### For Rheumatoid Arthritis:

The actual cause is not known. Risk factors include:

- ▪ Chronic inflammation of the membranes that line the joints
- ▪ Family traits
- ▪ Breakdown of the immune system

Treatment for arthritis includes:

- ▪ Exercise. This is very important. It prevents the muscles from shrinking. Your health care provider can plan an exercise program for your needs. One form of exercise that's effective and soothing is hydrotherapy. This is movement done in water.
- ▪ Medicines to help relieve pain and reduce inflammation. The medicines used most often are aspirin and other nonsteroidal anti-inflammatory drugs (NSAIDs). You can get some, such as ibuprofen, over-the-counter. Your doctor may prescribe other NSAIDs.

To Learn More, See Back Cover

**14. Bone & Muscle Problems**

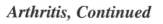

## *Arthritis, Continued*

Other medicines prescribed include:

- Corticosteroids
- Antirheumatic agents for rheumatoid arthritis
- Gold components for mild to moderate rheumatic arthritis
- Drugs that suppress the immune system. These are mostly used for rheumatoid arthritis.

- Physical therapy
- Surgery. Damaged joints can be repaired or replaced with artificial ones. Hip and knee joints are replaced most often. (See box on "Hip and Knee Joint Replacements" on page 263.)

### Self-Care:

- Follow a regular exercise program. Choose exercise routines that use all affected joints. Keep movements gradual, slow, and gentle. If a joint is inflamed, don't exercise it. Don't overdo it. Allow yourself sufficient rest. Focus on freedom of movement, especially in the water.

- Apply an over-the-counter cream with capsaicin to painful joints.

- Take an over-the-counter medicine for pain and swelling. (See "Pain relievers" in "Your Home Pharmacy" on page 43.)

- Don't do repeated activities that put too much stress on your joints. When you do such activities, like kneeling while you garden, use knee pads and take regular breaks.

- Lose weight if you are overweight.

- Beware of quacks. Because arthritis is so common and can be so painful, there are many products that promise to "cure" arthritis, but are not proven to work. Discuss over-the-counter products with your doctor before you take them. This includes glucosamine chondroiton, a popular product many people try.

### Contact Doctor When:

- Any of these problems last longer than 2 weeks:
  - Swelling in one or more joints
  - Early morning stiffness that lasts for more than an hour
  - Recurring pain or tenderness in any joint
  - Inability to move a joint normally
  - Redness or warmth in a joint

14. Bone & Muscle Problems

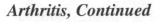

*Arthritis, Continued*

- • Unexplained weight loss, fever, or weakness combined with joint pain

- ▪ You have arthritis and your symptoms are not getting better with the pre-scribed treatment.

- ▪ You have side effects from your arthritis medicines, such as black, tarry stools, and/or stomach pain.

## For Information Contact:

Arthritis Foundation
1-800-283-7800
www.arthritis.org

## 89. Back Pain

### Prevention

Use proper lifting techniques to prevent back pain caused by muscular strain.

### The Dos and Don'ts of Lifting

Dos

- ▪ Wear good shoes with low heels, not sandals or high heels.

- ▪ Stand close to items you want to lift.

- ▪ Plant your feet squarely, shoulder width apart.

- ▪ Bend at the knees, not at the waist. Keep your knees bent as you lift.

- ▪ Pull in your stomach and rear end. Keep your back as straight as you can.

- ▪ Hold the object close to your body.

- ▪ Lift slowly. Let your legs carry the weight.

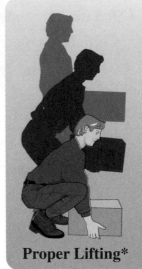

**Proper Lifting***

- ▪ Get help or use a dolly to move something that is too big or very heavy.

Don'ts

- ▪ Don't lift if your back hurts.

- ▪ Don't lift if you have a history of back trouble.

- ▪ Don't lift something that's too heavy.

- ▪ Don't lift heavy things over your head.

- ▪ Don't lift anything heavy if you're not steady on your feet.

- ▪ Don't bend at the waist to pick something up.

- ▪ Don't arch your back when you lift or carry.

- ▪ Don't lift too fast or with a jerk.

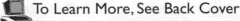 

**14. Bone & Muscle Problems**

### Back Pain, *Continued*

- Don't twist your back when you are holding something. Turn your whole body, from head to toe.

- Don't lift something heavy with one hand and something light with the other. Balance the load.

- Don't try to lift one thing while you hold something else. For example, don't try to pick up a briefcase while you are holding a grocery bag. Put the bag down, or lift the bag and the briefcase at the same time.

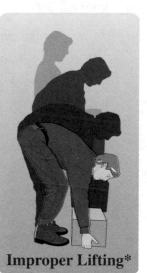

**Improper Lifting***

Other ways to prevent back pain are to develop and maintain good posture; lose weight, if you need to; exercise regularly; and sleep on a firm mattress.

## Signs & Symptoms

Back pain can be sharp, dull, acute, or chronic. There may also be swelling in the back area.

## Causes & Care

Causes of back pain include:

- Muscle strain of the lower back. This is a common cause.

- Back injury, such as a slipped or herniated disk, spinal fracture, etc.

- Osteoarthritis (see page 231)

- Osteoporosis (see page 259)

- Urinary tract infection (see page 186)

- Acute inflammation of the prostate gland (prostatitis) in men. (See "Prostate Problems" on page 331.)

- Cancer (rarely)

The goals of treatment are to treat the cause of the back pain; relieve the pain; promote healing; and avoid re-injury.

Self-care, on page 236, can be used for many cases of back pain.

When self-care is not enough, your doctor may prescribe:

- A stronger painkiller with or without codeine

- A muscle relaxant

- Therapy

- Surgery, when truly needed

14. Bone & Muscle Problems

## Back Pain, Continued

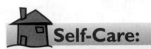
### Self-Care:

- Continue your regular activities as much as you can. Stop activities that increase pain, though. Rest the back if you must, but don't rest in bed more than 1 to 2 days, even if your back hurts a lot. Your back muscles can get weak if you don't use them or if you stay in bed longer than 1 to 2 days. Bed rest should only be used for persons with severe limitations (due mostly to leg pain).

- For the first 48 hours after back symptoms start, apply a cold pack to the painful area. Lie on your back with your knees bent. Put the cold pack under your lower back. Do this for 5 to 10 minutes at a time, several times a day. After 48 hours, apply heat. Use a moist heating pad, a hot-water bottle, hot compresses, a hot tub, hot baths, or hot showers. Use heat for 20 minutes at a time. Do this several times a day. Be careful not to burn yourself.

- Massage the back. This won't cure a backache, but can loosen tight muscles.

- If you need to, wear a brace or corset to support your back and keep it from moving too much.

- Take an over-the-counter medicine for pain and swelling. (See "Pain relievers" in "Your Home Pharmacy" on page 43.) Don't overdo it after taking a painkiller. You can hurt your back more. Then it will take longer to heal.

- Don't sit in one place too long . This strains your lower back.

- Sleep on a firm mattress.

- Don't sleep on your stomach. Sleep on your back or side, with your knees bent.

- Try some mild stretching and strengthening exercises (in the morning and afternoon) to make your stomach and back muscles stronger. (Consult your doctor before starting an exercise program.)

- The most important goal is to return to your normal activities as soon as it is safe. If your back pain is chronic or doesn't get better on its own, see your doctor. He or she can evaluate your needs. A referral may be given to a physical therapist, a physiatrist (a physical therapy doctor), an osteopath, or a chiropractor. Spinal manipulation, usually done by a chiropractor, uses the hands to apply force to "adjust" the spine. This can be helpful for some people in the first month of low back symptoms.

*Back Pain, Continued*

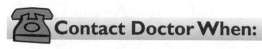 **Contact Doctor When:**

- The pain goes down the legs below the knee or the pain is severe.

- The pain increases when you move, cough, sneeze, lift, or strain.

- You have pain, burning, or itching when you pass urine, or bloody, cloudy, or dark urine.

- You have a fever or you vomit.

- You have sudden pain after being in a wheelchair or after a long stay in bed.

- You have painful red blisters on only one side of the back.

**♥ Get Immediate Care When:**

- You have extreme pain across your whole upper back that came on within 15 minutes for no reason.

- Your back pain occurs with "Heart Attack Symptoms" (see page 202).

- A neck, spine, back, or other serious injury or fall has occurred.

- The back pain is sudden and occurs with a "cracking" sound.

- You lose bladder or bowel control.

## Sciatica

Sciatica is inflammation of the sciatic nerve, which starts in the lower spine and goes down the back of the legs. Pressure on the nerve (from tight muscles, herniated disk, etc.) causes a sharp pain that can be felt in the buttock and may extend to the thigh, knee, or foot.

Treatment for mild sciatica is rest, heat, and over-the-counter medicine for pain. Physical therapy may be helpful. In some cases, surgery to repair a herniated disk may be needed.

# 90. Broken Bones

Bones in some senior citizens become thin with age and break easily due to osteoporosis. This is most common in women after menopause, but also can occur in some elderly men.

## Prevention

Prevent falls. (See "Use fall prevention measures" in the "Self-Care" section in "Osteoporosis" on page 262. See also "Home Safety Checklist" on page 23 and "Personal Safety Checklist" on page 24.)

**14. Bone & Muscle Problems**

*Broken Bones, Continued*

## Signs & Symptoms

There are 2 types of broken bones. Signs and symptoms depend on the type.

- Simple or closed fractures. The broken bone is not visible through the skin. There is not a skin wound near the fracture site.

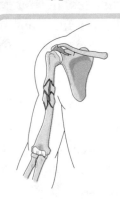

**Simple Fracture***

- Compound or open fracture. The bone can protrude through the skin or the skin has been cut due to the injury. This can cause bleeding. The wound will likely become infected without prompt and adequate medical care.

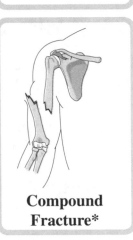

**Compound Fracture***

With either kind of break, the bone(s) can break in 1 or more places, each can be a partial or complete break.

These symptoms can occur in both types at the injured site:

- Pain. The pain gets worse with movement or when pressure is applied.
- Swelling and bruising
- Loss of function or feeling
- The area looks crooked, misshaped, or deformed.

Below the injured site, numbness and tingling can occur. The skin can be pale, blue, purple, or gray and feels colder than the skin on the uninjured limb.

## Causes & Care

- Falls and injuries
- Osteoporosis (see page 259). A hip, wrist, or spinal fracture is often the first sign of osteoporosis.
- Prolonged, repeated, or excessive stress placed on a bone

Treatment includes:

- First aid (see "Self-Care" on page 239)
- Medical care. This includes resetting the bone and wearing a splint or cast. Muscles and joints near the fracture site need to be exercised to prevent problems. {**Note:** Broken fingers, toes, and ribs don't require a cast.}
- Treatment for bleeding and shock may also be needed.

To Learn More, See Back Cover

*Broken Bones, Continued*

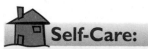

## Self-Care:

Before getting medical care:

- Immobilize the injured area. Make a splint:

  - Place rolled-up newspapers, an umbrella, etc., next to the injured area. Gently hold it in place with a necktie, strips of cloth, or a belt. Make the splint

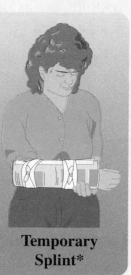

**Temporary Splint***

  long enough to extend past the joints above and below the break.

  - Or, lightly tape or tie an injured leg to the uninjured one, putting padding between the legs, if possible. Or, tape an injured arm to the chest, if the elbow is bent, or to the side if the elbow is straight, placing padding between the body and the arm.

  - Check the pulse in the limb with the splint. If you cannot find it, the splint is too tight. Loosen it.

- Check for swelling, numbness, tingling, or a blue tinge to the skin. If any of these signs occur, the splint is too tight. Loosen it right away to prevent permanent injury.

- For a broken arm, make a sling out of a triangular piece of cloth. Place the forearm in it and tie the ends around the neck so the

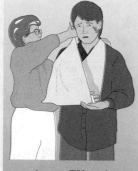

**Arm Sling***

  arm is resting at a 90-degree angle.

  - Keep the person quiet to avoid moving the injured area.

- Apply a cold compress to the injured area to help reduce swelling.

- Take acetaminophen for pain. Avoid aspirin if there is bleeding and in case surgery is needed.

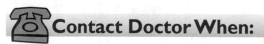

## Contact Doctor When:

You have a lot of pain or are not able to bear weight on the injured limb and/or there is a lot of bruising around the injury.

{**Note:** See "Immobilize the injured area" under "Self-Care" on this page.}

**14. Bone & Muscle Problems**

*Broken Bones, Continued*

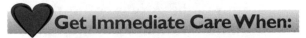

### Get Immediate Care When:

With a broken bone, any of these problems are present:

- A head, neck, and/or back injury. {**Note:** For a head, neck, and/or back injury, use extreme caution and do not move the victim. See "Head Injuries" on page 403 and "Neck/Spine Injuries" on page 408.}

- Severe bleeding and/or an open fracture occurs. {**Note:** See "First Aid for Major Bleeding" on page 389.}

- The bone broken is in the pelvis, hip, or thigh.

- The skin below the fracture is cold and blue; numbness occurs below the fracture; or any deformity occurs at the fracture site.

- Sweating, dizziness, thirst, or an ashen skin color occurs.

---

## Fractured Hip

A common broken bone in the elderly is a fractured hip. The bone broken is actually the head or neck of the thigh bone (femur).

### Signs & Symptoms

- Extreme pain when trying to walk

- Bruising, swelling, and tenderness in the hip area. Pain is often felt in the groin area.

- Crooked or misshaped hip. The leg looks shortened and/or rotated.

### Causes & Risk Factors

- A fall is the most common cause. See "Home Safety Checklist" on page 23 for ways to prevent falls.

- Osteoporosis (see page 259), lack of calcium in the diet or calcium imbalance

### Treatment

- Surgery is done to reconnect fractured bone parts.

- Prevention of blood clots, due to inactivity is very important for the first few weeks.

- Physical therapy

- Medicine for pain

- Rehabilitation which includes using a walker, then a cane, etc.

- Infection prevention and treatment, as needed

To Learn More, See Back Cover

14. Bone & Muscle Problems

# 91. Bursitis & Tendinitis

Bursitis and tendinitis share common symptoms, causes, and treatment. They differ in the part of the body affected.

Bursitis occurs when a bursa becomes inflamed. A bursa is a soft sac of liquid. It acts like a pillow or cushion to protect a joint, such as a shoulder, elbow, hip, or knee. It also eases joint movement.

Tendinitis is inflammation of a tendon. A tendon is a cord-like tissue that connects muscles to bone. "Tennis elbow," "trigger finger," and "golfer's shoulder," etc. can be due to tendinitis.

## Prevention

To prevent both bursitis and tendinitis:

- Stretch and warm up before activities that require joint movement, such as sports. Do stretching and strengthening exercises to keep your shoulder, neck, and arm muscles strong and flexible. One example is shown in the box to the right.

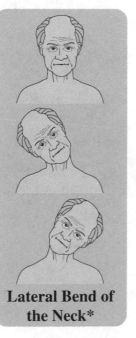

**Lateral Bend of the Neck\***

- Wear protective gear for sports. Wear shoes with good support and flexible soles.

- Wear a seat belt when riding in a car.

- Avoid injuries. (See "Use fall prevention measures" under "Self-Care" on page 262.)

- Avoid repeated activities that twist or put strain on a single joint. When you perform tasks over and over, use proper posture, proper equipment, and proper technique.

To prevent bursitis in the knees, use knee pads or cushions if you kneel a lot. Change positions and take breaks often.

## Signs & Symptoms

Signs and symptoms of both bursitis and tendinitis are:

- Pain and limited movement in the affected area

- Swelling

With bursitis, these symptoms may also be present:

- The affected area appears red, warm, or tender.

- Fever, if there is an infection

14. Bone & Muscle Problems

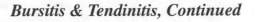

*Bursitis & Tendinitis, Continued*

With tendinitis, these symptoms may also be present:

- Tenderness that is often worse at night
- Muscle spasms
- The pain can be sudden and occur with a snapping sound if the Achilles tendon is ruptured.

## Causes, Risk Factors & Care

Causes for both bursitis and tendinitis are:

- A blow or injury
- Wear and tear and overuse of a joint, etc.
- Repetitive movements
- Calcium deposits in a tendon. For bursitis, the deposits are in the nearby tendon.

For bursitis, causes can also include: Arthritis, gout, and an infection.

Tendinitis can also be caused by lack of physical conditioning and not warming up muscles before exercising.

Most cases of bursitis and tendinitis can be treated with 2 weeks or less of self-care. When this is not enough, medical care may be needed.

Medical care includes:

- Corticosteroid injections (except for Achilles tendinitis)
- Surgery. For bursitis, the bursa can be removed. This is done only when medicines taken by mouth and/or by injection don't relieve bursitis symptoms. If a tendon is torn, surgery can be done to repair the tendon.

### Self-Care:

**For Bursitis:**

- When pain first appears, apply ice packs at 10 minute intervals (10 minutes on, 10 minutes off). Do this 3 to 4 times a day for 2 days.
- After 2 days, replace ice packs with heat. Try a heating pad set on low or a moist, warm washcloth over the affected joint. Do this for 15 to 20 minutes at a time, 3 to 4 times a day.
- Rest the painful joint for a few days.
- If bursitis is from an activity, do not return to the activity too quickly.
- Use a sling to rest an elbow.
- Remember "RIMS" (Rest, Immobilize, Maintain Mobility, Strengthen).

*Continued on Next Page*

**14. Bone & Muscle Problems**

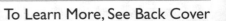

*Bursitis & Tendinitis, Continued*

*Self-Care, Continued*

- Take an over-the-counter medicine for pain and swelling. (See "Pain relievers" in "Your Home Pharmacy" on page 43.)

- To prevent stiffness, do stretching exercises. Begin by slowly moving the sore area. Be gentle, but try to reach a full range of movement.

- Ask your doctor to recommend exercises to prevent joint stiffness.

- Don't sleep on your arms

- Wear knee pads when you kneel, such as during gardening. Wear elbow pads if you do an activity in which you may bump your elbow.

**For Tendinitis:**

- Use **R.I.C.E.** (rest, ice, compression, and elevation).

  Rest. Rest the injured area as much as possible.

  Ice. Ice the injured area as soon as possible. Immediately putting ice on the injury helps to speed recovery because it not only relieves pain, but also slows blood flow, reducing internal bleeding and swelling.

- Put ice in a heavy plastic bag with a little water or use a bag of frozen vegetables. Wrap the ice pack in a towel before placing it on the injured area.

- Apply the ice pack to the injured area for 10 minutes. Reapply it every two hours and for the next 48 hours during the times you are not sleeping.

  Compression. Apply a snug elastic bandage to the injured joint. Numbness, tingling, or increased pain means the bandage is too tight. Remove the bandage every 3 to 4 hours and leave off for 15 to 20 minutes each time you do so.

  Elevation. Raise the injured body part above the level of the person's heart. Place it on a pillow, folded blanket, or stack of newspapers.

- Take an over-the-counter medicine to reduce the pain and inflammation. Acetaminophen eases muscle soreness, but does not help with inflammation. (See "Pain relievers" in "Your Home Pharmacy" on page 43.)

- Try liniments and balms. These provide a cooling or warming sensation. These ointments only mask the pain of sore muscles, though. They do not promote healing.

**14. Bone & Muscle Problems**

*Bursitis & Tendinitis, Continued*

### 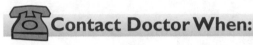 Contact Doctor When:

- You have any of these problems with bursitis:
  - You can't move the joint.
  - Fever of over 101°F
  - The area is very red or tender
  - The area is very swollen
- The same pain has occurred before or you have a history of arthritis.
- Bursitis or tendinitis symptoms started after an injury.
- Pain gets worse or persists after 2 weeks of using self-care.

## 92. Dislocations

A dislocation is a separation of the end of a bone and the joint it meets. Bones that touch in the joints sometime separate when they are overstressed.

Injuries related to dislocations include damage to the membrane lining the joint as well as tears to nearby muscles and ligaments.

## Prevention

- Protect a joint injured in the past by wrapping it with an elastic bandage or tape.
- Wear protective pads (shoulder, wrist, knee, etc.) when taking part in contact sports or in other activities in which you may fall or otherwise get injured.

## Signs & Symptoms

A dislocated joint is misshapen, very painful, and swollen. The skin around the area is discolored.

## Causes & Care

Causes include injuries from contact sports or falls, rheumatoid arthritis, and joints weakened by previous injury. Also force applied in the wrong direction can snap the ball of the upper arm bone out of the shoulder socket.

The shoulders are especially prone to dislocation injuries. Fingers, hips, ankles, elbows, jaws, and even the spine can be dislocated as well. A dislocated vertebrae in the spine often damages the spinal cord and can paralyze body parts lower than the injury site.

Do not try to put a dislocated bone back into its socket.

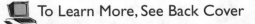 To Learn More, See Back Cover

## Dislocations, *Continued*

All dislocations need medical care. With treatment, you can usually expect the dislocated joint to function within 24 to 48 hours. Activity may need to be limited for the next 4 to 6 weeks, though, to give the injury enough time to heal.

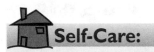

### Self-Care:

Seek help as soon as possible after the injury. The self-care tips below list things you can do for a dislocation before and after you get medical care.

Before Medical Care:

- Do not eat or drink anything. You may need anesthesia when your joint is put back into its socket.
- Immobilize the joint with a splint or sling.
- Ice the injured area (see below).

After Medical Care:

- Use R.I.C.E. (rest, ice, compression, and elevation) during the first 24 to 48 hours after the injury. (See R.I.C.E. on page 243.)

- Take an over-the-counter medicine for swelling and pain. Acetaminophen eases soreness, but does not help with inflammation. (See "Pain relievers" in "Your Home Pharmacy" on page 43.}

### Get Immediate Care When:

- An injury has occurred to the neck or spine. {**Note**: For a head, neck, and/or back injury, use extreme caution and do not move the victim. See "Head Injuries" on page 403 and "Neck/Spine Injuries" on page 408.}

- There is severe bleeding around the injury. (See "First Aid for Major Bleeding" on page 389.)

- Any of these problems are present:
  - An area is deformed
  - A limb is pale, cold, or numb
  - A limb is very painful and/or swollen or one that can't bear weight (See "Immobilize the injured area" under "Self-Care" on page 239.)

If none of the above apply, you probably do not have a dislocation. If you are not sure, contact your doctor.

14. Bone & Muscle Problems

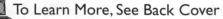

# 93. Foot Problems

You can get a number of foot problems as you age. Some are due to years of wear and tear on your feet. Others can be due to shoes that do not fit well or trimming your toenails too close to your skin. Circulation problems and diseases, such as diabetes, can lead to foot problems, too.

## Foot Problems Chart

| Signs & Symptoms | What It Could Be | What to Do |
|---|---|---|
| These problems appear in a matter of hours to a few days:<br>■ The skin of your foot or toe is gray to black in color.<br>■ You cannot feel sensation in your foot. | Gangrene | Get immediate care. |
| Pain from a fall or injury to your foot (not just a toe) with any of these problems:<br>■ Severe bleeding<br>■ Your foot is misshaped.<br>■ You can't move your foot.<br>■ Your foot looks blue or pale and is cold and numb.<br>■ Your foot is so painful and/or swollen that you can't put any weight on it. | Broken bone(s) in the foot (not just a toe) | Get immediate care. See "Broken Bones" on page 237. |
| Sudden onset of pain in your feet and legs. The skin on your feet changes colors to white, red, or blue. | Peripheral vascular disease | See "Peripheral Vascular Disease" on page 206. |

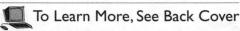

**14. Bone & Muscle Problems**

## Foot Problems, Continued

| Foot Problems Chart, Continued | | |
|---|---|---|
| **Signs & Symptoms** | **What It Could Be** | **What to Do** |
| Toes that turn white then red in response to cold. Tingling, numbness. | Frostbite, if occurs after cold exposure or cold feet | See "Frostbite" on page 400 and "Cold Hands & Feet" on page 118. |
| The bottom of the foot is red and swollen and feels warm and tender. | An infection called cellulitis | Contact doctor for an immediate appointment. |
| Cut or puncture from a dirty or contaminated object, such as a rusty nail or other object in the soil | Cut or puncture wound | Contact doctor. See "Cuts, Scrapes & Punctures" on page 120. |
| One or more of these problems with a foot wound:<br>■ Fever<br>■ Redness, tenderness, or warmth<br>■ Swelling<br>■ Pain<br>■ Pus | Infection | Contact doctor. |
| Severe pain in foot joint, often the big toe. The pain is not due to an injury. The joint hurts a lot when anything touches it. The area is red, swollen, and tender. | Gout | Contact doctor. See "Gout" on page 252. |
| Joint pain and morning stiffness in joints. Fatigue. | Rheumatoid arthritis | Contact doctor. See "Arthritis" on page 231. |

*Foot Problems Chart Continued on Next Page*

**14. Bone & Muscle Problems**

## Foot Problems, Continued

| Foot Problems Chart, Continued | | |
|---|---|---|
| **Signs & Symptoms** | **What It Could Be** | **What to Do** |
| Pain in only one toe after an injury to the toe | Broken toe or sprained toe | Contact doctor. |
| Open sores (ulcers) on the toes. Pain on the instep and cold pale skin color which improve with rest. | Buerger's Disease | Contact doctor. |
| Tenderness and pain under the heel bone | Heel spur | Contact doctor. |
| Moist, soft, red, or gray-white scales on the feet, especially between the toes. Cracked, peeling, dead skin area. Itching. Sometimes small blisters on the feet. | Athlete's foot | See "Athlete's Foot" on page 110. |
| White, brown, or yellow toenail. The nail can thicken, then get soft and weak. It may tear away from the nail bed or look deformed. | Toenail fungus | Contact doctor. |
| Painful growth on the ball or heel of the foot. Black pinholes or spots in the center. | Plantar warts | See "Warts" on page 147. |
| Thickened skin on the ball or heel of the foot. Usually no pain. | Calluses | See "Corns & Calluses" on page 119. |
| Discomfort, pain, tenderness, and/or redness under the corner of a toenail and nearby skin | Ingrown toenail | See "Ingrown Toenail" on page 129. |

 To Learn More, See Back Cover

## Foot Problems, Continued

| Foot Problems Chart, Continued | | |
| --- | --- | --- |
| **Signs & Symptoms** | **What It Could Be** | **What to Do** |
| Big toe points inward or outward. Bony bulge at side of big toe. Thickened skin. Possible fluid build-up near big toe. Stiffness or pain. | Bunion | See "Self-Care" for "Bunions" in this topic. |
| Thickened skin on tops of and between toes where rubbing is constant. Feels hard to the touch and looks round. Small, clear spot (hen's eye) may appear in the center. | Corns | See "Corns & Calluses" on page 119. |
| Pain between the heel and the ball of the foot usually brought on by walking or running or when weight is put on the foot | Plantar Fasciitis (irritation from ligaments and tissues in the foot arch) | See "Self-Care" for "Plantar Fasciitis" in this topic. |
| Red, sometimes fluid-filled sores, caused by shoes that rub the foot | Blisters | See "Self-Care" for "Blisters" in this topic. |
| Charley horse or muscle spasm in the foot, often at bedtime | Foot cramp | See "Self-Care" for "Foot Cramps" in this topic. |

*Foot Problems Chart Continued on Next Page*

14. Bone & Muscle Problems

*Foot Problems, Continued*

| Foot Problems Chart, Continued | | |
| --- | --- | --- |
| **Signs & Symptoms** | **What It Could Be** | **What to Do** |
| Curled or claw-like position in a toe (usually the 2$^{nd}$ toe). A corn forms on the top of the toe. Pain. | Hammertoe | See "Self-Care" for "Hammertoes" in this topic. |

{**Note:** With diabetes or circulation problems, contact your doctor for any foot problem.}

## Prevention

- Wear shoes that fit well. Don't wear shoes with pointed toes or ones that fit too tightly.
- Wash and dry your feet daily.
- Keep your feet moisturized.
- Inspect your feet daily for early signs of problems.
- Rest your feet by elevating them.
- Persons with diabetes and/or circulation problems need to take special care of their feet. Good foot care can prevent some foot infections. It may be necessary for a health care professional to cut the toenails.

## Self-Care:

**For Blisters:**

- Don't break a blister. If it breaks on its own, apply an antibacterial spray or ointment and cover with a bandage or sterile dressing.
- Don't cut away or pull off the broken blister's loose skin. This protects the new skin below it.

**For Bunions:**

- Don't wear high heels or shoes with narrow toes.

*Continued on Next Page*

To Learn More, See Back Cover

**14. Bone & Muscle Problems**

## Foot Problems, Continued

### Self-Care, Continued

- Wear sandals.
- Use moleskin or padding to separate overlapped toes.
- Try arch supports to reduce pressure.
- Use ring-shaped pads over a bunion.
- Cut out an old pair of shoes to wear in the house.
- Soak your feet in warm water.
- Take an over-the-counter pain reliever, if needed. (See "Pain relievers" in "Your Home Pharmacy" on page 43.)

### For Foot Cramps:

- Stretch the foot muscles.
- Pull the foot back into a flexed position.
- Push the foot into the floor.

### For Heel Spurs:

- Use a cushion or heel cup under the heel.
- Avoid prolonged standing.
- Lose weight, if overweight.
- Do not jog or run.
- Roll a tennis ball under ball of the foot.

- Put ice on the heel for 10 minutes. Remove it for 10 minutes. Repeat many times.
- Take an over-the-counter pain reliever, if needed. (See "Pain relievers" in "Your Home Pharmacy" on page 43.)

### For Hammertoes:

- Wear wide, roomy shoes.
- Massage the toes or get a foot rub.
- Changes shoes during the day. Try athletic shoes.
- Use small pads over the center toe to lessen pressure.

### For Minor Infections:

- Soak the foot in warm, soapy water for 20 minutes, 4 to 6 times a day. Pat the infected area dry. Use extra care if you have peripheral vascular disease. Make sure the water is not hot.
- Apply an over-the-counter antibiotic ointment, such as Neosporin. Cover with a sterile cloth or bandage.

### For Injuries:

Use R.I.C.E. (See R.I.C.E. on page 243.)

- For an injured toe, tape it to the toe next to it. Do this for 7 to 10 days.

*Continued on Next Page*

**14. Bone & Muscle Problems**

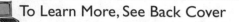

### Foot Problems, Continued

#### Self-Care, Continued

- Take an over-the-counter medicine to reduce inflammation and pain. (See "Pain Relievers" in "Your Home Pharmacy" on page 43.)

#### For Plantar Fasciitis:

- Rest the foot as much as you can.
- Use R.I.C.E. (See R.I.C.E. on page 243.)
- Take an over-the-counter medicine for pain and swelling. (See "Pain Relievers" in "Your Home Pharmacy" on page 43.)
- Wear shoes with a solid arch support.

#### For Plantar Warts:

- Try salicylic acid plasters or other over-the-counter products, such as Wart-Off. Follow package directions.
- Use cushions in shoes.
- Wash hands after touching warts to avoid re-infection.
- Wear sandals in the shower or public areas, such as pools.
- Do not pick at plantar warts.

See also, "Self-Care" for:

"Athlete's Foot" on page 110

"Cold Hands & Feet" on page 118

"Corns & Calluses" on page 119

"Cuts, Scrapes & Punctures" on page 121

"Ingrown Toenails" on page 130

"Splinters" on page 145

If self-care measures do not help or if your foot problem gets worse, contact your doctor.

## 94. Gout

Gout is a form of arthritis. It is most common in men older than 40. In women, it usually comes after menopause.

### Signs & Symptoms

- Excruciating pain and inflammation in a joint or joints. These symptoms come on suddenly and peak quickly.
- The affected area is swollen, red, or purplish in color. It feels warm and is very tender to the touch.
- Feeling of agonizing pain after even the slightest pressure, such as rubbing a sheet against the affected area
- Low-grade fever or chills and fever (sometimes)

14. Bone & Muscle Problems

To Learn More, See Back Cover

*Gout, Continued*

## Causes, Risk Factors & Care

When blood levels of uric acid rise above a certain level, thousands of hard, tiny uric acid crystals collect in the joints. These crystals act like tiny, hot, jagged shards of glass causing pain and inflammation. The crystals can collect in the tendons and cartilage, in the kidneys (as kidney stones), and in the fatty tissues beneath the skin. {**Note:** Crystals other than uric acid can cause some acute attacks similar to gout.}

Gout can strike any joint, but often affects the big toe. A gout attack can last several hours to a few days. Persons who have gout can be symptom-free for years between attacks. Gout triggers include:

- Mild trauma or a blow to the joint
- Drinking a lot of alcohol, especially beer
- Taking certain medications, such as aspirin, certain antibiotics, diuretics, and nicotinic acid
- Dehydration

Many conditions can mimic an acute attack of gout. These include infection, injury, and rheumatoid arthritis. See a doctor to diagnose the problem.

The first goal of treatment is to relieve the acute gout attack. The second goal is to prevent future attacks.

For immediate relief, your doctor will prescribe medicine, such as Colchicine, an antigout drug. For long-term relief, your doctor will prescribe medicine as needed to decrease uric acid production or to increase the excretion of uric acid from the kidneys.

### Self-Care:

Medical care is needed, but these self-care measures can help:

- Lose weight if you are overweight. Do not fast, though. This can raise uric acid levels.
- Limit alcoholic beverages.
- Drink plenty of fluids.
- Rest in bed, if you need to. Keep sheets and blankets from touching the affected joint.

### Contact Doctor When:

You have signs and symptoms of gout listed in this topic on page 252.

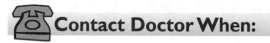

**14. Bone & Muscle Problems**

## 95. Leg Pain & Ankle Pain

Pain in the legs or ankles can range from mild to severe. The type and amount of pain depends on the cause. Common causes of leg and ankle pain in seniors are muscle cramps, arthritis, poor blood flow, and injuries.

### Leg Pain & Ankle Pain Chart

| Signs & Symptoms | What It Could Be | What to Do |
|---|---|---|
| Pain, redness (may have shades of red, purple, and blue), and swelling in the ankle or leg.  Bluish color in the toes. May be followed by severe shortness of breath that came on all of a sudden. May include coughing up blood or pink-frothed sputum. Chest pain. | Deep-vein thrombosis (DVT) with or without a blood clot to the lung | Get immediate care. See also "Phlebitis & Thrombosis" on page 207. |
| Swelling of both ankles at the same time. Shortness of breath. May have dry cough or cough with pink, frothy mucus. | Congestive heart failure | Contact doctor. See "Congestive Heart Failure" on page 197. |
| Leg muscle pain in one or both legs. Fatigue in the thighs, calves, and feet which improves with rest. Open sores on the lower leg, ankles, or toes. Weak or no pulse in the affected limb. Cold or numb feet. Pale, bluish-colored toes. | Peripheral vascular disease | See "Peripheral Vascular Disease" on page 206. |

To Learn More, See Back Cover

## Leg Pain & Ankle Pain, Continued

| Leg Pain & Ankle Pain Chart, Continued | | |
|---|---|---|
| **Signs & Symptoms** | **What It Could Be** | **What to Do** |
| Any of these signs with pain after a leg or ankle injury: A bone sticks out or bones in the injured limb make a grating sound; the injured limb looks deformed, crooked, or the wrong shape; a loss of feeling in the injured limb; and cold, blue skin under the affected injured area; the limb is very painful and/or swollen or one that can't bear weight, or inability to move the limb. | Broken bone or dislocation | See "Broken Bones" on page 237 and "Dislocations" on page 244. |
| Pain in the leg or ankle after an injury that <u>does not</u> keep you from moving the limb. | Sprain or strain; sport or other overuse injury | See "Sprains & Strains" topic on page 267. |
| Pain with fever, redness, tenderness, pus at a wound site. Red streak up the leg (rarely). | Infection | Contact doctor. Get an immediate appointment for red streak up the leg. |
| Sudden, severe pain in the knee or ankle joint, usually just on one side. The pain can be felt even when clothing is rubbed against the joint. The joint area is swollen, red or purplish in color, feels warm, and is very tender to the touch. | Gout | Contact doctor. See "Gout" on page 252. |

*Leg Pain & Ankle Pain Chart Continued on Next Page*

14. Bone & Muscle Problems

## Leg Pain & Ankle Pain, Continued

| Leg Pain & Ankle Pain Chart, Continued | | |
|---|---|---|
| **Signs & Symptoms** | **What It Could Be** | **What to Do** |
| Leg pain that radiates from the lower back. Pain or stiffness in the knees. Bowing of the legs or other bone deformity. Unexplained bone fractures. May have headache, dizziness, hearing loss, and/or ringing in the ears. | Paget's disease. This is a bone disorder that progresses slowly. Most persons with this disease do not develop symptoms. | Contact doctor. See "Care" and "Self-Care" for Paget's disease in this section. |
| Sharp pain from the buttocks down the leg. Numbness and tingling in the leg. | Sciatica | See "Sciatica" box on page 237. |
| Pain, stiffness, and swelling, usually in both knees or ankle joints. The joint looks deformed. Weakness and fatigue. Dry mouth and dry, painful eyes. | Rheumatoid arthritis | See "Arthritis" on page 231. |
| Pain, stiffness, and sometimes swelling of the knee or ankle joints. Often, the joint has gotten tender over months or years and may look enlarged or distorted. | Osteoarthritis | See "Arthritis" on page 231. |
| Leg or ankle pain with gradual loss of height; stooped posture; back-ache; and/or past bone fractures, especially in the wrists and hips. | Osteoporosis | See "Osteoporosis" on page 259. |

To Learn More, See Back Cover

## Leg Pain & Ankle Pain, Continued

| Leg Pain & Ankle Pain Chart, Continued | | |
| --- | --- | --- |
| **Signs & Symptoms** | **What It Could Be** | **What to Do** |
| Pain or itching in the legs with swollen and twisted veins that look blue and are close to the surface of the skin. The veins bulge and feel heavy. Swelling in the legs and ankles. | Varicose veins | See "Varicose Veins" on page 210. |
| Muscle or joint pain and chronic swelling of the knee joints that develop months or years after a deer-tick bite and a bulls-eye red rash with pale centers. | Lyme disease | See "Care" and "Self-Care" for Lyme disease in "Skin Rashes" on pages 142 and 144. |
| Pain and swelling around the knee joint. Pain gets worse with movement. Fever (maybe). | Bursitis | Follow guidelines for "Bursitis" on page 241. |
| Aches in leg muscles and joints with fever and/or chills; headache; dry cough; sore throat; and fatigue. | Flu | Follow guidelines for "Flu" on page 100. |
| Sudden, sharp, tightening pain in the leg, often the calf. The muscle feels hard to the touch. The pain subsides after a minute or so and the muscle relaxes. | Leg cramps | See "Prevention" and "Self-Care" for leg cramps in this topic. |

14. Bone & Muscle Problems

*Leg Pain & Ankle Pain, Continued*

## Prevention

### General Tips

- Get and stay at a healthy weight.

- Get regular exercise. This helps to keep ankle and leg muscles strong.

- Before you exercise, stretch and warm up your muscles. When you are done, cool them down.

- Protect your knees. Use knee pads when you garden or kneel. Always land on bent knees when jumping. Avoid deep knee bend exercises.

- Don't wear high-heeled shoes. Keep your shoes in proper shape.

- When you can, walk on grass instead of concrete.

- Take good care of your feet.

### To Prevent Leg Cramps:

- Get good sources of calcium and potassium. Good sources of calcium are nonfat milks, cheeses, and yogurts and calcium-fortified juices. Good sources of potassium are citrus fruits and juices, bananas, potatoes, bran cereals, and fish. Take calcium and potassium supplements as advised by your doctor.

- Drink plenty of water and other fluids. Limit drinks with caffeine. Avoid drinks with alcohol.

- Warm up your muscles before you exercise. Cool down your muscles when you are done.

- With your doctor's okay, wear elastic stockings while you are awake.

- Before you go to bed, stretch your calf muscles. Stand an arm's length away from a wall. Lean against it with the palms of your hands. Bend your left knee. Keep your right leg straight behind you. Keep both feet flat on the floor and your back straight. Lean forward. Feel your right calf muscle stretch. Hold the stretch as you count to 10 slowly. Repeat, switching leg positions.

- Take a warm bath before bed time.

- Sleep with loose-fitting blankets and night clothes. Keep your legs warm

- Ask your doctor about using quinine.

## Care

Self-care and medical care for leg and ankle pain depends on the cause. Find out what the cause could be from the "Leg and Ankle Pain Chart" on pages 254 to 257. Follow the guidelines for the suspected cause(s).

To Learn More, See Back Cover

## Leg Pain & Ankle Pain, Continued

For Paget's disease, most persons do not have symptoms bad enough to need treatment. Self-care measures in the next column can help persons with mild symptoms. Some persons may need prescribed medicines. These include anti-inflammatory drugs and calcitonin, which alters bone metabolism. Bone surgery may be needed to improve walking.

### Self-Care:

**For Pain, in General:**

- Take an over-the-counter medicine for pain. (See "Pain relievers" in "Your Home Pharmacy" on page 43.) If the pain is not better after a few doses, call your doctor.

- Use a heating pad (set on low), a hot pack, or a moist, warm towel on the area of pain. If the pain is due to an injury, don't use heat for 48 hours. Use R.I.C.E. (See page 243.)

**For Leg Cramps:**

- Sit with your leg flat on the floor. Pull your toes toward you. Point your heel away from you. Stretch the cramped muscle.

- Have someone massage the cramped muscle gently, but firmly.

- Apply a heating pad (set on low), a hot pack, or moist warm towel to the muscle cramp.

- Rub the muscle that is cramping. Rub upward from the ankle toward the heart. (**Note:** Do not rub a leg if you suspect phlebitis or thrombosis. See "Phlebitis & Thrombosis" on page 207.)

**For Paget's Disease:**

- If needed, take an over-the-counter medicine for pain. See "Pain relievers" in "Your Home Pharmacy" on page 43.

- Take other medicines as prescribed by your doctor.

- Get regular checkups to detect hearing loss.

## 96. Osteoporosis

Persons with osteoporosis suffer from a loss in bone mass and bone strength. Their bones become weak and brittle, which makes them more prone to fracture. Any bone can be affected by osteoporosis, but the hips, wrists, and spine are the most common sites.

14. Bone & Muscle Problems

*Osteoporosis, Continued*

One in 4 women over age 60 and nearly half of all people over age 75 suffer from osteoporosis.

## Prevention

To prevent or slow osteoporosis:

- Eat a balanced diet and get your recommended Adequate Intake (AI) for calcium every day. For persons 51 years and older, the AI for calcium is 1,200 milligrams per day. Women not on estrogen replacement therapy (ERT) should get 1,500 milligrams of calcium per day. To get your recommended calcium, choose high-calcium foods daily. Use the chart on page 261.

- Take calcium supplements, if necessary and advised by your doctor. Ask about taking Tums to get calcium.

- Get enough vitamin D every day. Good food sources are fortified milks and cereals, egg yolks, saltwater fish, and liver. You also get vitamin D from sunshine; 15 minutes of midday sunshine meets the daily need. Check with your doctor about taking a vitamin D supplement.

- Follow a program of regular, weight-bearing exercise at least 3 or 4 times a week. Examples include walking and aerobics. (A person with osteoporosis should follow the exercise program outlined by his or her doctor.)

- Don't smoke. This worsens osteoporosis and may negate the benefits of estrogen replacement therapy.

- Limit alcohol.

- Take medications as prescribed. This may include estrogen replacement therapy (ERT), alendronate, or raloxifene.

## Signs & Symptoms

Symptoms include:

- Gradual loss of height
- Rounding of the shoulders
- Back pain
- Stooped posture or dowager's hump

Osteoporosis can progress without any noticeable signs or symptoms. Often the first sign is a bone fracture of the hip, wrist, or spine.

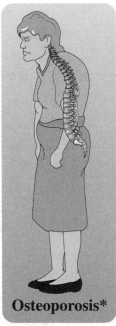

**Osteoporosis***

To Learn More, See Back Cover

**14. Bone & Muscle Problems**

*Osteoporosis, Continued*

## Calcium Chart

| Item | Amount | Mgs. of Calcium |
|------|--------|-----------------|
| Nonfat, plain yogurt | 8 ounces | 452 |
| Sardines, canned in oil with bones | 3 ounces | 371 |
| Collard greens, frozen chopped, cooked | 1 cup | 304 |
| Milk | 1 cup | 302 |
| Orange juice, calcium fortified | 6 ounces | 225 |
| Cheddar cheese | 1 ounce | 204 |
| Total cereal, dry | 1 cup | 200 |
| Spinach, cooked | 1 cup | 168 |
| Salmon, pink, canned with liquid and bones | 3 ounces | 167 |
| Broccoli, raw | 1 stalk | 158 |
| Tofu (if calcium is used in processing) | 3 ounces | 128 |
| Low-fat frozen yogurt | $1/2$ cup | 100 |
| Corn muffin made with milk, egg | 1 | 96 |
| Almonds | $1/4$ cup | 83 |
| Beans, canned with pork and tomatoes | 4 ounces | 76 |
| Chick peas (garbanzo beans), canned | 3 ounces | 75 |
| Low-fat cottage cheese | $1/2$ cup | 69 |
| Orange, fresh | 1 | 54 |
| Molasses | 1 teaspoon | 33 |

14. Bone & Muscle Problems

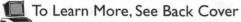

*Osteoporosis, Continued*

## Causes, Risk Factors & Care

The actual causes of osteoporosis are not known. Risk factors include:

- Being female. Women are 4 times more likely to develop osteoporosis than men because their bones are generally thinner and lighter and they have rapid bone loss at menopause or after the removal of both ovaries due to a sharp decline of estrogen.

- Having a thin, small-framed body

- Being Caucasian or Asian. African Americans and Hispanic Americans are at significant risk, too, though.

- Lack of physical activity, especially weight-bearing exercises, such as walking

- Lack of calcium

- Family traits

- Smoking cigarettes

- Alcoholism, which may damage bones. Heavy drinkers often have poor nutrition and are also more prone to fractures from falls.

- Taking certain medicines, such as corticosteroids and aluminum-containing antacids.

- Disorders, such as hyperthyroidism

There is no cure for osteoporosis. The focus of treatment is to prevent the disease (see "Prevention" on page 260), prevent further bone loss, and build new bone. Treatment includes:

- Medicines. These include: estrogen replacement therapy (ERT), calcitonin, and alendronate.

- Self-care measures listed below

### Self-Care:

- Follow measures under "Prevention" in this topic.

- Take medicines, as prescribed.

- Do the daily exercises approved by your doctor.

- Practice proper posture.

- Use fall prevention measures:
  - Use grab bars and safety mats, etc., in your tub and shower.
  - Use handrails on stairways.
  - Don't stoop to pick up things. Pick things up by bending your knees and keeping your back straight.
  - Wear flat, sturdy, nonskid shoes.
  - If you use throw rugs, make sure they have nonskid backs.
  - Use a cane or walker, if necessary.

*Continued on Next Page*

**14. Bone & Muscle Problems**

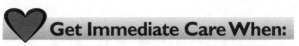

## Osteoporosis, Continued

### Self-Care, Continued

- See that halls, stairways, and entrances are well lit. Use night lights in hallways, bathrooms, etc.

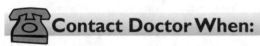

## Contact Doctor When:

- You have any signs or symptoms of osteoporosis on page 260.

- You need advice on estrogen replacement therapy (ERT) and other medicines.

## Get Immediate Care When:

After a fall, you are not able to get up or you have wrist, hip, or back pain.

## For Information Contact:

National Osteoporosis Foundations
1-202-223-2226
www.nof.org

Osteoporosis and Related Bone Disease National Resource Center
1-800-624-BONE (624-2663)
www.osteo.org

## FYI About Hip and Knee Joint Replacements

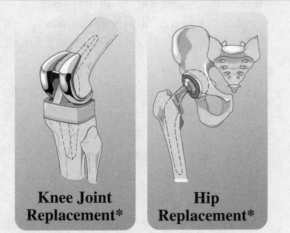

**Knee Joint Replacement***     **Hip Replacement***

Diseased parts of hip and knee joints can be replaced with new artificial parts. Before you agree to elective surgery, you should:

- Get a second opinion.

- Find out if nonsurgical therapies will take care of your needs. These include an exercise program to strengthen muscles in the joint area and improve the position of the joint; walking aids, such as a cane; medicines, such as nonsteroidal anti-inflammatory drugs (NSAIDs); and physical therapy.

- Weigh the benefits and risks of surgery specific to you. Hip replacement surgery may lead to problems for some persons. For example, people with severe muscle weakness or Parkinson's disease are more likely to damage or dislocate an artificial hip.

**14. Bone & Muscle Problems**

# 97. Shoulder Pain & Neck Pain

Shoulder pain and neck pain are common conditions in people over age 50. The pain can result from overuse and wear and tear on these areas of the body. Even swinging a golf club, cleaning windows, or reaching for a jar can strain and injure shoulder and neck muscles and tendons. This is especially true in people who are out of condition.

## Prevention

- To prevent tendinitis, see "Prevention" on page 241.

- To avoid injuries to the shoulder and neck, wear seat belts in vehicles and use protective gear when you take part in a sporting event.

- If you are out of condition, start to strengthen your muscles gradually. Slowly increase exercise intensity.

- Don't sleep on your stomach. You may twist your neck in this position.

- Sleep on a firm polyester pillow or use a special neck (cervical) pillow. Even a rolled towel under your neck can help.

- Practice good posture. Stand straight. Don't let your shoulders slump, your head droop, or your lower back slouch.

- When you carry things, such as a purse, switch from one hand or shoulder to the other.

- Keep the muscles in your shoulders strong and flexible to prevent injury. These exercises can help:

  - To stretch the back of your shoulder: Reach with one arm under your chin and place that hand across the opposite shoulder. Place the palm side of your other hand gently on the forearm and push the arm back. Hold for 15 seconds. Repeat 5 times. Switch sides.

  - Raise one arm and bend it behind your head to touch the opposite shoulder. Use the other hand to gently pull the elbow downward. Hold for 15 seconds. Repeat 5 times. Switch sides.

  - Holding light weights, lift your arms out horizontally and slightly forward. Keeping your thumbs toward the floor, slowly lower your arms halfway, then return to shoulder level. Repeat 10 times.

  - Sit straight in a chair. Flex your neck slowly forward and try to touch your chin to your chest. Hold for 10 seconds. Go back to the starting position. Repeat 5 times.

14. Bone & Muscle Problems

*Shoulder Pain & Neck Pain, Continued*

- Sit straight in a chair. Look straight ahead. Slowly tilt your head to the right, trying to touch your right ear to your right shoulder. Do not raise your shoulder to meet your ear. Hold for 10 seconds and straighten your head. Repeat 5 times on this side and then on your left side.

## Signs, Symptoms & Causes

- Poor posture and/or awkward sleeping positions. Sleeping on a soft mattress can give you a stiff neck when you wake up or when you sit or stand.

- Pinched nerve. This could be caused from arthritis or a neck injury. Pain from a pinched nerve usually runs down one side of the arm.

- Tension and stress can cause neck muscles to go into spasms.

- Accidents, falls, and/or injuries:

  - "Frozen shoulder." This can result from lack of use due to pain from an injury. The pain is severe with any movement. The shoulder joint is swollen.

  - Dislocated shoulder. See "Dislocations" on page 244.

- Torn rotator cuff. This is a tear in a tendon that holds the shoulder in place. Symptoms are pain at the top and outer sides of the shoulders, especially when you raise or extend your arm. You may also feel or hear a click when the shoulder is moved.

- Bursitis and tendinitis (see page 241)

- Arthritis (see page 231)

- A whiplash injury. This usually occurs when your motor vehicle is hit from behind or from some other jolt from behind. Symptoms are neck pain or stiffness that occurred within 24 hours of the jolt. You may also have a headache and a hard time walking.

- Infections. Swollen lymph nodes in the neck from an infection can cause pain, tenderness, and swelling.

- Heart attack. Pain can be felt in the shoulder or neck. (See "Heart Attack Warning Signs" on page 202.)

## Care

Treatment for neck and/or shoulder pain depends on the cause. Emergency medical care is needed for serious injuries; broken bones; heart attacks; and meningitis, an infection of the membranes that surround the brain.

Self-care can treat many less serious causes of neck and/or shoulder pain.

14. Bone & Muscle Problems

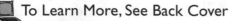

*Shoulder Pain & Neck Pain, Continued*

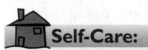

## Self-Care:

To treat arthritis, see "Arthritis" on page 231. To treat bursitis or tendinitis, see "Self-Care" in "Bursitis & Tendinitis" on pages 242 and 243.

### To Treat Neck Pain from a Whiplash Injury or Pinched Nerve:

See a doctor anytime your motor vehicle is hit from the rear because the accident can cause a whiplash injury. Treatment for this usually consists of using hot and cold packs, massage, exercises, sometimes a neck brace, and a pain reliever. After first checking with your doctor, do these things to ease neck discomfort:

- Rest as much as you can by lying on your back.

- Use cold and hot packs. See how to use them in R.I.C.E. on page 243.

- Improve your posture. When you sit, use a chair with a straight back. Make sure your buttocks go all the way to the chair's back. When you stand, pull in your chin and stomach.

- Use a cervical (neck) pillow or a rolled hand towel under your neck.

- Avoid activities that may aggravate your injury.

- Cover your neck with a scarf if you go outside when the weather is cold.

- Practice some of the stretching and strengthening exercises listed under the prevention section in this topic.

### For Pain:

- Take an over-the-counter medicine for pain and/or inflammation. (See "Pain relievers" in "Your Home Pharmacy" on page 43.)

- Take walks. Start with 3 to 5 walks a day each lasting 5 to 10 minutes. Gradually increase walking times.

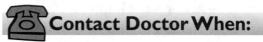

## Contact Doctor When:

- You have any of these problems:

  - Severe or persistent pain, swelling, or spasms in your shoulder

  - A shoulder that is painful and stiff and is very hard to move at all

  - Pain, tenderness, and limited motion in the shoulder

- The pain does not get better after 7 days of self-care.

- The neck or shoulder pain is severe enough to interfere with your sleep.

To Learn More, See Back Cover

**14. Bone & Muscle Problems**

### Shoulder Pain & Neck Pain, Continued

- Shoulder pain throbs or numbness goes down your shoulder or into your arm.
- A possible whiplash injury after being hit from behind
- Fever and redness or swelling around the shoulder

## ♥ Get Immediate Care When:

- A serious injury has occurred to the head or neck. (For a head, neck, or back injury, use extreme caution and do not move the victim. See "Head Injuries" on page 403 and "Neck/ Spine Injuries" on page 408.)
- Shoulder and/or neck pain occurs with heart attack or stroke symptoms (See "Heart Attack Warning Signs" on page 202 and "Stroke Warning Signs" on page 229.)
- You have all of these signs of meningitis: A stiff neck, fever, severe headache, nausea or vomiting, and confusion.
- You have any of these problems after an injury to the neck or shoulder:
  - You felt your shoulder pop out of place and pop back into place

- A burning, shooting pain or weakness in your shoulders
- Your shoulder looks misshapen.

# 98. Sprains & Strains

A sprain happens when you overstretch or tear a ligament (fibrous tissue that connects bones), a tendon (tissue that attaches a muscle to a bone), or a muscle. A strain occurs when you overstretch or overexert a muscle or tendon.

## Prevention

- Ease into any exercise program. Start off with things that are easy for you. Build up gradually.
- Before you exercise, warm up your muscles with slow easy stretches. Do this for all sports. Don't bounce.
- Don't overdo it. Stop if you feel pain.
- Cool down after hard exercise. Do the activity at a slower pace for 5 minutes.
- Wear the proper gear for the exercises you do.
- Follow safety measures to prevent slips and falls. (See "Fall prevention measures" under "Self-Care" in "Osteoporosis" on page 262; "Home Safety Checklist" on page 23; and the "Dos and Don'ts of Lifting" on page 234.)

**14. Bone & Muscle Problems**

*Sprains & Strains, Continued*

## Signs & Symptoms

- Pain
- Swelling

## Causes & Care

Sprains and strains are caused by falls and injuries, including sports injuries; twisting a limb; and overexertion.

Treatment for sprains and strains depends on the extent of damage. Self-care may be all that is needed for mild injuries. Severe sprains may require medical treatment. Some sprains require a cast. Others may need surgery if the tissue affected is torn.

### Self-Care:

- If the injury does not appear serious, use R.I.C.E. (see page 243).
- If you sprained a finger or hand, remove rings. (If you don't and your fingers swell up, the rings may have to be cut off.)
- If you have a badly sprained ankle, use crutches. They help keep weight off the ankle so it can heal.

- Take an over-the-counter medicine for pain and/or swelling. (See "Pain relievers" in "Your Home Pharmacy" on page 43.)

{**Note:** Call your doctor if the sprain or strain does not improve after using self-care for 4 days.}

### Contact Doctor When:

- Skin around the injury turns blue and/or feels cold and numb.
- Bad pain and swelling occurs or the pain gets worse.
- Pain is felt when you press along the bone near the injury.

### Get Immediate Care When:

- A strain or sprain occurred with great force from a vehicle accident or a fall from a high place.
- A bone sticks out or if bones in the injured part make a grating sound
- An injured body part looks crooked or misshapen.
- A loss of feeling occurs in the injured body part.
- You are unable to move or put weight on the injured part.

To Learn More, See Back Cover

## 99. Anemia

Anemia means that either your red blood cells or the amount of hemoglobin in your red blood cells is low. Hemoglobin is a protein that carries oxygen in your red blood cells.

There are many types of anemia. They include:

- Iron-deficiency anemia. This is the most common type.

- Folic-acid deficiency anemia. Folic acid is a B vitamin that is needed to make red blood cells.

- Vitamin $B_{12}$ deficiency anemia. One form of this is pernicious anemia.

- Anemia that results from a medical illness, such as an ulcer

## Prevention

### Ways to Get and Absorb Iron:

- Eat foods that are good sources of iron: Lean, red meats, liver, poultry, fish, and oysters; green, leafy vegetables; dried fruit; and iron-fortified cereals and wheat germ. {**Note:** Red meat not only supplies a good amount of iron, it also increases absorption of iron from other food sources.}

- Eat foods high in vitamin C, such as citrus fruits, tomatoes, and strawberries. Vitamin C helps your body absorb iron that is found in plant foods.

- If you drink tea, drink it between meals or add milk to your tea. The calcium in milk binds with the tannins. Tannins in tea inhibit iron absorption. (Herbal tea does not have tannins.)

- Avoid antacids with calcium, phosphates (which are found in soft drinks, beer, ice cream, etc.), and the food additive EDTA. These block iron absorption.

- Take a multivitamin and mineral supplement that your doctor advises. Senior multivitamin formulas have less iron than regular ones. {**Note:** High levels of iron in the blood may increase the risk for heart attacks.}

- If you take aspirin and/or other nonsteroidal anti-inflammatory drugs (NSAIDs), take them with food.

### Ways to Get and Absorb Folic Acid:

- Eat good food sources of folic acid every day. These include asparagus, brussels sprouts, spinach, romaine lettuce, collard greens, and broccoli. Other good sources are black-eyed peas, cantaloupe, orange juice, oatmeal, whole-grain cereals, wheat germ, and liver and other organ meats.

### Anemia, Continued

- Eat fresh, raw fruits and vegetables often. Don't overcook food. Heat destroys folic acid.

- Take the daily vitamin supplement your doctor suggests or prescribes.

- Don't smoke.

- Don't drink alcohol. It interferes with absorption of folic acid.

### Ways to Get Vitamin B$_{12}$:

- Eat animal sources of food. Good choices are lean meats, fish, poultry, and nonfat or low-fat dairy products. Some cereals also have vitamin B$_{12}$ added to them.

- Strict vegetarians (vegans) who eat no animal sources of food should get vitamin B$_{12}$ from a supplement or foods fortified with the vitamin.

## Signs & Symptoms

In general, signs and symptoms include:

- Tiredness

- Weakness

- Paleness. Paleness could be pale skin. Or paleness around the gums, nailbeds, or the linings of the lower eyelids.

- Shortness of breath

- Heart palpitations or rapid heartbeat

With iron-deficiency anemia, additional symptoms can occur. These include tiny cracks at the corner of the mouth; a smooth, sore tongue; brittle nails; and a hard time concentrating.

With severe folic-acid deficiency anemia, additional symptoms can occur. These include a sore, red tongue that looks glazed; appetite loss and weight loss; nausea and diarrhea; and swollen abdomen.

With severe vitamin B$_{12}$ deficiency anemia, additional symptoms can occur. These include chest pain on exertion; sore, red tongue that looks glazed; a hard time concentrating; appetite and weight loss; and nausea and diarrhea.

In advanced cases or vitamin B$_{12}$ deficiency anemia, these nervous system problems can occur:

- Numbness and tingling in the hands and feet

- Walking and balance problems

- Memory loss, confusion, dementia, or psychosis

To Learn More, See Back Cover

*Anemia, Continued*

## Causes, Risk Factors & Care

Iron-deficiency anemia is usually caused by blood loss in the stomach or intestines, such as with peptic ulcers or from conditions that lead to poor iron absorption. An example is chronic diarrhea from ulcerative colitis.

Folic-acid deficiency anemia usually occurs from not getting enough folic acid from foods and/or vitamin supplements. Elderly women who have poor diets are at risk for this.

Vitamin $B_{12}$ deficiency anemia is usually caused by the body's inability to absorb vitamin $B_{12}$ from food. It is very common among the elderly and can result from a lack of digestive acids and a substance called the intrinsic factor, which are needed to absorb vitamin $B_{12}$. Other causes are surgery that removes part or all of the stomach, and autoimmune problems that cause cells in the stomach's lining to shrink. Lack of vitamin $B_{12}$ in the diet is rarely the cause. Vitamin $B_{12}$ is found in animal foods. It is not in plant foods unless the vitamin is added to a food, such as some cereals.

Treatment for anemia depends on the type and what caused it. Your doctor can take blood tests and other tests to determine the cause. Folic-acid deficiency anemia is often treated with proper diet and folic acid supplements. Treatment for iron-deficiency anemia includes:

- A diet rich in iron and taking iron supplements. Take iron supplements only under your doctor's advice.

- Treatment for the underlying cause

Treatment for vitamin $B_{12}$ deficiency includes:

- Vitamin $B_{12}$ shots, usually taken once a month

- Large oral doses of vitamin $B_{12}$

Persons with severe anemia may need one or more blood transfusions.

{**Note:** All anemia in males and non-menstruating females needs to be checked out by a doctor. If you are diagnosed with iron-deficiency anemia, it is important to have an evaluation of your colon to rule out the presence of polyps, an early precursor to colon cancer.}

**15. Other Health Problems**

### Anemia, Continued

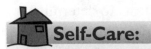

## Self-Care:

- Follow your doctor's treatment plan for the type of anemia you have.

- Follow the "Prevention" measures on pages 269 and 270, for the type of anemia you have.

- Take medicines and/or supplements as prescribed.

## Contact Doctor When:

- You feel faint or dizzy when you stand up or when you exert yourself.

- After repeated use of aspirin or other nonsteroidal anti-inflammatory drugs (NSAIDs), you have these signs:

  - Bloody, black, or tarry stools

  - Gnawing or burning pain in the abdomen

- You are female, still have menstrual periods and have any of these problems:

  - Vaginal bleeding between periods

  - Menstrual bleeding that has been heavy for several months

  - Bleeding 7 days or more every month

- You are female and have vaginal bleeding after reaching menopause.

- You have symptoms of anemia (paleness, tiredness, and weakness, etc.).

- You do not feel better after 2 weeks of treatment for anemia by your doctor.

## Get Immediate Care When:

You have blood in your stools or urine or black, tarlike stools, with lightheadedness, weakness, shortness of breath, and severe abdominal pain.

## For Information Contact:

National Heart, Lung, and Blood Institute
1-800-251-1222
www.nhlbi.nih.gov

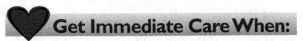

# 100. Cancer

Cancer refers to a broad group of diseases in which body cells become abnormal, grow out of control and are or become malignant (harmful). Cancer is the 2nd leading cause of death in the United States. About 1 in 3 of all Americans will develop some kind of cancer in their lifetime. The most common forms are cancer of the skin, lungs, colon and rectum, breast, prostate, urinary tract, and uterus.

## Prevention

Measures can be taken to lower the risk for certain forms of cancer.

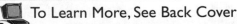

*Cancer, Continued*

**Dietary Measures:**

■ Reduce the intake of total dietary fat to no more than 30% of total calories and reduce the intake of saturated fat to less than 10% of total calories.

■ Eat more fruits, vegetables, and whole grains, especially:

• Broccoli and other cabbage-family vegetables, including cabbage and brussels sprouts. These contain cancer-fighting chemicals, such as sulforaphane antioxidants.

• Deep yellow-orange fruits and vegetables, such as cantaloupe, peaches, tomatoes, carrots, sweet potatoes and squash, and very dark-green vegetables, like spinach, greens, and broccoli for their beta-carotene and cancer-fighting chemical content

• Strawberries, citrus fruits, broccoli, and green peppers for vitamin C

• Whole-grain breads, cereals, fresh fruits and vegetables, and legumes for their dietary fiber content

■ Consume salt-cured, salt-pickled, and smoked foods only in moderation.

■ Drink alcoholic beverages only in moderation, if at all.

**Lifestyle Measures:**

■ Do not smoke or use tobacco products. Avoid secondhand smoke.

■ Limit your exposure to known carcinogens, such as asbestos, radon, and other workplace chemicals, as well as pesticides and herbicides.

■ Have x-rays only when necessary.

■ Limit your exposure to the sun's ultraviolet (UV) rays. When you are outdoors, wear sunscreen (applied often and that contains a sun protection factor [SPF] of 15 or higher) and protective clothing (sun hats, long sleeves, etc.). Wear sunglasses that protect your eyes from UV light.

■ Don't use sunlamps and tanning beds.

■ Reduce stress. Emotional stress may weaken the immune system, which fights off stray cancer cells.

## Signs & Symptoms

Cancer can be present without any signs or symptoms.

The symptoms in the chart on the next page are <u>not always</u> a sign of cancer. They can also be caused by less serious conditions. Only a doctor can make a diagnosis. Early cancer usually does not cause pain.

15. Other Health Problems

*Cancer, Continued*

## Cancer Warning Signs

- Change in bladder or bowel habits
- A sore that doesn't heal
- Unusual vaginal bleeding or rectal discharge or unusual bleeding from any part of the body
- Thickening or lump in the breast, testicles, or anywhere else
- Indigestion or difficulty swallowing
- Obvious change in a mole or wart
- Nagging cough or hoarseness that lasts longer than 3 weeks

Symptoms of specific cancers depend on the type of cancer; the stage the cancer is in; and whether or not the cancer has spread to other parts of the body. This is called metastasis.

## Causes, Risk Factors & Care

Exactly what causes all cancers is not known. Evidence suggests that cancer could result from complex interactions of:

- Viruses
- A person's genetic makeup and immune status
- Other risk factors, such as:
  - Exposure to the sun's ultraviolet rays, nuclear radiation, x-rays, and radon
- Use of tobacco and/or alcohol (for some cancers)
- Use of certain medicines, such as DES (a synthetic estrogen)
- Polluted air and water
- Dietary factors, such as a high-fat diet; specific food preservatives, such as nitrates and nitrites; charbroiling and chargrilling meats
- Exposure to a variety of chemicals, such as asbestos, benzenes, vinyl chloride, wood dust, some ingredients of cigarette smoke, etc.

## Cancer, Continued

In many cases, cancer is curable. Early detection and proper treatment increase your chances for surviving cancer. Early detection is more likely if you:

- Know the warning signs for cancer (see page 274) and report any of them to your doctor if they occur.

- Do regular self-exams, such as monthly breast self-exam if you are a women, and a testicular self-exam, as directed by your doctor, if you are a man. {**Note:** Men can also get breast cancer and should check with their doctor for signs to look for.}

- Look for any noticeable changes in warts or moles or for any wounds that have not healed.

- Get routine tests that can help detect early signs of cancer. (See the "Common Health Tests & When to Have Them" on page 35.) Examples are a digital rectal exam, sigmoidoscopy, and stool blood test. For women they also include pap tests, breast exams, and mammograms.

If and when cancer is diagnosed, treatment will depend on the type of cancer, the stage it is in, and your body's response to treatment.

In general, cancer treatment includes one or more of the following:

- Surgery to remove the cancerous tumor(s) and clear any obstruction to vital passageways caused by the cancer

- Radiation therapy

- Chemotherapy

- Possibly biological therapy, hormonal therapy, or stem cell or bone marrow transplant

{**Note:** To find out about clinical trials (research studies) for specific types of cancer, call the Cancer Information Service listed on the next page.}

### Self-Care:

{**Note:** Medical treatment, not self-care, is needed to treat cancer. Follow the self-care guidelines as advised by your doctor as part of your treatment plan.}

### 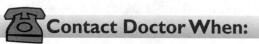 Contact Doctor When:

- You have one or more warning signs of cancer listed on page 274.

- You need regular check-ups and cancer screening tests and exams. (See "Common Health Tests & How Often to Have Them" on page 35. You may need to have some tests sooner or more often. Follow your doctor's advice.)

15. Other Health Problems

*Cancer, Continued*

## For Information Contact:

Cancer Information Service
1-800-4-CANCER (422-6237)
www.nci.nih.gov
www.cancertrials.nci.nih.gov
(for information on clinical trials)

American Cancer society
1-800-ACS-2345 (227-2345)
www.cancer.org

# 101. Diabetes

Diabetes is often called "having too much sugar." It is really too much sugar (glucose) in the blood and not enough in the body's cells. Glucose needs to get into the cells to be used for energy. Insulin is the hormone needed for glucose to get from the blood into the cells. Diabetes results when: No insulin is made; not enough insulin is made; or when the insulin made is not used properly.

Two forms of diabetes are:

- **Type 1.** With this type, the pancreas gland either makes no insulin or very small amounts. This type most often has its onset in children and young adults, but can happen at any age.

- **Type 2.** The pancreas still makes insulin, but does not make enough or the body does not use insulin the right way.

## Prevention

Maintain your ideal body weight. Many cases of Type 2 diabetes can be prevented by not being overweight.

## Signs & Symptoms

Diabetes can be a very serious, life-threatening condition. The signs and symptoms of possible new onset diabetes, as well as those in a known diabetic who becomes ill, should be taken very seriously.

The words **CAUTION** and **DIABETES** identify signs and symptoms.

- **C**onstant urination
- **A**bnormally increased thirst
- **I**ncreased hunger
- **T**he rapid loss of weight
- **E**xtreme irritability
- **O**bvious weakness and fatigue
- **N**ausea and vomiting

- **D**rowsiness
- **I**tching
- **B**lurred vision

To Learn More, See Back Cover

### Diabetes, Continued

- **E**xcessive weight
- **T**ingling, numbness, or pain in the arms and legs
- **E**asy fatigue
- **S**kin infections

Also, in women, repeated vaginal yeast infections can be an early sign of diabetes.

In Type 1 diabetes, symptoms tend to come on quickly. In Type 2, symptoms tend to come on more slowly. Diabetes can be present without any symptoms.

The American Diabetes Association and the National Institutes of Health (NIA) advise that you get a test to screen for diabetes every 3 years starting at age 45. This is to detect and treat diabetes early.

## Causes, Risk Factors & Care

Factors tied to Type 1 diabetes are:

- A family history of Type 1 diabetes
- A virus that has injured the pancreas gland
- A problem that has destroyed cells in the pancreas gland that make insulin

Risk factors for Type 2 diabetes are:

- Being overweight, especially if you are over age 40.

- Family history of diabetes. This is when one or more of your relatives (mother, father, aunt, uncle, brother, sister, or grandparent) have diabetes.

- Being female with a past history of gestational diabetes and/or having had a baby who weighed more than 9 pounds.

- Being of a certain ethnic descent. African Americans, Hispanics, Native Americans, and Asians are more prone to diabetes.

With the exception of weight loss in some cases of Type 2 diabetes, there is no cure for diabetes. Treatment will depend on the type and severity of the disease. Both forms require a treatment plan that maintains normal, steady blood-sugar levels. This plan includes:

- Proper diet and exercise to meet your specific needs. Weight loss can actually cure some cases of Type 2 diabetes. Even if weight loss does not completely cure it, it will lessen its severity.

- Regular monitoring of blood sugar levels, especially for Type 1 diabetes

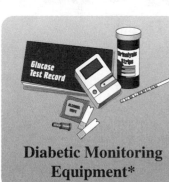

**Diabetic Monitoring Equipment***

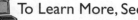
15. Other Health Problems

## Diabetes, Continued

■ Medicine: Persons with Type 2 diabetes may need to take oral medicines if proper diet, exercise, and weight control do not keep blood sugar levels within normal range. Sometimes insulin is needed for Type 2 diabetics. All Type 1 diabetics need insulin.

■ With either type of diabetes, routine care and follow-up treatment are important. Careful control of blood sugar levels can allow a person with diabetes to lead a normal, productive life. It can also prevent serious complications. These include damage to nerves and blood vessels. These damages can lead to many health problems, such as infections and injuries, heart disease, stroke, kidney disease, and blindness.

### Self-Care:

■ Do not smoke.

■ Follow the diet prescribed by your health care provider. In general, you will need to:

  • Lose weight if you are overweight.

  • Eat regular meals at regular times. You may be given a meal plan for breakfast, lunch, dinner, and snacks. You may be told to count carbohydrates in everything you eat. Books, booklets, and food labels list carbohydrate amounts.

  • Have 20 to 35 grams of dietary fiber per day. Strictly limit saturated fats and not have more than 300 milligrams of cholesterol every day.

  • Limit alcohol as advised by your doctor.

■ Work with your doctor to develop an exercise program that works for you.

■ When you exercise, carry something with you to eat or drink that has sugar. Examples are fruit juice, 6 or 7 hard candies, and 3 glucose tablets.

■ Find out if you should carry a glucagon emergency kit with you. Your doctor needs to prescribe this.

■ Test your blood glucose with a home monitoring device. Test as often as your health care provider advises.

■ If told to, monitor your urine ketones. This tests your urine, not your blood.

*Continued on Next Page*

**15. Other Health Problems**

## Diabetes, Continued

### Self-Care, Continued

- Keep a journal of your blood glucose levels, your food intake, and the exercises you do. Share your journal with your doctor.

- Buy and wear a medical alert tag. Get one from a drug store or from: MedicAlert Foundation International 1-800-344-3226 www.medicalert.org

- Take good care of your feet.

  - Check your feet every day. Inform your doctor of any problem.

  - Keep your feet clean.

  - Wear shoes and slippers that fit your feet well.

  - Don't go barefoot.

  - Cut toenails straight across. Do not cut close to the skin. Have a foot doctor cut your toenails, if advised.

- Take good care of your skin and protect it from damage.

  - Keep your skin clean.

  - Avoid cuts, scrapes, punctures, etc. Treat any skin injury right away.

  - Don't get sunburn. Use sunscreen when in the sun.

- Wear gloves in cold weather or when you do work that may injure your hands.

- Schedule an eye exam at least once a year.

- When you travel, plan, in advance, for your needs.

  - Locate one or more medical care facilities where you are going before you leave home.

  - Carry your self-care supplies with you. Make sure you take your medications; snacks and quick sugar sources; self-testing equipment; glucagon emergency kit, if you have one, etc.

  - If traveling by plane, ask for a special meal at least 24 hours ahead of time and/or bring foods that fit your meal plan(s).

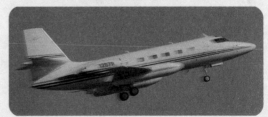

- If you get sick, follow the plans worked out ahead of time with your doctor for self-testing of blood sugar and ketones; what to eat and drink; and how to adjust insulin or oral pills.

15. Other Health Problems

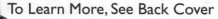

## Diabetes, Continued

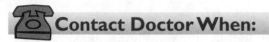 **Contact Doctor When:**

- Signs of low blood sugar (see box below) do not respond to having a sugar source, such as $^1/_2$ cup of fruit juice, 3 glucose tablets, or 6 to 7 regular hard candies. Contact your doctor without delay. If the diabetic loses consciousness, get immediate care.

- You have a change in mental status or low blood sugar signs (see box below) occur more often.

- Blood glucose tests are higher or lower than they should be despite following your treatment plan.

- You need an eye exam to check for signs of preventable complications.

- You have diabetes and any of these problems:
  - Signs and symptoms of an infection (redness, pain, pus, warm feeling at the site, and fever). See also, "Urinary Tract Infections" on page 186.
  - A wound that does not heal, any foot problem, troublesome dry skin, or a splinter that you cannot remove
  - Vomiting, rectal problems, or loss of bladder control
  - Any illness that makes it hard to keep your blood sugar under control

- You do not have diabetes, but have one or more signs and symptoms of diabetes, listed on page 276, or need to schedule a screening test for diabetes.

| **Signs of Low Blood Sugar (Hypoglycemia)** | |
|---|---|
| - Shaky feeling; weakness; dizziness | - Numbness around the mouth |
| - Sweating; cold, clammy skin | - Sudden mood changes; confusion |
| - Hunger | - Seizures and/or loss of consciousness |

| **Signs of High Blood Sugar (Hyperglycemia)** | |
|---|---|
| - Urinating often; extreme thirst | - Rapid breathing |
| - Dry, itchy skin | - Feeling very sleepy; confusion |
| - Fruity breath odor | - Loss of consciousness. Can result in diabetic coma. |

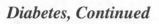 To Learn More, See Back Cover

15. Other Health Problems

*Diabetes, Continued*

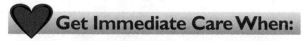 Get Immediate Care When:

Any of these problems occur with diabetes:

- With ketones in the urine with Type 1 diabetes, these signs of very high blood sugar (hyperglycemia):
  - Tiredness
  - Fruity breath odor
  - Dry, flushed skin
  - Nausea and/or vomiting
  - Hard time breathing, usually short, deep breaths
  - Lethargy. Can't be roused.
- These signs of very high blood sugar (hyperglycemia) without ketones in the urine with Type 2 diabetes:
  - Extreme thirst
  - Very high blood glucose levels
  - High fever
  - Vision loss
  - Lethargy, confusion
- Passing out

{**Note:** These symptoms usually come after an illness, such as the flu, that has caused dehydration. If these symptoms are present, drink water while seeking immediate care.}

Also, it is wise and safe to take some food at the same time just in case the symptoms are of low blood sugar rather than high. If the blood sugar is high, the little bit of extra calories will do no extra harm. In general, persons with diabetes learn to tell when their blood sugar is too low.

## For Information Contact:

American Diabetes Association
1-800-232-3472
www.diabetes.org

## 102. Fatigue

Fatigue is being very, very tired. Often, it is a symptom of another health problem.

### Signs & Symptoms

- Feeling drained of energy
- Feeling exhausted
- Having a very hard time doing normal activities
- Having low motivation
- Feeling inadequate
- Having little desire for sex

15. Other Health Problems

*Fatigue, Continued*

## Causes & Care

Causes that need medical care include anemia, depression, heart disease, low thyroid, lupus (the systemic type), and chronic fatigue syndrome (the fatigue lasts for 6 months or more).

Other physical causes include lack of sleep, poor diet, side effects from allergies or chemical sensitivities, being in hot, humid conditions, and prolonged effects of the flu or a bad cold.

Possible emotional causes are burnout, boredom, a major life change, like divorce or retirement.

Treatment depends on the cause(s) of the fatigue. For example, iron supplements can help with the fatigue that results from iron-deficiency anemia. It is important to keep track of any other symptoms that take place with the fatigue, so both physical and emotional causes can be identified and dealt with.

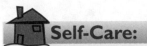

## Self-Care:

- Eat better. Eating too little or too much is hard on your body. Don't skip breakfast. Eat whole-grain breads and cereals and raw fruits and vegetables every day. It may help to eat 5 to 6 light meals a day instead of 3 large ones.

- Get more exercise. Exercise can give you more energy. It can calm you, too. Take a walk outdoors, if you can.

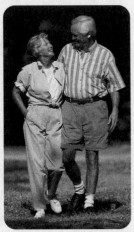

- Cool off. Being in a hot environment can drag you down. Drink plenty of water.

- Rest and relax. Get a good night's sleep. Relax during the day, too. Practice deep breathing or meditation.

- Change your routine. Try to do something new and interesting every day. If you already do too much, make time for some peace and quiet.

- Lighten your work load. Assign tasks to others when you can. Ask for help when you need it.

*Continued on Next Page*

**15. Other Health Problems**

To Learn More, See Back Cover

### Fatigue, Continued

*Self-Care, Continued*

- Do something for yourself. Do things that meet only your needs, not just those of others.
- Avoid too much caffeine and alcohol. Don't abuse drugs.

## ☎ Contact Doctor When:

- Any of these problems occur with the fatigue:
  - Chest pain with exertion
  - Shortness of breath
  - Loss of weight or appetite
  - Yellow skin and/or eyes (jaundice)
  - Blurry or double vision
  - Vomiting a lot
  - Feeling anxious and not being able to calm down
  - Swelling in the legs
  - Swollen lymph glands
  - Sore throat
  - Headache
  - Painful swelling in the neck, armpit, or groin

- Fever
- Night sweats
- Excessive thirst and/or urination
- The fatigue started only after taking a new medicine or a change in dose of a medicine.
- For women, the fatigue came with menopause or after menopause.
- Fatigue occurs for no apparent reason, has lasted for more than 2 weeks, and has kept you from doing your usual activities.

## ♥ Get Immediate Care When:

Any of these problems occur with the fatigue:

- "Heart Attack Warning Signs" (see page 202)
- "Stroke Warning Signs" (see page 229)

## 103. Fever

Fever is one way the body fights an infection or illness. It helps speed up the body's defense actions by increasing blood flow. A fever in an older person can sometimes cause more problems than in younger persons. A high fever, for example, can put an extra strain on the heart. This could trigger heart failure for an older person with heart disease.

15. Other Health Problems

***Fever, Continued***

Fevers are also more likely to cause delirium or disorientation in older adults than in younger persons.

## Prevention

- Avoid very hot conditions.
- Drink plenty of fluids.
- To fight off infections, eat well, get plenty of rest, and exercise on a regular basis. Also, get recommended immunizations (see page 36).

## Signs & Symptoms

- Your skin feels warm.
- You may sweat.
- Your temperature is higher than 100°F.

Normal body temperature ranges from 97°F to 100°F. You can take your temperature using a mercury, digital, or ear thermometer. A rectal reading is one degree higher than one by mouth or ear.

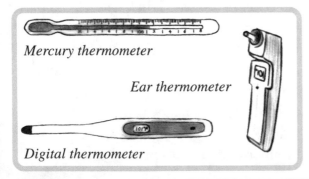

*Mercury thermometer*

*Ear thermometer*

*Digital thermometer*

The body can lose some of its ability to generate a fever as it ages. Also, a temperature reading of 97°F to 98°F or lower could be a sign of an infection in an older person. Even if you don't have a fever, look for other signs of infections. These include: Redness, swelling, pain, and/or pus at the infection site; headache; restlessness; and confusion.

## Causes & Care

Fever is a sign of another problem, such as an infection.

Body temperature changes throughout the day. It is usually lowest in the morning and highest in the late afternoon and evening.

Other factors that can affect your temperature reading include:

- Wearing too much clothing, if you're overdressed enough to raise your body temperature
- Exercise
- Hot, humid weather
- Taking your temperature by mouth after you drink a hot liquid, like tea

**15. Other Health Problems**

## Fever, Continued

If having a fever up to 102°F causes you no harm or discomfort and you have no other medical problems, you may not need to treat the fever. If the fever makes you uncomfortable, is 102°F or higher, or if you are frail or have a medical condition, you should treat it. Treatment includes self-care and taking an antibiotic for a bacterial infection, if needed.

### Self-Care:

- Drink at least $1^1/_2$ to 2 quarts of liquids every day. This includes water, fruit juice, etc. Check with your doctor first, though, if you have kidney disease or congestive heart failure.

- Take a sponge bath with tepid (about 70°F) water (not alcohol).

- Take an over-the-counter medicine to reduce fever. (See "Pain relievers" in "Your Home Pharmacy" on page 43.)

- Don't wear too many clothes or use too many blankets.

- Don't do heavy exercise.

- For high fevers, put cold packs or cool wash cloths on the neck, groin, and under the armpits.

### Contact Doctor When:

- Your temperature is higher or lower than normal and you have any of these problems:
  - Ear pain
  - Persistent sore throat
  - Vomiting
  - Diarrhea
  - Abdominal pain
  - Urinary pain, burning or frequency
  - Pain over eyes or cheeks
  - Skin rash or skin that is red and swollen or has areas of pus

- A fever is present after recent surgery or with a chronic illness, such as heart disease, lung disease, kidney disease, cancer, or diabetes.

- Your temperature is 101°F or higher and you are frail or in poor health.

- The fever exceeds 102°F (101°F in a person over 60) or has lasted more than 4 days despite efforts to reduce it.

### Get Immediate Care When:

- A fever is present with: Rapid heartbeat; no sweating; confusion; and/or loss of consciousness (after being in a hot place). These are signs of a heatstroke.

15. Other Health Problems

### Fever, *Continued*

- A high fever occurs with a stiff neck, headache, lethargy, nausea and vomiting. These are signs of meningitis.

- You have a temperature of 102°F or higher with these symptoms:

  - Chest pain that gets worse when you breathe in

  - Shortness of breath

  - A cough with phlegm that may have blood

  - Rapid breathing

  - Fatigue and abdominal pain

  - Bluish nails and lips (sometimes).

  These could be signs of bacterial pneumonia.

## 104. Headaches

Headaches are one of the most common health complaints.

### Prevention

- Keep a headache diary of when, where, and why the headaches seem to start.

- Be aware of early symptoms. Try to stop the headache as it begins.

- Exercise on a regular basis.

- Keep regular sleeping times

- Don't smoke. If you smoke, quit.

- Cut down on salt.

- Avoid excess alcohol. Alcohol can lead to a "hangover" headache.

## Signs, Symptoms & Causes

Symptoms vary depending on the type.

### For Tension or Muscular Headaches:

- A dull ache in your forehead, above your ears, or at the back of your head

- Pain in your neck or shoulders

Most headaches are this type.

Common causes of tension headaches are tense or tight muscles in the face, neck, or scalp; stress; and concentrating hard for long periods of time.

### For Migraine Headaches:

- One side of your head hurts more than the other.

- You feel sick to your stomach or vomit.

- You see spots or zigzag flashes of light.

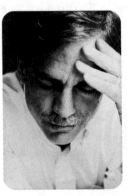

To Learn More, See Back Cover

### Headaches, Continued

- Light hurts your eyes, noise bothers you, your ears ring, and/or your face is pale.

- After the headache, some people have a drained feeling with tired, aching muscles. Others feel great after the headache goes away.

Migraines can occur with or without an aura. An aura is when a person sees spots or flashing lights for 10 to 15 minutes or his or her face becomes numb. Ten percent of all migraines are this type; 90% occur without an aura.

Migraine headaches happen when blood vessels in your head open too wide or close too tight.

### For Cluster Headaches:

- Sharp, burning, and intense pain, on one side of the head. The pain can be so severe, that you can't lie down or keep still.

- Pain in or on the sides of your eyes; watery eyes

- Pupils that look smaller; droopy eyelids

These headaches attack in groups, every day for a week or more at a time. They usually start at night and can last from 15 minutes to 3 hours. They can interrupt sleep. Or they can start during the hours that you are awake. Cluster headaches usually occur once or twice a year, usually in older men. People in the same family tend to get cluster headaches.

### For Sinus Headaches:

- Pain in your forehead, cheekbones, and nose that is worse in the morning

- Increased pain when you bend over or touch your face

- Stuffy nose

A sinus headache occurs when fluids in the nose aren't able to drain well and a buildup of pressure occurs in the sinuses. A cold, allergies, dirty or polluted water, and airplane travel can cause a sinus headache.

### Other Causes of Headaches:

- Some medications, such as nitroglycerin.

- Reading a lot, especially in dim light and eating or drinking something very cold, such as ice cream. {**Note:** To prevent ice cream headaches, warm the ice cream for a few seconds in the front of your mouth.}

- Hunger or sensitivity to certain foods and drinks. (See box on the next page.)

15. Other Health Problems

## Headaches, Continued

■ A symptom of a health condition. Example are allergies, high blood pressure, low blood sugar, infections, and shingles.

Less often, a headache can be a symptom of a serious health problem that needs immediate attention. Examples are acute glaucoma, stroke, and **giant cell (temporal) arteritis**. This is chronic inflammation of certain blood vessels, often in the temple region.

### Foods and Drinks That May Cause Headaches

■ Alcohol, especially red wine

■ Bananas (if more than $1/2$ banana daily)

■ Caffeine (from coffee, tea, colas, some medicines, chocolate). Caffeine withdrawal.

■ Citrus fruits (if more than $1/2$ cup daily)

■ Cured meats (like hot dogs, ham, etc.)

■ Chicken livers, pate

■ Foods with MSG (monosodium glutamate), such as soy sauce, meat tenderizers, seasoned salt

■ Hard cheeses like aged cheddar, etc.

■ Nuts and peanut butter

■ Onions

■ Sour cream

■ Vinegar

■ Brewer's yeast

■ Broad beans, lima beans, fava beans, snow peas

■ Figs, raisins, papayas, avocados

■ Sauerkraut, preserved, marinated, or pickled foods, such as herring

■ Sourdough bread

## Care

Self-care can be used for headaches caused by tension, fatigue, and/or stress. The Food and Drug Administration (FDA) has approved over-the-counter Excedrin Migraine to treat migraine headaches.

Headaches that are symptoms of other health conditions are relieved when the condition is treated with success.

Prescribed medicines can be used to treat migraine and cluster headaches.

In addition, biofeedback has helped many people who have suffered from headaches.

To Learn More, See Back Cover

*Headaches, Continued*

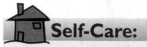 **Self-Care:**

- Rest in a quiet, dark room with your eyes closed.

- Rub the base of your skull with your thumbs. Work from the ears toward the center of the back of your head. Also, rub gently along the side of your eyes. Gently rub your shoulders, neck, and jaw.

- Take a warm bath or shower.

- Place a cold or warm washcloth, whichever feels better, over the area that aches.

- Take an over-the-counter medicine for pain. Take it right away. Use one(s) that your doctor advises.

- Relax. Picture a calm scene in your head. Meditate or breathe deeply.

- Notice if certain things, such as smoke, or fluorescent lights trigger headaches. Try to stay away from the things that seem to bring on headaches.

**Contact Doctor When:**

- Your vision was disturbed before the headache began.

- You have any of these problems with the headache:
  - A boring or burning pain in the skin of the temple region(s) of your head
  - Scalp tenderness
  - Reddened skin at your temples

- Headaches come at the same time of day, week, or month.

- A headache started after you took a new medicine.

**Get Immediate Care When:**

A headache occurs with any of these problems:

- A serious head injury or a blow to the head that cause severe pain, enlarged pupils, vomiting, confusion, or lethargy

- Seizure(s) or passing out

- Severe pain in and around one eye

- Blurred or double vision

- Talking differently

- A headache started all of a sudden and is the worst one you have had.

- Feeling confused or acting like a different person

- A problem moving your arms or legs

- Fever, stiff neck, <u>and</u> nausea or vomiting

**15. Other Health Problems**

*Headaches, Continued*

- You've had a headache for more than 2 to 3 days, and the pain keeps increasing.
- Severe throbbing pain that occurred suddenly in one or both temples.
- You feel sick and/or your scalp is sensitive to the touch.

## For Information Contact:

National Headache Foundation
1-800-843-2256
www.headaches.org

# 105. Hepatitis

Hepatitis is an inflammation of the liver. With hepatitis, the liver has trouble screening poisons from the bloodstream, and can't regulate bile. Bile is a liquid made in the liver. It is stored in the gallbladder. It is sent to the small intestine to help digest fats.

## Signs & Symptoms

Signs and symptoms depend on the cause. Some persons have no symptoms. When symptoms first occur, they are much like those of the flu: Fatigue, fever, appetite loss, nausea and vomiting, and joint pain.

Later, symptoms include jaundice, dark urine, and pale, clay-colored stools.

## Causes & Care

- One or more types of viral hepatitis. (See "Viral Hepatitis Chart" on page 291.)
- Some immune system disorders. One example is Wilson's disease. With this, too much copper is stored in the liver and other body organs.
- Chronic alcohol or drug use
- Reaction to certain medications. One example is long-term use or an overdose of acetaminophen. This is especially true for heavy drinkers.
- In some cases, the cause is not known.

Treatment will vary on the type of hepatitis and how severe it is.

- For viral forms, see the "Treatment" sections in "Viral Hepatitis Chart" on pages 291 to 293.
- For immune system disorders, treatment for the disorder is needed.
- For chronic alcohol or drug use, the use of the substance must be stopped. This may require a program of "detox" – to withdraw the substance slowly or to use an antidote for the substance.
- For chemical exposure and medication reactions, the use of the causative substance must be stopped.

*Hepatitis, Continued*

## Viral Hepatitis Chart

### Hepatitis A

**How You Get It**

Contact with food, water, or something contaminated by the feces of a person with this virus or eating contaminated oysters or clams. It takes about 2 weeks for you to actually get sick. You are contagious for 1 to 2 weeks before you feel sick and for the first week or so of the illness.

**Prevention**

Hepatitis A vaccine. Get this if you are going to a foreign country where the virus is widespread. If so, wash your hands often, drink boiled water, and don't eat unpeeled or uncooked fruits or foods rinsed with water. The virus can also be prevented if you get special antibodies within 2 weeks of exposure.

**Treatment**

Rest. Drink plenty of fluids. Don't drink alcohol or use any drugs or medicines that affect the liver, such as acetaminophen. One to 2 months of these self-care measures are enough to treat nearly everyone who gets this type.

### Hepatitis B

**How You Get It**

From direct contact with infected blood or bodily fluids from a person with this virus. Examples are sharing drug needles or having sex with an infected person.

**Prevention**

Get 3 doses of Hepatitis B vaccine. These are currently given to children and teenagers. They are also recommended for high risk persons: Health care workers who are exposed to blood and bodily fluids; IV drugs users; persons with multiple sex partners; and persons living with someone who has the virus.

*Viral Hepatitis Chart Continued on Next Page*

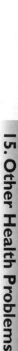

15. Other Health Problems

## Hepatitis, Continued

### Hepatitis B, Continued

**Treatment**

Rest. Drink plenty of fluids. Don't drink alcohol or use any drugs or medicines that affect the liver, such as acetaminophen. For chronic cases, your doctor may prescribe medication. While most people with this type recover, up to 10% can become chronic. (The person can spread the infection even though he or she has no symptoms.) This type can lead to cirrhosis of the liver and liver failure in some persons. Practice safe sex. (See "Prevention" on page 360.) Don't use IV drugs. Sexual partner(s) of infected persons should be tested for the virus even if they have no symptoms.

## Hepatitis C

**How You Get It**

Sharing drug needles, sexual contact, and from blood transfusions given before 1992, if the blood contained the virus.

**Prevention**

There is no vaccine. Practice safe sex (see page 360) and don't use IV drugs. Don't share razors or toothbrushes. Ask that sterilized equipment be used for acupuncture, ear piercing, etc.

**Treatment**

Rest. Drink plenty of fluids. Don't drink alcohol or use any drugs or medicines that affect the liver, such as acetaminophen. For chronic cases, your doctor may prescribe medication. Most people with this type recover. The virus can become chronic, though. It can also cause chronic liver damage, cirrhosis of the liver, and liver cancer.

## Hepatitis D

**How You Get It**

You can have this type if you are already infected with Type B and/or you share drug needles or have sexual contact with an infected person. This type is not common in the U.S.

 To Learn More, See Back Cover

## Hepatitis, Continued

| Hepatitis D, Continued | |
|---|---|
| **Prevention** | **Treatment** |
| Hepatitis B vaccine for persons who do not already have Type B hepatitis. Practice safe sex. (See "Prevention" on page 360). Don't use IV drugs. | Rest. Drink plenty of fluids. Don't drink alcohol or use any drugs or medicines that affect the liver, such as acetaminophen. Medication helps some infected persons. |

### Hepatitis E

| **How You Get It**<br><br>Contact with food, water, or something contaminated with feces of an infected person. Not common in the U.S; more common in Africa and India.<br><br>**Prevention**<br><br>No vaccine. If you are going to a foreign country where this virus is wide- | spread, wash your hands often, drink boiled water, and don't eat unpeeled or uncooked fruits or foods rinsed with water.<br><br>**Treatment**<br><br>Rest. Drink plenty of fluids. Don't drink alcohol or use any drugs or medicines that affect the liver, such as acetaminophen. |
|---|---|

### Self-Care:

- Rest.
- Drink at least 8 glasses of fluids a day.

- Avoid alcohol and any drugs or medicines that affect the liver, such as acetaminophen.
- Follow a healthy diet. Take vitamin and mineral supplements as advised by your doctor.

*Hepatitis, Continued*

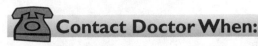

## Contact Doctor When:

- The whites of your eyes and/or your skin looks yellow.

- You have dark urine and pale stools.

- You have any signs or symptoms of hepatitis (see page 290), especially if you have been exposed to the illness.

- You have repeat symptoms of hepatitis and you have had it before.

## Get Immediate Care When:

The person with hepatitis has confusion, excessive sleepiness, or can't be roused.

# 106. HIV/AIDS

HIV stands for human immunodeficiency virus. AIDS, acquired immune deficiency syndrome, is caused by HIV. HIV destroys the body's immune system leaving a person unable to fight off diseases. The virus also attacks the central nervous system causing mental and neurological problems.

About 10% of all new AIDS cases are now in people age 50 and older. In the last few years, new AIDS cases rose faster in middle-age and older persons than in persons under 40.

## Prevention

Some day a cure for AIDS may exist. For now, prevention is the only protection.

- See "Prevention" in "Basic Facts About STDs" on page 360.

- Don't have sex with people who are at high risk for contracting HIV:

  - Persons with multiple sex partners or who inject illegal drugs

  - Partners of persons infected or exposed to HIV

  - Persons who have had multiple blood transfusions, especially before 1985, unless tested negative for HIV

- Don't share needles and/or "the works" with anyone. This includes illegal drugs, such as heroin, steroids, insulin, etc. Don't have sex with people who use or have used injected illegal drugs.

- Don't share personal items that have blood on them, such as razors.

15. Other Health Problems

*HIV/AIDS, Continued*

## Signs & Symptoms

Early symptoms of HIV/AIDS:

- Fatigue
- Loss of appetite
- Chronic diarrhea
- Weight loss
- Persistent dry cough
- Fever
- Night sweats
- Swollen lymph nodes

Persons with AIDS fall prey to many diseases such as skin infections, fungal infections, tuberculosis, pneumonia, and cancer. These "opportunistic" infections are what lead to death in an AIDS victim. When HIV invades the brain cells, it leads to forgetfulness, impaired speech, trembling, and seizures.

## Causes & Care

HIV is spread when body fluids, such as semen and blood pass from an infected person to another person. For the most part, the virus is spread by sexual contact or by sharing drug needles and syringes.

In older people, sexual activity is the most common cause of HIV infection. The second one is blood transfusions given before 1985, if the blood contained HIV. Since 1985, blood screening tests are done on donated blood. This makes it highly unlikely that you'd get HIV from current blood transfusions.

Certain activities are likely to promote contracting HIV. High-risk activities include:

- Unprotected anal, oral, and/or vaginal sex except in a monogamous relationship in which neither partner is infected with HIV. "Unprotected" means without using condoms alone or with other latex or polyurethane barriers. When used correctly, every time and for every sex act, these provide protection from HIV. Though not 100% effective, they will reduce the risk. Male latex condoms are preferred. The Reality female condom may also offer protection. Particularly high-risk situations are having sex:
  - When drunk or high
  - With multiple or casual sex partners
  - With a partner who has had multiple or casual sex partners
  - With a partner who has used drugs by injection or who is bisexual

15. Other Health Problems

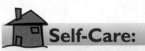

## *HIV/AIDS, Continued*

- When you or your partner has signs and symptoms of a genital tract infection

- Sharing needles and/or "the works" when injecting any kind of drugs

You cannot get HIV from donating blood, touching, hugging, or social (dry) kissing with a person with HIV. You cannot get HIV from a cough, sneeze, tears, or sweat, using a hot tub, public telephone or restroom.

You can get screening tests for HIV at doctors' offices, clinics, and health departments. You can also use a home collection test and counseling service called *Home Access*. Look for this test kit in drug stores, national retail stores, public health clinics, etc. You can also buy a *Home Access* test kit by phone. Call: 1-800-HIV-TEST (448-8378).

Current treatments for HIV/AIDS include:

- Medications. There are many older drugs, such as AZT, and newer ones, such as protease inhibitors and ones known as "Nukes" and "non-Nukes." These drugs are often used in multidrug combinations.

- Treating infections, such as giving antibiotics for pneumonia.

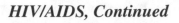 **Self-Care:**

Medical care, not self-care alone, is needed to treat HIV/AIDS. Self-care measures include:

- Taking steps to reduce the risk of getting infections and diseases:
  - Get adequate rest
  - Get proper nutrition
  - Take vitamin supplements as suggested by your doctor
- Getting emotional support:
  - Join a support group for persons infected with HIV
  - Ask your family and friends for support. Let them know how they can help you.

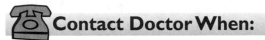 **Contact Doctor When:**

- You test positive for HIV.

- You have early signs and symptoms of HIV/AIDS listed on page 295.

- You need screening tests for HIV. Do this when:
  - You have been told that a present or past sexual partner with whom you have had sexual relations, without using condoms, has HIV.

To Learn More, See Back Cover

**15. Other Health Problems**

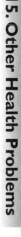

## HIV/AIDS, *Continued*

- You engaged in high risk activities for getting infected with HIV (see "Causes and Care" on page 295).

- You want to get tested for HIV for "peace of mind."

## For Information Contact:

AIDS Information Hotline
1-800-342-AIDS (342-2437)
www.cdcnac.org

# 107. Insomnia

In general, adults need 5 to 9 hours of sleep a day. You should get as many hours of sleep as you have normally needed to feel rested and refreshed the next day. As you age, the number of hours may be spread out over the day, but you still need just as much sleep.

## Signs & Symptoms

- Having trouble falling asleep

- Waking up in the middle of the night

- Waking up too early and not being able to get back to sleep

- Fatigue or feel drowsy during the day because of lack of sleep

## Causes & Care

- Too much caffeine or having it before bedtime

- Going to bed with a full bladder

- Too much noise when you fall asleep. This includes a snoring partner.

- A lack of physical exercise

- Lack of a sex partner

- Side effects of some medicines, such as stay-awake pills

- Emotional stress

- Depression or anxiety

- Sexual problems, such as impotence

- **Restless leg syndrome (RLS)**. This is a condition which results in involuntary jerking movement of the legs

- Any condition, illness, injury, or surgery that causes pain and/or discomfort which interrupts sleep. Examples are arthritis and hot flashes.

- Asthma, allergies, and early-morning wheezing

- An overactive thyroid gland

- Heart or lung conditions that cause shortness of breath when lying down

15. Other Health Problems

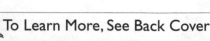

## Insomnia, Continued

When the problem that causes insomnia is found and treated, the insomnia usually goes away. Self-care may be enough to help you get a good night's sleep. If needed, your doctor may refer you to a sleep disorders clinic.

### Self-Care:

- Avoid caffeine in all forms after noon. Caffeine is in coffee, tea, chocolate, colas and some other soft drinks. Check labels for caffeine content in over-the-counter medicines.

- Avoid long naps during the day.

- Don't have more than 1 alcoholic drink at dinner time and during the evening. Check with your doctor about using any alcohol if you are taking medicines.

- Have food items rich in the amino acid L-tryptophan, such as milk, turkey, or tuna fish before you go to bed. Do not take L-tryptophan supplements, though. Eating foods with carbohydrates such as cereal, breads, and fruits may help as well.

- Get regular exercise, but not within a few hours of going to bed.

- Before bedtime take a warm bath or read a book or do some type of repetitive, calm activity. Avoid things that hold your attention, such as watching a suspense movie.

- Make your bedroom comfortable. Create a quiet, dark atmosphere. Use clean, fresh sheets and pillows and keep the room temperature neither too warm nor too cool.

- Ban worry from the bedroom. Don't rehash the mistakes of the day as you toss and turn.

- Get into a regular bedtime routine. For example, lock or check doors and windows. Brush your teeth. Read.

- Count sheep! Picturing a repeated image may bore you to sleep.

- Listen to recordings made especially to help promote sleep. Look 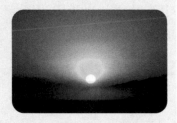 for them at a library or bookstore.

- Ask your doctor about taking Melatonin, an over-the-counter product. Take as directed by your doctor.

*Continued on Next Page*

 To Learn More, See Back Cover

*Insomnia, Continued*

### Self-Care, Continued

- If you've tried to fall asleep, but are still awake after 30 minutes, get up and sit quietly in another room. Do this for about 20 minutes. Then go back to bed. Repeat this as many times as you need to until you are able to fall asleep.

- Check with your doctor before you take an over-the-counter sleeping pill or pain reliever with added medicine for sleep, such as Tylenol PM. If your doctor does prescribe sleep medicine, make sure you take it as directed. Also, don't take anyone else's sleeping pills.

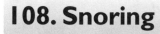

## Contact Doctor When:

- You get side effects, like dizziness, hallucinations, confusion, etc., from prescribed sleeping pills.

- You have trouble falling or staying asleep due to pain or discomfort from an illness or injury, or the need to wake up to use the bathroom.

- Insomnia occurred after taking medication.

- You have had insomnia for 3 or more weeks, with or without using self-care.

# 108. Snoring

Snoring is the sound heard when the airway is blocked during sleep. Persons who sleep on their backs are more likely to snore because the tongue falls back toward the throat and partly closes the airway. Nine out of 10 snorers are men and most of them are age 40 or over.

Snoring can be a nuisance or a signal of a serious health problem, sleep apnea.

## Signs & Symptoms

**For Snoring:**

Loud sounds and snorting sounds, usually while sleeping on the back

**For Sleep Apnea:**

- Loud snoring and snorting sounds while sleeping on the back

- Repeated periods when breathing stops 10 or more seconds during sleep. This usually happens for 20 to 30 seconds at a time. It can last up to 1 to 2 minutes at a time.

- Problems during waking hours due to lack of deep sleep, such as sleepiness, exhaustion, hard time concentrating, irritability, and depression or other mental changes.

- Morning headache

15. Other Health Problems

*Snoring, Continued*

## Causes, Risk Factors & Care

- Enlarged tonsils and adenoids
- Obesity
- Nasal allergies or deformities
- Smoking, heavy drinking, and/or over-eating (especially before bedtime), or any use of alcohol and/or sedatives
- Sleep apnea is more common in men than in women. It especially affects men who are middle-aged and older.
- An obstructed airway. This is more common as people age, especially those who are obese or who have smoked for many years.
- A chronic respiratory disease
- Hormonal changes from menopause, in women

Self-care treats most cases of snoring and some cases of sleep apnea. When this is not enough, treatment includes:

- Medications. Examples are certain antidepressants and hormones.
- A prescribed breathing device. A mask is worn over the mouth and nose. Air is forced through the mask to keep the airway open.

- Surgery to remove tissue in the throat that causes the airway to close up

### Self-Care:

- Sleep on your side. Prop an extra pillow behind your back so you won't roll over. Try sleeping on a narrow sofa for a few nights to get used to staying on your side.
- Sew a large marble or tennis ball into a pocket on the back of your pajamas. The discomfort it causes may prompt you to sleep on your side.
- If you must sleep on your back, raise the head of the bed. Put bricks or blocks between the mattress and box springs. Or buy a wedge especially made to be placed between the mattress and box spring to elevate the head section.
- Lose weight, if overweight
- Don't drink alcohol or eat a heavy meal within 3 hours of bedtime.
- If necessary, take an antihistamine or decongestant before you go to bed to relieve nasal congestion. {**Note:** Older men should check with their doctor before taking these medicines. They can give older men urinary problems.}

*Continued on Next Page*

To Learn More, See Back Cover

**15. Other Health Problems**

*Snoring, Continued*

*Self-Care, Continued*

- Get rid of allergens in the bedroom, such as dust, down-filled (feathered) pillows, and bed linen.

- Try over-the-counter "nasal strips." These keep the nostrils open and lift them up, keeping nasal passages unobstructed.

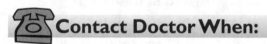

## Contact Doctor When:

- Signs and symptoms of sleep apnea occur during working hours:
  - Sleepiness or chronic daytime drowsiness
  - Irritability
  - Falling asleep while driving or working
  - Poor memory, lack of concentration
  - Loss of sex drive
  - Headaches

- Repeated periods of stopped breathing occur for 10 seconds or longer during sleep. (Someone else notices this.)

- Snoring persists despite using self-care.

# 109. Thyroid Problems

The thyroid is a small, butterfly-shaped gland located just in front of the windpipe (trachea) in your throat. Its normal function is to produce hormones needed to convert food to energy, regulate growth and fertility, and maintain body temperature.

## Signs & Symptoms

**Hypothyroidism** occurs when the thyroid gland does not make enough thyroid hormone. Signs and symptoms are:

- Fatigue and excessive sleeping
- Dry, pale skin
- Deepening of the voice
- Dry hair that tends to fall out
- Unexplained weight gain
- Frequently feeling cold
- Puffy face (especially around the eyes)
- Heavy and/or irregular menstrual periods, if still menstruating
- Poor memory
- Constipation
- Enlarged thyroid gland

**15. Other Health Problems**

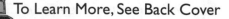

*Thyroid Problems, Continued*

**Hyperthyroidism** occurs when the thyroid produces too much thyroid hormone. Two common forms are Graves' disease and toxic multinodular goiter. Signs and symptoms are:

- Tremors, nervousness
- Mood swings
- Weakness, diarrhea
- Heat intolerance
- Shortened menstrual periods, if still menstruating
- Unexplained weight loss
- Fine hair (or hair loss)
- Rapid pulse, heart palpitations
- Bulging eye or eyes
- Enlarged thyroid gland

{**Note:** In elderly persons symptoms for this can be more like ones for hypothyroidism.}

## Causes, Risk Factors & Care

### For Hypothyroidism:

- Autoimmune disorders
- Removal of the thyroid gland.
- Treating the thyroid gland with radioactive iodine for hyperthyroidism

- Persons who are over 50 years old, very overweight, or female are at a greater risk for hypothyroidism.

### For Hyperthyroidism:

- Autoimmune disorders
- Family traits
- Too much iodine in the diet

Medical care, not self-care, is needed to treat thyroid problems. Hypothyroidism is treated with iodine and/or medicine to supplement thyroid hormones. Hyperthyroidism treatment varies. It includes surgical removal of the thyroid, radioactive iodine, and/or medicine to stop overproduction of thyroid hormones. Some treatments result in the need to take thyroid medicine from then on and follow-up care.

## ☎ Contact Doctor When:

- You have signs and symptoms of hypothyroidism or hyperthyroidism listed on page 301 and this page.

- You need to schedule thyroid testing. Ask your doctor about this. {**Note:** The American College of Physicians (ACP) recommends that all women over age 50 have a thyroid function test even if they do not have thyroid disease symptoms.}

To Learn More, See Back Cover

**15. Other Health Problems**

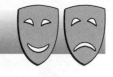

Everyone, regardless of age, race, sex, or economic status, is subject to emotional upsets. You can feel down, angry, or anxious in response to a variety of things. Feelings like these can come and go quite often. When these feelings are disturbing, interfere with daily life, and/or linger for weeks or months, they may signal a problem that needs professional help.

Many people do not seek mental health services because of the "stigma" of having an "emotional" problem. Society tends to view mental health issues differently from medical ones. When someone breaks a leg, has chest pains, or needs to get a prescription, they'll see a doctor. When they feel depressed or have a problem with alcohol, though, they may be embarrassed to seek help. Many people view these conditions as "weaknesses" that they should be able to handle themselves. Unfortunately, this view keeps them from getting professional care that can help them deal with and/or treat these conditions.

To recognize a problem and get help is not a sign of weakness. It is a sign of strength.

# 110. Alcohol Problems

About 15% of elderly persons living at home drink too much. How much is too much? The National Institute on Alcohol Abuse (NIAA) recommends that older adults drink no more than 1 drink per day. (See "Use Alcohol Wisely" on page 21. It lists examples of 1 serving of different drinks.) Anything more than this is too much. Persons with certain medical conditions and/or who take medicines

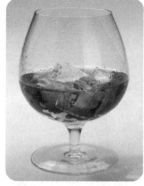

that interact with alcohol may need to abstain from alcohol.

This topic will help you figure out if you have a drinking problem. It will help you decide when to get help.

## Prevention

- Talk to persons who will listen to your feelings without putting you down.

- Seek help for mental health problems, such as depression.

- Learn how to relax without alcohol.

*Alcohol Problems, Continued*

- Contact your Employee Assistance Person (EAP) at work or your doctor. He or she can help evaluate your risk level and help you get treatment.

- Visit a self-help meeting for alcohol users, such as Alcoholics Anonymous (AA). See first hand the problems that alcohol has caused others.

## Signs & Symptoms

### For Alcohol Abuse:

Alcohol abuse leads to one or more of these problems in a 12-month period:

- Failure to fulfill work or home duties

- Drinking at times that puts you or others in danger, such as when driving a car

- Legal problems from using alcohol, such as getting arrested for drunk driving

- Drinking continues, even though it causes or worsens problems with others

### For Alcohol Dependence or Addiction:

- Cravings for alcohol. The need is as strong as the need for food and water.

- Being unable to stop using alcohol or losing control over it

- The need for more alcohol to get "high"

- Withdrawal symptoms when alcohol is stopped. These include:
  - Tremors of the hand or face
  - Chills, sweating
  - Nausea, vomiting
  - Fatigue, depression
  - Anxiety, panic, being very edgy
  - Insomnia
  - Blackouts
  - Acting "spaced out"

- Withdrawal symptoms go away when alcohol is taken.

- Alcohol is found hidden.

- Behavior changes, such as an abrupt change in mood or attitude and temper flare-ups that are not usual

## Causes, Risk Factors & Care

- Increased use and tolerance of alcohol

- Family history of alcohol abuse. You are about 4 times more likely to be an alcoholic if one of your parents is; and 10 times more likely if both parents are.

- Mental health problems, such as depression and anxiety

- Prolonged fatigue or stress

## Alcohol Problems, Continued

- Prolonged use of prescribed pain pills
- Ongoing financial or family problems

Drinking problems in older adults are often neglected by families, doctors, and the public. Symptoms of drinking problems can be mistaken for other conditions common in the elderly, such as depression. Alcoholism is a serious condition that needs treatment. Treatment includes taking part in a self-help group, such as AA, or a "rehab" center, and/or counseling. Older persons tend to do better in counseling programs that focus on social relationships. Medications, such as Naltrexone, which blocks the craving for alcohol and the pleasure of getting high, may be prescribed.

### Self-Care:

**Use Alcohol Wisely:**

- Know your limit and stick to it. You may choose not to drink at all.
- When you have a drink, drink slowly. Set it down between sips. Don't keep it in your hand.
- Avoid persons whose drinking habits provoke you to drink too much.

- Some prescribed drugs and alcohol do not mix. Some mixtures can be fatal. Don't have alcohol with prescribed drugs if the drug's label or your doctor or pharmacist tells you not to. Ask your doctor how much, if any, alcohol you can have if you take any prescribed drugs.
- Use less alcohol and more mixer in your drink. After you have 1 drink with alcohol, drink ones without it.
- Eat when you drink. Food helps to slow alcohol absorption.
- If you drink when you eat out, order your drink with, not before, your meal.
- Don't drink and drive. Designate a driver who will not be drinking.
- Coffee or fresh air cannot make you sober. To get sober, stop drinking.

### Contact Doctor When:

- You or a loved one has answered "Yes" to one or more of these "**CAGE**" questions:
  - Have you ever felt your should **C**ut down on your drinking?
  - Have people **A**nnoyed you by criticizing your drinking?
  - Have you ever felt bad or **G**uilty about your drinking?

*Alcohol Problems, Continued*

- Have you ever had a drink to steady your nerves or to get rid of a hang-over (**E**ye opener)?

{**Note:** Even if all 4 **CAGE** questions had "No" answers, there could still be a problem. Some people say, "But I only drink beer." This doesn't mean they don't have an alcohol problem.}

- You or a loved one has one or more signs and symptoms of alcohol abuse listed on page 304.

- You or a loved one has started drinking again after quitting.

### ♥ Get Immediate Care When:

- Signs of alcohol overdose occur. These are no breathing or very slow breathing; stupor; seizures; and/or coma. {**Note:** This could be from too much alcohol. It could also be from mixing alcohol and prescribed drugs.}

- Hallucinations, seizures, tremor, or delirium occur due to alcohol withdrawal.

- The person who has been drinking threatens to harm himself or herself or someone else.

## For Information Contact:

Al-Anon Family Group Headquarters and Alateen
1-800-356-9996
www.Al-Anon-Alateen.org

Alcohol and Drug Abuse Helpline
1-800-ALCOHOL (252-6465)
www.adcare.com

# III. Anxiety

Anxiety is a feeling of dread, fear, or distress over a real or imagined threat to your mental or physical well-being. A certain amount of anxiety is normal. It can alert you to seek safety when you are in physical danger. Anxiety is not normal, though, when there is no apparent reason for it or when it overwhelms you and interferes with your day-to-day life.

## Signs & Symptoms

- Rapid pulse and/or breathing rate
- Racing or pounding heart
- Dry mouth, shortness of breath
- Sweating, trembling
- Faintness
- Numbness/tingling of the hands, feet, or other body part

### *Anxiety, Continued*

- Feeling a "lump in the throat"
- Stomach problems
- Insomnia

## Causes & Care

Anxiety can result from a side effect of some medicines and a withdrawal from nicotine, alcohol, drugs, or medicines, such as sleeping pills.

Anxiety can be a symptom of a medical condition, such as a heart attack, an overactive thyroid gland, or low blood sugar (hypoglycemia).

Anxiety can also be a symptom of a number of illnesses known as anxiety disorders. These include:

- Phobias. These are irrational fears of specific situations, activities, or objects.
- Panic disorder. With this, a person has repeated panic attacks, brief episodes of acute anxiety that come on all of a sudden when there is no real danger. A person having a panic attack may rush to an emergency room because they think they are having a heart attack or feel like they are going to die.

- Obsessive-compulsive disorder. With this, the sufferer has persistent, involuntary thoughts (obsessions) and does repeated acts, such as washing his or her hands (compulsions).

- Post-Traumatic Stress Disorder. With this, a person re-experiences a traumatic past event, like a wartime event, robbery, or accident. Symptoms include nightmares, flashbacks of the event, excessive alertness, and emotional numbness to people and activities.

Self-care (see below) treats mild anxiety that does not interfere with daily living.

When this is not enough treatment includes medication, counseling, and treating any medical condition which causes the anxiety.

Self-help groups, such as Agoraphobics in Motion (AIM) can also be a part of treatment.

## Self-Care:

- Look for the cause of the stress that results in anxiety. Deal with it using stress management. (See "Self-Care" in "Stress" on page 323.)

- Lessen your exposure to things that cause you distress.

*Continued on Next Page*

## Anxiety, Continued

### Self-Care, Continued

- Talk about your fears and anxieties with someone you trust, such as a friend, spouse, minister, etc.

- Eat healthy foods. Eat at regular times. Don't skip meals.

- If you are prone to low blood sugar episodes, eat 5 to 6 small meals per day instead of 3 larger ones. Avoid sweets on a regular basis, but carry a source of sugar, such as a small can of orange juice, with you at all times. This will give you a quick source of sugar in the event you do get a low blood sugar reaction.

- Get regular exercise.

- Limit or avoid caffeine.

- Avoid nicotine and alcohol.

- Avoid medicines that have a stimulating effect, such as over-the-counter diet pills and stay awake pills.

- Don't "bite off more than you can chew."

- Help others. This may help you overcome or forget about your anxiety.

- Do a relaxation exercise daily, such as biofeedback or meditation.

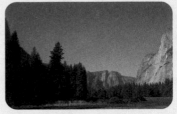

- Rehearse for events that are coming up about which you have felt anxious in the past or think will cause anxiety. Imagine yourself feeling calm and handling the situation well.

## Contact Doctor When:

- With anxiety, you have excessive hair growth; round face and puffy eyes; skin changes (reddening, thinning, and stretch marks); and high blood pressure.

- With anxiety, you have a rapid heartbeat, hyperactivity, weight loss, muscle weakness, tremors, bulging eyes, and feeling hot or warm all the time.

- You have been through or seen a traumatic event and you suffer from any of these problems:

  - Nightmares, night terrors, and/or flashbacks of the event

  - Lack of concentration, poor memory, sleep problems

### Anxiety, Continued

- Feelings of guilt for surviving the event
- Startled easily by loud noises or anything that reminds you of the event
- Lack of interest in the activities and people you once enjoyed

■ Your anxiety occurs only when you don't eat or when you do too much physically, especially if you are diabetic.

■ Your anxiety occurs only after taking an over-the-counter or prescribed medicine, or withdrawing from medication, nicotine, alcohol, or drugs.

■ You have recurrent panic attacks that come when you don't expect them and have 1 or more of these problems:
  - Continued concern about having more attacks
  - Worry about what will happen as the result of a panic attack, such as losing control, or "going crazy"
  - A change in things you normally do because of past panic attacks

■ You avoid situations or places that you think will provoke a panic attack.

■ You use alcohol or drugs to help you deal with situations that provoke the thought of another panic attack.

■ Anxiety is keeping you from doing the things you want to do every day.

### Contact Doctor or Counselor When:

■ Any of the following keep you from doing your daily activities:
  - Checking something over and over again, such as seeing if the door is locked
  - Repeated, unwanted thoughts, such as worrying you could harm someone
  - Repeated, senseless acts, such as washing your hands over and over again

### Get Immediate Care When:

Any symptoms of a heart attack are present with the anxiety. See "Heart Attack Warning Signs" on page 202.

### For Information Contact:

National Mental Health Association
1-800-969-NMHA (969-6642)
www.nmha.org

16. Mental Health Conditions

# 112. Codependency

Codependency is when a person becomes the "caretaker" of an addicted or troubled individual. The individual can be addicted to alcohol, drugs, or gambling or be troubled by a physical or emotional illness. Codependents can be this individual's spouse, lover, child, parent, sibling, coworker, or friend.

## Signs & Symptoms

The codependent:

- Enables or allows the person to continue his or her self-destructive or troubled behavior. The codependent denies that the person has a problem.

- Rescues or makes excuses for the person's behavior

- Takes care of all household and financial chores

- Rationalizes that the person's behavior is normal by simply letting it take place. The codependent may take part in the same behavior as the addicted or troubled individual.

- Acts like a hero, or becomes the "super person" to preserve the family image

- Blames the person and makes him or her the scapegoat for all problems

- Withdraws from the family and acts like he/she doesn't care

## Causes, Risk Factors & Care

A person is more likely to become codependent if he or she:

- Puts other people's wants and needs before his or her own

- Is afraid of being hurt and/or rejected by others or hurting others' feelings

- Has low self-esteem or has a self-esteem tied to what is done for others

- Places too many expectations on him or herself and others

- Feels overly responsible for others' behaviors and feelings

- Does not think it is okay and normal to ask for help

Most codependents do not realize they have a codependency problem. They think they are actually helping the troubled person, but they are not.

Admitting to the problem is the first step in treatment. Self-care and counseling treat codependency. For many people, the self-care is not easy to do without the help of a counselor.

To Learn More, See Back Cover

*Codependency, Continued*

### 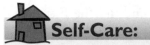 Self-Care:

- Read books on codependency. You can find these in the library and bookstores. You may find you identify with what you read and gain understanding.

- Focus on these 3 <u>C</u>'s:
  - You did not <u>c</u>ause the other person's problem.
  - You can't <u>c</u>ontrol the other person.
  - You can't <u>c</u>ure the problem.

- Don't lie, make excuses, or cover up for the person's drinking, drug, or other problem. Admit that this way of living is not normal and that the abuser or troubled person has a real problem and needs professional help.

- Refuse to come to the person's aid. Every time you bail the abuser out of trouble, you reinforce their helplessness and your hopelessness.

- If you or your children are being physically, verbally, or sexually abused, do not allow it to go on. Get help. For information contact: National Domestic Violence Hotline 1-800-799-SAFE (799-7233) www.ndvh.org

- Join a support group for codependents. Examples are self-help groups for family and friends of substance abusers, such as Al-Anon and Alateen. For information contact: AL-ANON Family Group Headquarters 1-800-356-9996 www.alanon.alateen.org

- Continue with your normal family routines. For example, include the drinker when he/she is sober.

- Focus on your own feelings, desires, and needs. Vent negative thoughts in healthy ways. Begin to do what is good for your own well-being.

- Allow others to express their feelings openly. Show them 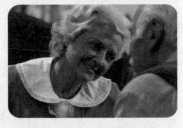 how by expressing your own feelings.

- Set limits on what you will and won't do. Be firm and stick to your limits.

- Engage in new experiences and interests. Find diversions from your loved one's problem.

- Take responsibility for yourself and others in the family to live a better life whether your loved one recovers or not.

*Codependency, Continued*

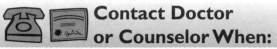

## Contact Doctor or Counselor When:

You do 3 or more of the following:

- You think more about another person's behavior and problems than about your own life.

- You feel anxious about the addicted or troubled person's behavior and constantly check on them to try to catch them in their bad behavior.

- You worry that if you stop trying to control the other person, that he or she will fall apart.

- You blame yourself for this person's problems.

- You cover up or "rescue" this person when they are caught in a lie or other embarrassing situation related to their addiction or other problem.

- You deny that this person has a "real" problem with drugs, alcohol, etc. and become angry and/or defensive when others suggest there is an addiction or other substance abuse problem.

# 113. Depression

Depression is more than just the blues or the blahs. It is a medical illness. It is just as much an illness as diabetes and heart disease. Depression is not a sign of being weak. It is not the person's "fault." Depression is not a normal part of aging, but is a common problem in older adults.

Depression makes a person less able to manage life. It affects a person's mood, mind, body, behaviors.

Depression may worsen or even cause other medical problems.

## Signs & Symptoms

A person who is depressed:

- Feels sad, hopeless and helpless
- Feels guilty and/or worthless
- Thinks negative thoughts
- Has lost interest in life, including sex

Other signs and symptoms are:

- Changes in eating or sleeping patterns
- Fatigue. Loss of energy or enthusiasm
- A hard time concentrating or making decisions
- Ongoing physical symptoms, such as headaches

To Learn More, See Back Cover

***Depression, Continued***

- Crying spells
- Thoughts of suicide or death

In older persons, these usual symptoms of depression may be replaced by dizziness, confusion, refusal to eat or drink, paranoia, and/or a loss of mental status.

As a person ages, the signs of depression are much more likely to be dismissed as moods of "old age." The symptoms can mimic ones of other conditions, too.

## Causes & Care

- Some types of depression run in families.
- Brain chemical imbalances
- Life changes, such as divorce, retirement, and the death of a loved one
- Hormonal changes, such as that which comes with menopause
- Medical illness, surgery, or a disability
- Problems with others
- Worries about money
- Abuse of drugs. This includes alcohol and some medicines.
- Seasonal Affective Disorder (SAD). This is a lack of natural sunlight between late fall and spring.

- A side effect of medicines, such as a type to treat high blood pressure.
- Low self-esteem
- Holiday "blues"
- Isolation from others or being in a nursing home

Most likely, depression is caused by a mix of family traits; brain chemical factors; emotional factors; and other factors, such as a medical illness or alcohol abuse.

In some people, certain things that occur in life may bring on depression. Examples are extreme stress and grief. In others, depression occurs even when life is going well.

Only about 3% of depressed older adults get treatment for depression. Treatment includes medicine(s), especially antidepressants; psychotherapy; or both.

A special kind of light therapy may be used for persons who have mild or moderate depression that comes in the fall and winter.

Self-care may be all that is needed for mild depression. Self-care measures are also helpful with medical treatment.

Persons who are depressed should not self-diagnose, though.

**16. Mental Health Conditions**

## *Depression, Continued*

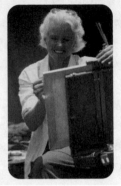

### Self-Care:

- Discuss all medicines you take with your doctor or pharmacist. Ask if what you take could lead to depression. When prescribed medicine for depression, take it as prescribed. Let your doctor know about side effects.

- Ask your doctor about St. John's Wort, an over-the-counter herb. It may be useful for mild to moderate depression.

- Don't use drugs. Limit alcohol. Too much alcohol and the use of other drugs can cause or worsen depression. Drugs and alcohol can also make medicines for depression work less. Harmful side effects can happen when alcohol and/or drugs are mixed with medicine.

- Eat healthy foods. Eat at regular times.

- Exercise regularly.

- Relax. Listen to soft music. Take a warm bath or shower. Do relaxation exercises. Read a good book.

- Talk to someone who will let you express the tensions and frustrations you are feeling.

- Be with positive people.

- Help someone else. This will focus your attention away from yourself.

- Do something different. Join a social group. Take a class, etc.

- Take a vacation that you will enjoy.

- Take on a new project. Do something you enjoy and that lets you express yourself. Write, paint, sing, etc.

- Laugh. Watch funny shows, etc.

### Contact Doctor When:

- You have had a lot less interest or pleasure in almost all activities most of the day, nearly every day for at least 2 weeks.

- You have been in a depressed mood most of the day nearly every day and have had any of the symptoms that follow for at least 2 weeks:

  - You feel slowed down or restless. You are not able to sit still.

  - You feel worthless or guilty.

  - You have changes in appetite. You lose or gain weight.

  - You have thoughts of death or suicide.

To Learn More, See Back Cover

## Depression, Continued

- You have problems concentrating or thinking. It is hard to remember things or make decisions.

- You have trouble sleeping or you sleep too much.

- You have a loss of energy or you feel tired all the time.

- You have headaches.

- You have aches and pains.

- You have stomach and/or bowel problems.

- You have sexual problems.

- You feel negative or hopeless.

- You are worried or anxious.

- Depression has hindered your daily activities for more than 2 weeks.

- You have withdrawn from normal activities for more than 2 weeks.

- The depression comes with dark, cloudy weather or winter months. It lifts when spring comes.

- You are feeling depressed now and one or more of these things apply:

  - You have been depressed before and did not get treatment.

  - You have been treated for depression in the past and it has come back.

- You have taken medicine for depression in the past.

- You have depression from a medical problem, taking over-the-counter or prescribed medicine, or alcohol or drug abuse.

- During holiday times you withdraw from family and friends or you dwell on past holidays to the point that it interferes with your present life.

### ♥ Get Immediate Care When:

You just tried to commit suicide or are planning ways to commit suicide.

### For Information Contact:

National Mental Health Association
1-800-969-NMHA (969-6642)
www.nmha.org

# 114. Drug Abuse & Dependence

Drug problems result from drug abuse and/or dependence. The drugs can be:

- Illegal drugs, such as cocaine

- Inhalants. These are vapors from substances, such as glue, solvents, and paints, that are used to get "high."

*Drug Dependence & Abuse, Continued*

- Some prescribed legal drugs. These include painkillers, muscle relaxants, stimulants, tranquilizers, etc.

Misuse of prescribed drugs is more common in seniors than using illegal drugs.

## Prevention

### To Prevent Problems with Prescribed Medicines:

- Use medicines only as prescribed.
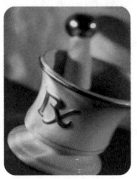
- Discuss the effects of taking more than one medicine and/or taking medicine with alcohol with your doctor and pharmacist. Have your prescriptions filled at the same pharmacy. The pharmacist can check for harmful drug interactions.

- Don't increase the dose of a medicine or take it more often than prescribed, unless advised by your doctor.

- Don't use medicine prescribed for someone else.

- Don't mix drugs with alcohol, driving, or operating machines. These combinations can be fatal.

- Ask your doctor about the risks of addiction when he or she prescribes sleeping pills or sedatives; tranquilizers; and/or strong pain relievers. Find out how long you should take these medicines. Ask if there are ways to treat your problem without them.

- Find out how to gradually reduce the usage of a medicine to avoid harmful side effects.

### To Prevent Problems with Illegal Drugs:

- Try to stay out of situations where drugs are available.

- If your friends insist that you take drugs in order to socialize with them, just say NO!

- Learn as much as you can about the harmful effects of drugs.

- Visit a self-help meeting for drug users, such as Cocaine Anonymous (CA). See first hand the problems that drugs have caused others.

- Contact your doctor or your Employee Assistance Person (EAP) at work, if available to you. He or she can help evaluate your risk level and help you get treatment.

- Talk to persons who will listen to your feelings without putting you down.

To Learn More, See Back Cover

*Drug Dependence & Abuse, Continued*

- Seek help for mental health problems, such as depression or chronic anxiety. Do this before they lead to drug problems.

- Don't take part in risky behaviors if you have been taking drugs. Examples are unsafe sex, sharing needles, or using non-sterile needles.

- Learn how to relax without drugs. Develop healthy interests. Take part in leisure activities.

## Signs & Symptoms

### For Drug Abuse:

- Failure to fulfill work or home obligations

- Legal problems, such as getting arrested for disorderly conduct

- Physical harm that results from car accidents, etc.

- Relationship problems, such as arguments or physical fights

- Drugs are found or items used to take drugs are found. Examples are:

  - Glass pipes used to smoke drugs

  - Straws used to sniff drugs

  - Needles used to inject drugs

- Withdrawal symptoms (see below)

### For Drug Dependence:

- Cravings for the drug

- Need for increased amounts of the drug to get the desired effect

- Withdrawal symptoms when the drug is stopped:

  - Tremors of the hand or face

  - Chills, sweating

  - Nausea, vomiting

  - Fatigue, depression

  - Anxiety, panic

  - Being very edgy

  - Insomnia

  - Blackouts

  - Acting "spaced out"

  - Hallucinations

  - Delirium

- Behavior changes. These include:

  - Being late or absent for work, often on Mondays and Fridays.

  - Abrupt change in mood or attitude

  - Temper flare-ups that are not usual

  - Asking for money, more than usual, from family and friends. Stealing.

  - Being secretive about actions and things that are owned

*16. Mental Health Conditions*

***Drug Dependence & Abuse, Continued***

- Being with a new group of people, especially with those who use drugs

- Having problems dealing with others

A person can abuse a drug without becoming addicted to it. Addicts, however, usually have distress and the daily problems that result from drug abuse.

## Care

The first step is to admit there is a problem. Often, the person who has the problem does not see the harm that it causes. Other persons around him or her see the problem first. Knowing how harmful drug abuse and dependence are can help a person seek treatment.

The treatment for drug dependence and abuse varies and depends on the drug(s) being used and the person's needs. Types of treatment include:

- Emergency medical care. This may be needed for drug overdoses or for violent or out-of-control behaviors.

- Medical treatment for physical problems due to the use of a drug(s) and/or for proper care and supervision from drug withdrawal

- Counseling

- Support groups, such as Narcotics Anonymous (NA), Cocaine Anonymous (CA), and Alcoholics Anonymous (AA). (See places to contact on pages 306 and 319.)

### Self-Care:

- Follow "Prevention" measures listed on page 316.

- Follow treatment guidelines from your doctor.

- Take part in a support group, if needed.

### Contact Doctor or Counselor When:

Three or more of the following have applied in the last 12 months due to drug abuse:

- More of a drug was needed to get intoxicated or to reach a desired effect.

- Withdrawal symptoms, listed on page 317, occurred when the drug was stopped or less was taken.

- The drug or one similar to it was needed to relieve or avoid withdrawal symptoms.

- The drug was needed in larger amounts often or was taken over a longer period of time than you intended.

### *Drug Dependence & Abuse, Continued*

- Failure to cut down or control the use of a drug

- A lot of time was spent doing things necessary to get the drug, use the drug, or recover from its effects.

- Important social, work, or leisure activities were given up or done less often so the drug could be taken.

- The drug was continued even though it resulted in physical or psychological problems or made these problems worse.

One or more of the following occurred in the last 12 months due to drug use:

- Taking part in situations that could cause physical harm while under the influence of a drug, such as driving or operating a machine

- Legal problems, such as getting arrested for disorderly conduct

- Relationship problems due to the effects of the drug, such as physical fights or arguments with others

## Get Immediate Care When:

A drug overdose has occurred. Possible signs include:

- The victim is not breathing and has no pulse.

- The victim is unconscious.

- The victim is hallucinating, confused, convulsing, breathing slow and shallow, and/or slurring their words.

- The person's personality is suddenly hostile, violent, and aggressive.

## For Information Contact:

Alcohol and Drug Abuse Helpline
1-800-ALCOHOL (252-6465)
1www.adcare.com

National Cocaine Hotline
1-800-COCAINE (262-2463)
www.drughelp.org

## 115. Grief/Bereavement

Grief is a deep sadness or sorrow that results from a loss. The loss can be from something big or small. It can be from something positive or negative.

Bereavement is a process of grieving most often linked with the death of a loved one.

## Signs & Symptoms

### Stages of Grief

- Shock. The person feels dazed or numb.

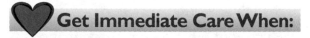

**16. Mental Health Conditions**

*Grief/Bereavement, Continued*

- Denial and searching. The person:
  - Is in a state of disbelief
  - Asks questions such as, "Why did this happen?" or, "Why didn't I prevent this?"
  - Looks for ways to keep their loved one or loss with them
  - Thinks he or she sees or hears the deceased person
  - Begins to feel the reality of the event
- Suffering and disorganization. The person:
  - Has feelings, such as guilt, depression, anxiety, loneliness, fear, and/or hostility
  - May place blame on everyone and everything
  - May get physical symptoms, such as headaches, stomachaches, constant fatigue, and/or shortness of breath
  - Withdraws from routine and social contacts
- Recovery and acceptance. The person:
  - Begins to look at the future instead of focusing on the past
  - Adjusts to the reality of the loss
  - Develops new relationships
  - Develops a positive attitude

The normal period of grieving the loss of a loved one lasts from 1 to 3 years, but could take longer.

## Causes & Care

Examples of things that cause grief include:

- A new or lost job, a promotion, demotion or retirement
- Relationships, such as getting divorced or having a child leave home
- An illness, injury and/or disability
- The death of a family member or friend, loss of property, or moving to a new place

There are many factors that shape a person's response to a loss, such as death. These factors include:

- Age and gender
- Health
- How sudden the loss was
- Cultural background
- Religious beliefs
- Financial security
- Social network
- History of other losses or traumatic events

Each of these factors can add to or reduce the pain of grieving.

To Learn More, See Back Cover

## Grief/Bereavement, Continued

Understanding the normal stages of grief, the passage of time, and self-care treat most cases of grief. When these are not enough, professional counseling can help.

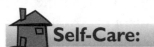

### Self-Care:

- Eat regular meals.

- Get regular physical exercise, such as walking.

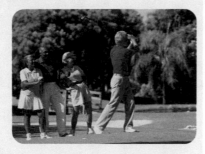

- Allow friends and family to assist you. Tell them how you really feel. Don't hold your feelings inside. Visit them, especially during the holidays, if you would otherwise be alone. Traveling during the holidays may also be helpful.

- Try not to make major life changes, such as moving during the first year of grieving.

- Join a support group for the bereaved. People and places to contact include churches or synagogues, funeral homes, and hospice centers.

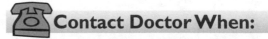

### Contact Doctor When:

You have any of these problems after a reasonable amount of time has passed since the loss. The time will vary from person to person and with the type of loss.

- You are thinking about suicide.

- You abuse medicines and/or alcohol to feel better or to "numb" your pain.

- You are not able to cope day-to-day.

- You are not taking care of your own health.

- You have ongoing problems, such as insomnia, excessive crying, depression, feelings of guilt, etc.

- You place extreme stress on your marriage, your children, and/or others.

- You have refused to sort through the deceased's belongings.

### Get Immediate Care When:

You attempt suicide or make plans for suicide.

## For Information Contact:

Grief Recovery Helpline
1-800-445-4508

Resources to Help With Grief
212-759-4050
www.christophers.org/grief

**16. Mental Health Conditions**

## 116. Stress

Stress is the way you react to any change in the status quo (good, bad, real, or even imagined). Stress can make you more productive. It can also help you respond to situations that threaten your safety, such as a fire.

High levels of stress, though, can make you less productive. When left unchecked, stress can lead to a number of health problems. These include headaches, heartburn, back or neck pain, high blood pressure, and a lowering of your body's immune system.

### Prevention

Practice good health habits.

- Eat healthy foods. Avoid foods high in fat and sugar. Eat at regular times. Don't skip meals.

- Limit caffeine. It causes anxiety and increases the stress response.

- If you drink alcohol, have no more than 1 drink a day. One drink is: 12 oz. of regular beer or 5 oz. of wine or $1^1/_2$ oz. of 80 proof distilled spirits (whiskey, gin, etc.)

- Drink 8 to 10 glasses of water each day.

- Check with your doctor about taking vitamin and mineral supplements. This is especially true for ones labeled "stress tablets" or "stress formulas." In general, a multivitamin and mineral supplement that gives 100% of RDAs is safe. Do not take vitamins and minerals that give more than 10 times the RDA unless your doctor tells you to. High doses of some nutrients, such as vitamin $B_6$, can be harmful. Focus first on healthy foods.

- Get enough sleep and rest.

- Get regular exercise.

- Balance work and play. Plan some time for hobbies and recreation. Plan one or more vacations during the year.

- Prevent burnout.

  - Pay attention to any signals your body is sending. Insomnia and overeating may be signs of burnout.

  - Make goals that you can reach. Think in terms of long-range goals, not just day-to-day problems.

  - Treat yourself to something special from time to time. A pleasant break, a change of scenery, etc. can reduce some of the resentment that often leads to burnout.

  - Meditate. Do deep-breathing exercises.

To Learn More, See Back Cover

## Stress, Continued

- Take charge. Although you can't control other people's actions, you can control your response to what comes your way.
- Don't try to please everyone. You can't.

# Signs & Symptoms

Physical symptoms of stress are: Increased heart rate and blood pressure, rapid breathing, and tense muscles.

Emotional reactions include irritability, anger, losing your temper, and lack of concentration.

# Care

Prevention and self-care measures deal with most cases of stress. When these are not enough, counseling and/or medical care may be needed.

## Self-Care:

- Count to 10 when you're so upset you want to scream. This gives you time to reflect on what's bothering you and helps to calm you down.
- Have a warm cup of herbal tea.

- Own a pet. Studies show that having a pet, such as a dog or cat, appears to buffer the effects of stress on health.

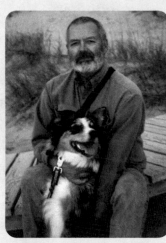

- Get rid of or manage your exposure to things that cause stress.
- Budget your time. Make a "to do" list. Prioritize your daily tasks. Don't over-schedule or commit to doing too much.
- View changes as positive challenges.
- Find ways to learn acceptance. Sometimes a difficult problem is out of control. When this happens, accept it until changes can be made.
- Talk about your troubles with a friend, relative, clergy member.
- Escape for a little while. Watch a movie, visit a museum, etc.
- Laugh a lot. Keep a sense of humor.
- Take a warm shower or bath.
- Listen to music that you find soothing in a quiet, calm environment.

*Continued on Next Page*

*16. Mental Health Conditions*

## Stress, Continued

### Self-Care, Continued

■ Reward yourself with little things that make you feel good. Add to your stamp collection, buy a flower, etc. Give yourself some "me" time.

■ Help others.

■ Have a good cry. Tears can help cleanse the body of substances that form under stress. Tears also release a natural pain-relieving substance from the brain.

■ Practice deep breathing:

  • Sit in a chair, arms at your sides, legs uncrossed.

  • Note any tension in your muscles.

  • Put one hand on your chest and the other hand on your abdomen.

  • Take in a breath slowly and deeply through your nose. Allow your abdomen to expand and push up your hand. After your abdomen is full of air, allow your chest to expand, pushing up your other hand. This is one long, steady breath.

  • Hold the air in for 3 seconds.

  • Purse your lips and exhale through your mouth. Make a relaxing, whooshing sound.

  • Continue to take long, slow, deep inhales through your nose and let out long, slow exhales through your mouth.

  • Focus on the sound and feeling of deep breathing. Continue for 3 to 5 minutes.

### Contact Doctor or Counselor When:

■ You often have anxiety, nervousness, crying spells, or confusion about how to handle your problem.

■ You abuse alcohol and/or drugs (illegal or prescription) to deal with stress.

■ You have been a part of a traumatic event in the past (e.g., wartime event, airplane crash, rape, or assault) and you now experience any of these problems:

  • Flashbacks (reliving the stressful event), painful memories, nightmares

  • Feeling easily startled and/or irritable

  • Feeling "emotionally numb" and detached from others and the outside world

16. Mental Health Conditions

*Stress, Continued*

- Having a hard time falling asleep and/or staying asleep

- Anxiety and/or depression

■ You suffer from a medical illness that you are unable to cope with or that leads you to neglect proper treatment.

■ You withdraw from friends, relatives, and coworkers.

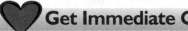 **Get Immediate Care When:**

■ You are so distressed that you make plans for suicide or have recurrent thoughts of suicide or death.

■ You have impulses or plans to commit violence.

## 117. Suicidal Thoughts

A lot of people think about suicide or say things like, "I wish I was dead" at times of great stress. For most people, these thoughts are a way to express anger, and other emotions. They may not, in and of themselves, be a sign of a problem.

Suicidal threats and attempts are a person's way of letting others know that he or she needs help. Suicide attempts and/or threats should never be taken lightly or taken only as a "bluff." Most people who threaten and/or attempt suicide more than once usually succeed if they are not stopped.

Here are some facts on suicide:

■ It is the 8th leading cause of death in the U.S. It is the 5th leading cause of death in persons over age 65. Adults over age 65 have the highest rate of suicide.

■ It is more common in men than in women. Women attempt suicide 3 times more often than men, but men die from suicide 4 times more often than women. White men die from suicide more often than black men.

■ More deaths occur from suicides than from homicides every year.

### Prevention

■ Know the warning signs for suicide. See "Contact Doctor or Counselor When" section in this topic.

■ Take courses that teach problem solving, coping skills, and suicide awareness. Call your local hospital and community centers to find out where you can take these courses.

**16. Mental Health Conditions**

### Suicidal Thoughts, Continued

- Get help for emotional and/or physical problems that lead to thoughts of or attempted suicide, such as depression (see page 312).

- Keep firearms, drugs, and other means to commit suicide away from potential victims.

## Signs, Symptoms & Causes

Suicidal thoughts could be a signal for help if they:

- Don't go away or occur often

- Lead to suicidal threats, gestures, or attempts

- Are a symptom of a medical illness or mental health condition, such as:

  - Depression (see page 312). Up to 70% of persons who die from suicide have suffered from depression right before their deaths.

  - Bipolar disorder (manic depression). This is a mood disorder with mood swings from elation and/or euphoria to severe depression. Suicide can take place during either a manic or depressive episode.

  - Schizophrenia. This is a group of mental disorders in which there are severe disturbances in thinking, mood, and behavior. The sufferer has delusions, hallucinations, disordered thinking, and/or inappropriate emotions.

  - Grief/bereavement (see page 319). A person may find it hard to go on living without their loved one or may want to be with him or her in death.

## Care

Emergency care and hospitalization is necessary after an attempted suicide. Persons with suicidal thoughts should seek medical treatment.

### Self-Care:

If you are having thoughts of suicide:

- Let someone know. Talk to a trusted family member or friend. If it is hard for you to talk directly to someone, write your thoughts down. Let someone else read them.

- Call your local crisis intervention or suicide prevention hotline. Look in your local phone book or call the operator for the number. Follow up with a visit to your doctor or local mental health center, if told to do so.

To Learn More, See Back Cover

## *Suicidal Thoughts, Continued*

### ☎ 📋 Contact Doctor or Counselor When:

- You have thoughts of suicide and any of these conditions: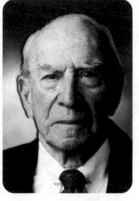

  - Depression

  - Manic depression

  - Schizophrenia

  - Any other mental health or medical condition

- Thoughts of suicide came as a result of taking, stopping, or changing the dose of a prescribed medicine or using drugs and/or alcohol.

- You have thoughts of suicide with signs and symptoms of depression (see page 312).

- With thoughts of suicide, you have recently done 1 or more of the following:

  - Given away favorite things, cleaned the house, and gotten legal matters in order

  - Purchased or gotten a weapon or pills that could be used for suicide

- Given repeated statements that indicate suicidal thoughts, such as, "I want to be dead," "I don't want to live anymore," or, "How does a person leave their body to science?"

- Made suicidal gestures, such as stood on the edge of a bridge, cut your wrists with a dull instrument, or driven recklessly on purpose

- Suicidal thoughts have come as a result of an upset in life, such as a separation; a divorce; death of a loved one or other loss, such as the loss of a job; rejection, or being ridiculed.

- You have thoughts of suicide and have a family history of death by suicide.

### ♥ Get Immediate Care When:

- You attempt suicide. Call 911!

- You are making plans for suicide.

- You have repeated thoughts of suicide or death.

### For Information Contact:

National Mental Health Association
1-800-969-NMHA (969-6642)

# Chapter 17. Men's Health

17. Men's Health

## 118. Impotence

Impotence is **erectile dysfunction**. It occurs when a man is not able to have or maintain an erection to complete intercourse. Almost all men have temporary periods when this occurs. This is not impotence. Impotence is when this occurs in 25% or more attempts. With impotence, the penis does not get enough blood flow to keep the penis rigid enough for satisfying intercourse.

The chances of impotence increase as men age, but this is not a natural part of aging. Impotence is a common problem, though. More than 30 million men in the U.S. have some form of failure to have or maintain an erection.

## Signs & Symptoms

One or more of the following occur in 25% or more of attempts:

- Not being able to get an erection
- Having an erection that is too brief, weak, or painful for satisfying sexual intercourse
- Having an erection, but it loses its strength upon penetration

## Causes & Care

Impotence is a symptom or secondary condition of other conditions.

### Physical Conditions

One or more of these problems account for about 85% of cases:

- Diabetes
- Blood vessel diseases
- Spinal cord injuries
- Some prostate or pelvic surgeries
- Multiple sclerosis
- Kidney or liver disease
- Hormone deficiencies
- Smoking, alcohol, and/or drug abuse
- Side effect of some prescribed drugs. Examples are water pills, beta blockers, major tranquilizers, tricyclic antidepressants, and lipid-lowering drugs.

### Psychological Causes

These account for about 10% of cases. Examples are:

- Stress, including job stress
- Money or relationship problems
- Grief
- Depression or anxiety
- Low self-esteem

To Learn More, See Back Cover

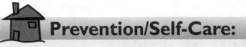

## *Impotence, Continued*

Not being able to perform adds to the problem. Suspect a psychological cause if you have erections during sleep or as you wake up from sleep.

### Unknown Causes

These account for about 5% of cases.

Seek medical care. A doctor, often a urologist, can diagnose the cause and prescribe treatment. Treatment includes:

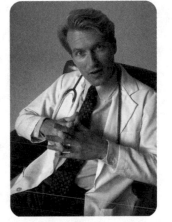

- Treating any medical condition that results in impotence

- Medicine, such as Viagra. Only take Viagra as prescribed by your doctor. Let your doctor know if you are taking any other medicines, especially nitroglycerin and other heart medicines.

- Penile implant or injections

- A vacuum pump device

## Prevention/Self-Care:

- Don't smoke.
- Don't use street drugs.
- Don't have more than 1 alcoholic drink a day.
- Relax. Manage stress.
- Get plenty of rest.
- Share your thoughts, fears, and needs with your partner.
- Don't focus on just performance. Find pleasure in hugging, kissing, and caressing your partner.
- If you have diabetes or other medical conditions, follow your treatment plan.

## Contact Doctor When:

- You need a consult to rule out, diagnose, and/or treat medical conditions which may cause impotence.
- Impotence began after taking prescribed medicine.
- Impotence began after prostate or other surgery or trauma to the pelvis.
- You want information on medical ways to treat impotence.

## For Information Contact:

Impotence Center
www.wellweb.com/impotent

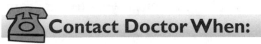

17. Men's Health

# 119. Jock Itch

Jock itch gets its name because an athletic supporter worn, then stored in a locker, and then worn again without being washed, provides an environment in which fungi, which cause jock itch, thrive.

## Prevention

- Don't wear garments that fit tightly. Wear boxers, not briefs.

- Change underwear after tasks that leave you hot and sweaty.

- Shower soon after a workout. Dry the groin area well.

- Apply talc or other powder to the groin area.

- Wash workout clothes after each wearing.

- Sleep in the nude or in a nightshirt.

- Don't use antibacterial (deodorant) soaps.

## Signs & Symptoms

Redness, itching, and scaly patches of skin occur on the skin of the groin, scrotum, and/or thigh areas.

## Causes, Risk Factors & Care

Jock itch is usually caused by a fungal infection. It can also result from a bacterial infection or be a reaction to chemicals in clothing, irritating garments, or medicines that you take. Jock itch is more likely to occur after taking antibiotics.

Self-care treats jock itch.

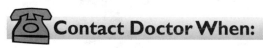

### Self-Care:

- Follow prevention tips in this topic.

- Use an over-the-counter antifungal cream, powder, or lotion. Examples are ones with clotrimazole, such as Lotrimin; with miconazole, such as Micatin; and with tolnaftate, such as Tinactin. Follow package directions.

### Contact Doctor When:

You have symptoms of jock itch that last more than 2 weeks despite using self-care.

To Learn More, See Back Cover

# 120. Prostate Problems

The prostate gland is a male sex gland. It makes a fluid that forms part of semen, the white fluid that contains sperm. The prostate is about the size of a walnut. It is located below the bladder and in front of the rectum. The prostate surrounds the upper part of the urethra, the tube that empties urine from the bladder.

Prostate problems are common in men 50 and older. Prostate problems include:

- Prostatitis. This is an infection or inflammation of the prostate. It can be an acute or chronic problem. With chronic prostatitis, an infection comes back again and again.

- Enlarged prostate. This is called benign prostatic hyperplasia (BPH). Most men get this with aging.

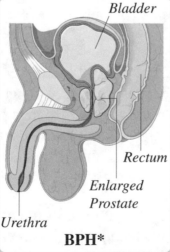

Bladder

Rectum

Enlarged Prostate

Urethra

**BPH\***

- Prostate cancer. This is the second most common form of cancer among American men. Lung cancer is first.

## Signs & Symptoms

### For Prostatitis:

- Pain and burning when you urinate
- Pain with orgasm
- Strong urge to urinate
- Urinating often, even during the night
- A hard time starting to urinate or emptying your bladder all the way
- Pain in the lower back and/or between the scrotum and anus
- May have blood in the urine, fever, chills

There is usually no fever with chronic prostatitis and other symptoms are usually milder than with an acute infection.

### For an Enlarged Prostate:

- Increased urge to urinate
- Urinating often, especially during the night
- Delay in onset and/or slow stream of urine flow
- Not emptying the bladder all the way
- Not being able to urinate at all (rarely)

These symptoms indicate that the prostate gland has enlarged enough to obstruct the flow of urine. Sometimes BPH causes a urinary tract infection (UTI). Over time, a few men might have bladder or kidney problems or both.

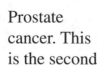

*Prostate Problems, Continued*

### For Prostate Cancer:

Prostate cancer may have no symptoms until it is advanced. When symptoms occur, they include:

- Symptoms of an enlarged prostate (see page 331)
- Blood in the urine
- Swollen lymph nodes in the groin area
- Impotence
- Pain in the hips, pelvis, ribs, or spine

## Causes & Risk Factors

### For Prostatitis:

Bacterial infection. With the chronic form, the infection comes back again and again. Sometimes, urine tests may not show bacteria, but a prostate exam can confirm an infection.

### For Enlarged Prostate:

- Normal aging. More than half of men in their 60s have BPH. Up to 80 percent of men in their 70s and 80s may have BPH.
- Prostate infections can increase the risk.

### For Prostate Cancer:

- Aging. The chances increase rapidly after age 50. About 80% of all cases occur in men over age 65.
- Race. African American men are twice as likely to get prostate cancer as Caucasian American men.
- Family traits. Having a father or brother with prostate cancer doubles the risk.
- Diet. A diet high in fat and dairy products and low in fruits and vegetables may increase the risk. Fruits and vegetables with the plant chemical, lycopene (in tomatoes, watermelon, etc.) may help lower the risk.

## Care

Your doctor can diagnose prostate problems with a physical exam and tests.

Men 50 years of age and older should have a digital rectal exam every year to screen for prostate cancer. Other tests that a doctor might order are a prostate-specific antigen (PSA) blood test and a transrectal ultrasound (TRUS). Men should discuss the need for these tests with their doctor.

Treatment for prostate problems depends on which problem is present.

### For Prostatitis:

Treatment is antibiotics and self-care.

To Learn More, See Back Cover

*Prostate Problems, Continued*

### For an Enlarged Prostate:

Treatment varies. Options include:

- Watchful waiting. This is getting no treatment, but having regular exams to see if your BPH is causing problems or getting worse.

- Medications. One type helps relax the smooth muscle of the bladder neck and prostate. Another type causes the prostate to shrink.

- Surgery. There are many types and many new procedures. Check with your doctor for one(s) best suited for your needs.

Prostate surgery can result in problems, such as impotence and/or incontinence. It is important to discuss the benefits and risks of these operations with your doctor. Most men who undergo surgery have no major problems.

### For Prostate Cancer:

Treatment depends on many factors. These include the patient's age and general health and whether the cancer has spread beyond the prostate.

- Watchful waiting. If the cancer is growing slowly, treatment may not be needed right away, but the man should be closely monitored by his doctor. Men who are older or have another serious illness may choose this option.

- Surgery. There are many types.

- Radiation therapy

- Hormonal therapy

More than one type of treatment may be used.

### Self-Care:

### For an Enlarged Prostate:

- Stay sexually active.

- Avoid taking over-the-counter medicines with antihistamines.

- Avoid dampness and cold temperatures.

### For Prostatitis:

- Take antibiotics as prescribed.

- Rest until fever and pain are gone.

- Take an over-the-counter medicine for pain and swelling, if needed. (See "Pain relievers" in "Your Home Pharmacy" on page 43.)

*Continued on Next Page*

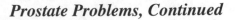

## Prostate Problems, Continued

### Self-Care, Continued

**For Both an Enlarged Prostate and Prostatitis:**

- Take warm baths.

- Don't let the bladder get too full. Urinate as soon as the urge arises. Relax when you urinate.

- When you take long car trips, stop often to urinate.

- Limit coffee, alcohol, and spicy foods.

- Drink 8 or more glasses of water every day, but don't drink liquids before going to bed.

- Reduce stress.

- Don't smoke. If you smoke, quit.

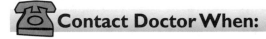
## Contact Doctor When:

- You have any signs or symptoms listed for prostatitis on page 331; enlarged prostate on page 331, or prostate cancer on page 332.

- You have a diagnosis of a prostate cancer or an enlarged prostate, and your symptoms are getting worse.

- You have symptoms of prostatitis that: Don't improve after 3 days of treatment; get worse during treatment; or come back after treatment.

- You need to schedule screening tests for an enlarged prostate and prostate cancer.

## For Information Contact:

American Foundation for Urologic Disease
1-410-468-1800
www.afud.org

Cancer Information Service
1-800-4-CANCER (422-6237)
www.nci.nih.gov

To Learn More, See Back Cover

## 121. Breast Lumps, Cancer, & Self-Exam

# Breast Lumps

Feeling a lump or lumps in your breast(s) can be scary. For a lot of women, the first thought is cancer. The good news is that 80 to 90% of breast lumps are not cancerous.

## Signs, Symptoms & Causes

- Solid tumors. These include:
  - Lipomas. These are fatty tumors that can grow very large. They are usually benign.
  - Fibroadenomas. These lumps are round, solid, and movable and are usually benign.
  - Cancerous lumps. Often, these are firm to hard masses that do not move when felt. They are often an irregular shape.
- Cysts (sometimes called fibrocystic breast disease). These cysts:
  - Are fluid filled sacs
  - Are painful and feel lumpy or tender
  - Can occur near the surface of the skin of the breast and/or be deep within the breast. This second type may need to be tested with a biopsy to make sure it is benign.

- Nipple-duct tumors. These tumors occur within the part of the nipple that milk flows through and cause a discharge from the nipple. These tumors should be surgically removed.

In rare instances, there can be a bloody discharge from the nipple which could indicate cancer.

# Breast Cancer

Breast cancer is the most common form of cancer among women. It accounts for 30% of cancers women get. Each year, there are approximately 175,000 new cases of breast cancer and 43,000 deaths from it. Only lung cancer causes more cancer deaths among women.

## Signs & Symptoms

Breast cancer often develops without signs and symptoms. This is why early screening for breast cancer is needed. See also "Signs, Symptoms, & Causes" under "Breast Lumps" on this page.

## Causes & Risk Factors

Breast cancer results from malignant tumors that invade and destroy normal tissue. When these tumors break away and spread to other parts of the body, it is called metastasis. Breast cancer can spread to the lymph nodes, lungs, liver, bone, and brain.

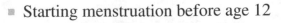

### *Breast Lumps, Cancer, & Self-Exam, Continued*

For women, the risk of breast cancer increases as women get older. The National Cancer Institute (NCI) has given the following statistics for women's chances of developing breast cancer:

| By Age | Chances |
|--------|---------|
| 25 | 1 in 19,608 |
| 30 | 1 in 2,525 |
| 35 | 1 in 622 |
| 40 | 1 in 217 |
| 45 | 1 in 93 |
| 50 | 1 in 50 |
| 55 | 1 in 33 |
| 60 | 1 in 24 |
| 65 | 1 in 17 |
| 70 | 1 in 14 |
| 75 | 1 in 11 |
| 80 | 1 in 10 |
| 85 | 1 in 9 |
| Ever | 1 in 8 |

Other risk factors for breast cancer include:

- Personal history of breast lesions, especially ductal carcinoma in situ (DCIS) and lobular carcinoma in situ (LCIS)
- Never giving birth or having a first fullterm pregnancy after age 30
- Starting menstruation before age 12
- Family history of breast cancer for a woman whose mother, sister, or daughter has had the disease.
- Having familial cancer genes, such as BRCA1 or BRCA2
- Having had breast biopsies, especially if the biopsy showed a change in breast tissue known as atypical hyperplasia
- Having European Jewish ancestry
- Race. White women have a greater risk than African American women. African Americans with breast cancer are more likely to die from it, though.

To estimate your risk for breast cancer, ask your doctor or contact the National Cancer Institute (see page 340) about The Breast Cancer Risk Assessment Tool.

## Detection

- Mammograms. (See "Common Health Tests & How Often to Have Them" on page 35.) Have mammograms at facilities that are accredited by the American College of Radiology (ACR). Call The National Cancer Institute (see page 340) to find ones in your area.
- Clinical breast exams. These are breast exams by a doctor or nurse.
- Breast self-exam (see page 339)

To Learn More, See Back Cover

18. Women's Health

*Breast Lumps, Cancer, & Self-Exam,*
*Continued*

If a lump or other problem is found, additional tests can check for cancer.

## Care

Finding and treating the cancer early is vital. Treatment is based on the type, size, and location of the tumor. It also depends on the stage of the disease and individual factors you may have. One or more of these methods are used:

- Surgery. There are many options. Ask your doctor about the benefits and risks for each type of surgery and decide together which option is best for you.
- Chemotherapy
- Radiation therapy
- Hormonal therapy
- Stem cell or bone marrow transplant
- Clinical trials or research studies for breast cancer

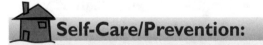

## Self-Care/Prevention:

### For Cystic Breasts:

- Do a breast self-exam monthly or as advised by your doctor. See "Breast Self-Exam (BSE)" on page 339.

- Get to and stay at a healthy body weight.
- Follow a low-fat diet.
- Get regular exercise. This can stimulate circulation to your breasts.
- Avoid caffeine in: Beverages (coffee, colas, and drinks with chocolate); foods (chocolate); and medicines (appetite suppressants, some pain relievers, such as Extra Strength Excedrin, etc.)
- Limit salt and sodium intake to prevent fluid buildup in the breasts.
- Don't smoke and don't use nicotine gum or patches.
- Take an over-the-counter pain reliever. (See "Pain relievers" in "Your Home Pharmacy" on page 43.)
- Wear a bra that provides good support. You may want to wear it while you sleep, too.

### For Breast Pain:

- Apply warm heat (heating pad set on low, or hot water bottle) for 30 minutes, then an ice pack for 10 minutes. Repeat as often as needed.
- If advised by your doctor, take vitamin supplements.

*Continued on Next Page*

**18. Women's Health**

*Breast Lumps, Cancer, & Self-Exam, Continued*

## Self-Care, Continued
### For Breast Cancer:

- Do a breast self-exam monthly or as advised by your doctor. See "Breast Self-Exam (BSE)" on page 339.

- Schedule a mammogram as advised by your doctor.

- Check with your doctor about taking the prescribed medicine, tamoxifen.

- Eat a variety of fruits and vegetables and whole grains and cereals.

- Eat vegetables with sulforaphane, a plant chemical that may help protect against breast cancer. Examples are broccoli, cabbage, cauliflower, and brussels sprouts.

- Avoid unnecessary x-rays. Wear a lead apron when you get dental and other x-rays not of the chest.

- Limit your alcohol intake to 1 drink per day, if any.

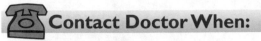

## Contact Doctor When:

- You see or feel any lumps, thickening, or changes of any kind.

- You notice dimpling, puckering, retraction of the skin, or a change in the shape or contour of the breast.

- Your nipples become drawn into the chest or inverted totally, change shape, or become crusty from a discharge.

- You have a nonmilky discharge when you squeeze the nipple of either breast or both breasts.

- You have breast pain or a constant tenderness.

- You normally have lumpy breasts (already diagnosed as being benign by your doctor), but now notice any new lumps or have any lumps that have changed in size or you are concerned about having "benign" lumps.

- You have a family history of breast cancer, especially in your mother, sister, or daughter, even if you don't notice any problems when you examine your breasts. Your doctor can counsel you about a preventive and screening program that suits your needs.

To Learn More, See Back Cover

*Breast Lumps, Cancer, & Self-Exam, Continued*

## Breast Self-Exam (BSE)

Do a breast self-exam (BSE) once a month. Do it at the same time each month to learn what is normal for you. If you menstruate, the best time to do a BSE is 2 or 3 days after your period stops. If you have gone through menopause, do a BSE the same day of each month, such as the first day of the month.

Some lumpiness or thickening in the breasts is normal. Your "job" isn't just to find lumps, but to notice if there are any changes. If you have questions, ask your doctor. Don't self-diagnose.

### BSE Is a Three-Step Process:

1. In the shower
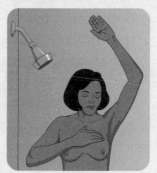
   - Put one of your hands behind your head. With your fingers flat, gently move the pads of your fingers over every part of each breast. Use your right hand for the left breast; your left hand for the right breast.

   - Check for any thickenings, lumps, or knots.

2. In front of a mirror: Hold your arms 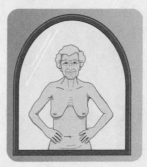 at your sides. Raise your arms over your head. In both positions, look for changes in the shape of the breasts; swelling; dimpling; or changes in the nipples.

3. Lying down: Put a pillow under your right shoulder. 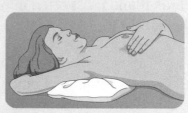 Place your right hand behind your head. With the fingers of your left hand held flat, press your right breast gently in small circular motions around an imaginary clock.  Start at 12 o'clock, then move to 10 o'clock, etc. until you get back to 12 o'clock. Each breast will have a normal ridge of firm tissue. Then move in 1 inch toward the nipple. Keep circling to examine every part of your breast including the nipple. Repeat with the left breast. Finally, squeeze the nipple of each breast gently. Check for a clear or bloody discharge.

18. Women's Health

*Breast Lumps, Cancer, & Self-Exam, Continued*

## For Information Contact:

National Cancer Institute
1-800-4-CANCER (422-6237)
www.nci.nih.gov

# 122. Cervical Cancer

Cancer of the cervix, the lower, narrow part of the uterus, can occur at any age, but is found most often in women over the age of 40.

Cervical cancer accounts for about 4% of all cancers found in women. Each year, about 15,000 women in the United States learn that they have this type of cancer.

## Signs & Symptoms

An abnormal Pap test can be an early sign of cervical cancer. There are often no symptoms, though, especially in the early stages. In very late states, symptoms are:

- Vaginal bleeding or spotting between periods
- Vaginal bleeding after intercourse
- Watery or thick vaginal discharge that may have an odor
- Pain in the pelvic area

Symptoms in the final stages are:

- Anemia
- Appetite and weight loss
- Pain in the abdomen
- Leakage of urine and feces through the vagina

## Causes, Risk Factors & Care

Certain risk factors have been identified that increase the chance that cells in the cervix will become abnormal or cancerous. It is believed, in many cases, that cervical cancer develops when 2 or more of these risk factors act together:

- Having a history of the sexually transmitted human papilloma virus (HPV). There are many types of this virus. Some types put women at greater risk than others. {**Note:** Not all women who are infected with HPV get cervical cancer and the virus is not present in all women who have it.}
- Having had frequent sexual intercourse before age 18
- Having multiple sex partners. The more partners, the greater the risk.
- Having sex partners who began having sexual intercourse at a young age; have had many sexual partners; or were previously sexually active with women who had cervical cancer.

To Learn More, See Back Cover

## Cervical Cancer, Continued

- Having had a sex partner with HPV
- Smoking
- Being the daughter of a mother who took a drug known as DES during pregnancy. This drug was used from about 1940 to 1970, mostly to prevent miscarriages.
- Having a weakened immune system

If cervical cancer is found early, most women can be cured. To find it early, have Pap tests and pelvic exams as often as your doctor advises. Also ask your doctor about testing for STDs, especially if you or your sex partner have multiple sex partners.

Treatment will depend on the exact diagnosis. The precancerous form of cervical cancer is known as **dysplasia**. This can be treated with laser therapy, conization (removal of a portion of the cervix), or cryotherapy (freezing). For cervical cancer, surgery, radiation therapy, and/or chemotherapy is needed.

### Self-Care:

- Schedule and have Pap tests and pelvic exams as often as advised.

- Take measures to prevent getting HPV and other sexually transmitted diseases (STDs). (See "Prevention" in "Basic Facts About STDs" on page 360.)
- Get checked for HPV if your doctor advises. Tell your partner or partners to get tested, too.
- Avoid douching. If you do, don't do so more than once a month.
- Don't smoke. If you smoke, quit.

### Contact Doctor When:

- You have a leakage of urine and feces through the vagina; pain in the abdomen; anemia; and appetite and weight loss.
- You have any of these problems:
  - Constant vaginal bleeding or vaginal bleeding after menopause
  - Spotting between periods or bleeding after intercourse
  - Pelvic pain
  - Thick or watery vaginal discharge
- You have 2 or more risk factors for cervical cancer listed on page 340 and you have not had a Pap test and pelvic exam for more than a year.
- It is time for your periodic Pap test and pelvic exam.

18. Women's Health

*Cervical Cancer, Continued*

## For Information Contact:

National Cancer Institute
1-800-4-CANCER (422-6237)
www.nci.nih.gov

# 123. Hormone Replacement Therapy (HRT)

Hormone replacement therapy (HRT) gives prescribed hormones: estrogen, progester-one, or progestin (a progesterone-like substitute). Estrogen without progesterone or progestin is Estrogen Replacement Therapy (ERT). It is usually prescribed for women who have had their uterus removed.

Hormone replacement can be given in many forms:

- Pills
- Estrogen patches
- Estrogen vaginal creams
- Internal devices, such as the vaginal ring, Estring.

You and your doctor can choose the form of HRT and the schedule of taking it.

### Benefits of HRT

- Lowers the risk of heart disease. The longer it is taken, the greater the benefit. Heart disease is a major health risk to postmenopausal women.

- Slows bone density loss. The risk of osteoporosis fractures is reduced by 25 to 50% while you take HRT.

- Relieves hot flashes

- Reduces thinning of the vaginal lining

- Reduces sagging of the pelvic muscles

- Improves spirits in someone with mild depression

- Improves cholesterol levels

- Improves bladder function. This can help with incontinence.

- May lower the risk of colon cancer

- May lower the risk of Alzheimer's disease

### Risks of HRT

The greatest fear with HRT is the possible increased risks of breast and uterine cancer. There is no increased risk for uterine cancer if progesterone is given with estrogen. The risk of breast cancer may increase slightly after 5 to 8 years of HRT. The risk for these cancers may increase with certain health conditions. Examples are high blood pressure, diabetes, stroke, and migraines. Also, HRT increases the risk for blood clots.

To Learn More, See Back Cover

## *Hormone Replacement Therapy (HRT), Continued*

### Side Effects of HRT May Include:

- Weight gain or bloating
- Headaches
- Vaginal bleeding
- Breast tenderness
- Depression

### Should You Take HRT?

Many experts believe that the benefits of HRT may be greater than the risks. Before you decide about HRT, discuss the possible benefits, risks, and side effects with your doctor. The decision should be based on:

- Your age and stage of menopause you are in. If you are in perimenopause, your doctor may advise you to take an oral contraceptive and then switch to HRT after menopause.
- Your personal health history and risk factors for heart disease, osteoporosis, breast cancer, etc.
- Your symptoms
- An understanding of the risks and benefits of HRT

If you are taking hormones, you should have regular medical checkups. The American College of Obstetricians and Gynecologists recommends that all women taking HRT get a medical checkup every year. At that time, the doctor or nurse should read your blood pressure, give you pelvic and breast exams, and order a mammogram to check for breast cancer.

### If You choose Not to Take HRT or are Advised Against It:

- Follow "Self-Care" measures in "Menopause" on page 345.
- Follow "Prevention" and "Self-Care" measures in "Osteoporosis" on pages 260 and 262.
- Have regular checkups with your doctor.
- Ask about medicine alternatives, such as Raloxifene or other "designer estrogens."

## 124. Menopause

Menopause ("the change of life") is when a women's menstrual periods have stopped for 1 whole year. In general, it occurs between the ages of 45 and 55. It can, though, occur as early as 35 or as late as 65 years of age. It can also result from the surgical removal of both ovaries.

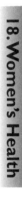

18. Women's Health

*Menopause, Continued*

## Signs & Symptoms

Most of the following signs and symptoms occur in perimenopause, a time span of about 4 years before menopause. Some occur after menopause. Signs and symptoms vary from woman to woman.

**Physical Signs and Symptoms:**

- Hot flashes. These are sudden waves of heat that can start in the waist or chest and work their way to the neck and face and sometimes the rest of the body. They can occur as often as every 90 minutes. Each one can last from 15 seconds to 30 minutes; 5 minutes is average. Seventy-five to 80% of women going through menopause have hot flashes.

- Irregular periods. Periods can get shorter and lighter for 2 or more years. Periods can stop for a few months and then start up again and be more widely spaced. They can bring heavy bleeding and/or the passage of many small or large blood clots.

- Vaginal dryness. This results from hormone changes. The vaginal wall also becomes thinner. These problems can make sexual intercourse painful or uncomfortable and can lead to irritation and increased risk for infection.

- Loss of bladder tone which can result in stress incontinence (leaking urine when you cough, sneeze, laugh, or exercise)

- Headaches, dizziness

- Skin and hair changes. The skin is more likely to wrinkle. {**Note:** Sun exposure and smoking cause skin changes more than menopause does.} Growth of facial hair, but thinning of hair in the temple region can occur.

- Muscles lose some strength and tone.

- Bones become more brittle, increasing the risk for osteoporosis.

- The risk for a heart attack increases when estrogen levels drop.

**Emotional Changes:**

- Irritability, mood changes

- Lack of concentration, difficulty with memory

- Tension, anxiety, depression

- Insomnia which may result from hot flashes that interrupt sleep

## Causes & Care

Hormone changes that come with aging cause menopause. The body makes less estrogen and progesterone.

18. Women's Health

## Menopause, *Continued*

Treatment for the symptoms of menopause varies from woman to woman. Self-care may be all that is needed. Hormone replacement therapy (HRT) can reduce many of the symptoms of menopause. Each woman should discuss the benefits and risks of HRT with her doctor. For the vast majority of women, the benefits far outweigh the risks. (See "Hormone Replacement Therapy (HRT)" on page 342.)

Medication to treat depression and/or anxiety may be prescribed in some women. Also, certain sedative medicines can help with hot flashes.

## Self-Care:

### For Hot Flashes and Night Sweats:

- Wear lightweight, cotton clothes. When you sleep: Have changes of nightwear ready; instead of blankets, use only a top sheet; keep the room cool.
- Limit or avoid beverages with caffeine or alcohol. Avoid rich and/or spicy foods.
- Don't eat a lot of food at one time.

- Drink cool water when you feel a hot flash coming on and before and after exercise. Avoid hot drinks.
- Have 1 to 2 servings per day of a food made with soy (soybeans, soy milk, tofu, miso, etc.).
- Keep cool: Open a window; lower the thermostat; use air conditioning and/or fans.
- Relax. Meditate, etc.

### For Vaginal Dryness and Painful Intercourse:

- Don't use deodorant soaps or scented products in the vaginal area.
- Use a water soluble lubricant, such as K-Y Jelly, Replens, etc. Avoid oils or petroleum-based products.
- Use a prescribed estrogen cream for the vagina.
- Keep sexually active.
- Don't use antihistamines, unless truly needed.

### To Deal with Emotional Symptoms:

- Get regular exercise.
- Talk to women who have gone through menopause.

*Continued on Next Page*

18. Women's Health

## Menopause, Continued

### Self-Care, Continued

- Manage stress.
- Use massage therapy.
- Relax. Meditate, do yoga, etc.
- Eat healthy. Check with your doctor about taking vitamin/mineral supplements.

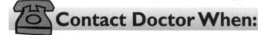 **Contact Doctor When:**

- You have any of these problems:
  - Heavy bleeding with your periods
  - Bleeding between periods
  - Passing many small or large blood clots, which leave you pale and very tired
- You have symptoms that are severe or occur often enough to interfere with your normal activities.
- Menstrual periods have begun again after not having a period for 6 months.
- You want advice on HRT and taking vitamin E.
- You have side effects, if on HRT.
- You no longer have regular menstrual periods and need advice to prevent getting pregnant.

## For Information Contact:

National Women's Health Information Center

1-800-994-WOMAN
www.4women.gov

# 125. Ovarian Cancer

The ovaries are two almond-sized organs on either side of the uterus. Growths can form in, on, or near the ovaries.

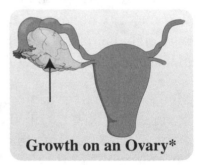

**Growth on an Ovary***

For the most part, tumors in the ovary are benign. Malignant tumors are ovarian cancer. This type of cancer occurs most often between the ages of 50 and 75, but can occur at any age.

## Signs & Symptoms

Often there are no symptoms in the early stages. In many cases, the cancer has spread by the time it is found. When symptoms appear, they are vague intestinal problems, so are often ignored. They include:

- Discomfort or pain in the lower abdomen or pelvis

To Learn More, See Back Cover

### Ovarian Cancer, Continued

- Feeling full, even after a light meal
- Fluid build-up in the abdomen. A woman may notice that her waistline is getting bigger and her clothes don't fit in the waist area for no apparent reason.
- Gas, indigestion, nausea
- Weight loss
- Vaginal bleeding

## Causes, Risk Factors & Care

Ovarian cancer may result from constant activity in the cells in the ovaries that increases the possibility of genetic mutation. This is more apt to occur when regular ovulation is not interrupted by pregnancy, breast-feeding, or taking birth control pills. Risk factors for ovarian cancer are:

- Not having children or having had them at an older age
- Not ever taking birth control pills
- Going through menopause after age 55
- Family history of ovarian, colon, breast, prostate, or lung cancer
- Personal history of breast, uterine, colon, or rectal cancer
- Being Caucasian

There is no completely reliable test for ovarian cancer. Ways to detect it include yearly pelvic and rectal exams and an ultrasound. A CA-125 blood test can be done, but is more useful in detecting the progression of ovarian cancer in women who have the disease.

When cancer is found, treatment includes:

- Surgery. The ovaries, uterus, and fallopian tubes are removed. If the cancer has spread, the surgeon removes as much of the cancer as possible.
- Chemotherapy
- Radiation therapy

### Self-Care:

**Note:** Medical care, not self-care, is needed to treat ovarian cancer.

### Contact Doctor When:

- You have 1 or more warning signs of ovarian cancer listed in this topic.
- You need to schedule yearly pelvic and rectal exams.
- You have a family history of ovarian, colon, breast, prostate, or lung cancer. This is especially true if your mother, sister, or daughter has had ovarian cancer.

18. Women's Health

### Ovarian Cancer, Continued

- You have a personal history of breast, uterine, or rectal cancer.

## For Information Contact:

National Cancer Institute
1-800-4-CANCER (422-6237)
www.nci.nih.gov

## 126. Uterine Cancer

The uterus (womb) is a hollow, pear-shaped organ in a female's lower abdomen between the bladder and the rectum. Cancer of the uterus most often affects the endometrium, the lining of the uterus, so is also called endometrial cancer. It is the most common reproductive cancer in women. Most women diagnosed with uterine cancer are between the ages of 50 and 70. When found and treated early, though, more than 90% of cases can be cured.

## Signs & Symptoms

- Abnormal bleeding, spotting, or discharge from the vagina is the most common symptom.

- Any vaginal bleeding or spotting after menopause. The bleeding can begin as a watery, blood-streaked discharge. Later it can contain more blood.

**Note:** Some cases of uterine cancer can be detected by a Pap test, but this is used to detect cervical cancer. Even if you have had a recent normal Pap test, see your doctor if you have post menopausal vaginal bleeding.

Cancer of the uterus does not often occur before menopause. It can occur around the time menopause begins, though. When bleeding stops and starts up again, let your doctor know. If you are on hormone replacement therapy, you may have regular cyclic bleeding.

## Causes, Risk Factors & Care

The risk for uterine cancer is greater if you have had increased exposure to estrogen from one or more of the following:

- Late menopause or early menstruation

- Irregular periods or ovulation

- Polycystic ovarian disease. The ovaries become enlarged and contain many cysts due to hormone imbalances.

- Obesity. Women who are obese make more estrogen.

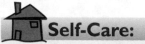

### *Uterine Cancer, Continued*

- Estrogen replacement therapy (ERT). (See "Hormone Replacement Therapy (HRT)" on page 342.) {**Note:** Estrogen-only replacement therapy increases the risk slightly for uterine cancer. This is why hormone replacement with estrogen and progesterone is often recommended.}

Other risk factors include:

- A history of infertility
- A history of endometrial hyperplasia. This is abnormal thickening of the endometrium.
- A history of breast, colon, or ovarian cancer
- Diabetes

Treatment includes one or more of the following:

- Surgery. Most women have a total hysterectomy. This removes the uterus, cervix, fallopian tubes, and ovaries.
- Radiation therapy
- Chemotherapy
- Hormonal therapy

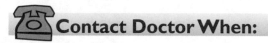

## Self-Care:

Medical care, not self-care, is needed for uterine cancer.

## Contact Doctor When:

- You have any signs and symptoms of uterine cancer listed on page 348.
- You need to schedule your yearly pelvic exam.

## For Information Contact:

National Cancer Institute
1-800-4-CANCER (422-6237)
www.nci.nih.gov

## 127. Vaginal Problems

A number of vaginal problems occur in women over age 50. Often, the problems are due to changes in the vagina that come with menopause. These include:

- Vaginal dryness
- Thinning of the walls of the vagina
- Loss of elasticity in the muscles in the vagina
- Shrinkage of the labia (external genitals that cover and protect the opening of the vagina)

18. Women's Health

### Vaginal Problems, Continued

These changes can lead to common vaginal problems, such as:

- Pain during and after intercourse
- Vaginitis – vaginal swelling, irritation, and/or infections. (See "Vaginal Problems Chart" below.)

Less common vaginal problems in women over 50 are:

- Sexually transmitted diseases (STDs). (See "STDs Chart" on page 362.)
- Cancer of the vagina, which is rare.

- Abnormal vaginal bleeding (unless still menstruating or on hormone replacement therapy (HRT)

It is common for menstrual periods to be irregular for several years before menopause. This is normal vaginal bleeding. For premenopausal women, the most common causes of abnormal vaginal bleeding, in this order, are: Not ovulating; malignancy; pregnancy; endometriosis; and benign tumors. The most common cause after menopause is malignancy.

The chart below lists signs and symptoms of vaginal problems and what to do about them. {**Note:** All vaginal bleeding that occurs after menstruation has stopped should be evaluated by your doctor.}

## Vaginal Problems Chart

| Signs & Symptoms | What It Could Be | What to Do |
|---|---|---|
| Vaginal bleeding with:<br>- A known bleeding disorder and you also have blood in your urine or stool<br>- Heavy vaginal bleeding after taking a clot dissolving drug for a heart attack or stroke | Hemorrhage | Get immediate care. |

*Vaginal Problems Chart Continued on Next Page*

To Learn More, See Back Cover

18. Women's Health

## Vaginal Problems, Continued

| Vaginal Problems Chart, Continued | | |
|---|---|---|
| **Signs & Symptoms** | **What It Could Be** | **What to Do** |
| Vaginal bleeding after trauma to the abdomen, pelvis, or vagina or vaginal bleeding with any of these problems:<br>▪ Dizziness and very heavy bleeding (you saturate more than 1 full sized pad in an hour's time)<br>▪ Pale and moist skin and a decreased level of consciousness<br>▪ Extreme shortness of breath or a very hard time breathing<br>▪ Severe abdominal pain | Internal injury | Get immediate care. |
| Vaginal bleeding with 2 or more of these problems:<br>▪ Abdominal tenderness and/or bloating<br>▪ Pain in the pelvis or back<br>▪ Pain during intercourse<br>▪ Skin on your abdomen feels sensitive<br>▪ Vaginal discharge with abnormal color or odor<br>▪ Change in menstrual flow, if still menstruating<br>▪ Fever, chills | Pelvic Inflammatory Disease (PID). This is an infection of the uterus, fallopian tubes, and/or ovaries. | Contact doctor. |

*Vaginal Problems Chart Continued on Next Page*

18. Women's Health

## Vaginal Problems, Continued

| Vaginal Problems Chart, Continued | | |
| --- | --- | --- |
| **Signs & Symptoms** | **What It Could Be** | **What to Do** |
| Vaginal bleeding after menopause (unless on estrogen replacement therapy (ERT) | Infection of the cervix, uterus, or vagina. Cervical, uterine, or vaginal cancer. | Contact doctor. Follow guidelines in "Cervical Cancer" on page 340 and "Uterine Cancer" on page 348. |
| Abnormal vaginal bleeding with: <br>• Mild itching and burning around the vagina <br>• Burning or pain when urinating or urinating more often <br>• A vaginal discharge with abnormal color <br>• Abdominal discomfort | Gonorrhea or similar sexually transmitted disease (STD) | Contact doctor. See "Gonorrhea" on page 364. |
| Sores and/or painful blisters in the genital area and sometimes on the thighs or buttocks | Genital herpes | Contact doctor. See "Genital Herpes" on page 362. |
| • Vaginal itching, burning, and redness <br>• Greenish-yellow vaginal discharge <br>• Burning or pain when urinating | Trichomoniasis | Contact doctor. See "Trichomoniasis" on page 366. |

*Vaginal Problems Chart Continued on Next Page*

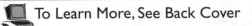 To Learn More, See Back Cover

## Vaginal Problems, Continued

### Vaginal Problems Chart, Continued

| Signs & Symptoms | What It Could Be | What to Do |
|---|---|---|
| ▪ Mild vaginal irritation or burning<br>▪ A watery, grayish white, or yellow vaginal discharge with a fishy odor | Bacterial vaginosis. This is an infection from one or more types of bacteria that may or may not be sexually transmitted. | Contact doctor. |
| Vaginal dryness, irritation, itching, and burning | Atrophic vaginitis. This is caused by a decrease in estrogen. | Contact doctor. See "Care" for "Atrophic Vaginitis" on page 354. |
| ▪ Itching, irritation, and redness around the vagina<br>▪ Thick, white vaginal discharge that looks like cottage cheese and may smell like yeast<br>▪ Burning and/or pain when urinating or with sex | Vaginal yeast infection | Use self-care. (See "Care" and "Self-Care/Prevention" for "Vaginal Yeast Infections" on page 354. |
| Itching and redness in the outer genital area without other symptoms | Vaginitis from contact dermatitis | Use self-care. See "Care" and "Self-Care/Prevention" for "Contact Dermatitis in the Vaginal Area" on pages 354 and 355. |

18. Women's Health

*Vaginal Problems, Continued*

## Care

Medical treatment depends on the cause.

### For Atrophic Vaginitis:

Use a prescribed estrogen cream or prescribed estrogen pills.

### For Bacterial Vaginosis:

Use a prescribed antibiotic cream or gel or prescribed antibiotic pills.

### For a Vaginal Yeast Infection:

It is important, though, to make sure that you have the right problem diagnosed. A burning sensation could be a symptom of a urinary tract infection caused by bacteria, which requires an antibiotic. Antibiotics will not help yeast infections. They make them worse. Trichomoniasis mimics yeast infections, too. (See "Trichomoniasis" on page 366.)

Chronic vaginal infections can be one of the first signs of diabetes, sexually transmitted diseases, or HIV in women.

Self-care measures treat most vaginal yeast infections. Your doctor can prescribe a vaginal cream or suppositories or an oral antifungal medicine, such as Diflucan.

### For a Severe Case of Contact Dermatitis in the Vaginal Area:

Use an ointment prescribed by your doctor.

Other medical treatments are treating the specific cause, such as STDs (see page 362), cervical cancer (see page 340), and uterine cancer (see page 348).

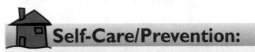

## Self-Care/Prevention:

### For a Vaginal Yeast Infection or Bacterial Vaginosis:

- Bathe or shower often. Clean the inside folds of the vulva. Dry the vaginal area well.

- Wipe from front to back after using the toilet.

- Wear all-cotton underwear.

- Don't wear garments that are tight in the crotch.

- Change underwear and workout clothes right away after sweating.

- If you still menstruate, use unscented tampons or sanitary pads and change them often.

- Don't use bath oils, bubble baths, feminine hygiene sprays, or perfumed or deodorant soaps.

*Continued on Next Page*

18. Women's Health

## Vaginal Problems, Continued

### Self-Care/Prevention, Continued

- Don't sit around in a wet bathing suit.

- Shower after you swim in a pool to remove the chlorine from your skin. Dry the vaginal area well.

- Eat well. Include foods that contain live cultures of "lactobacillus acidophilus," such as yogurt. If you can't tolerate yogurt, take an over-the-counter product that contains lactobacillus acidophilus.

- Let your doctor know if you tend to get yeast infections whenever you take an antibiotic. He or she may have you also take a vaginal antifungal agent.

### When You Have a Vaginal Yeast Infection:

- Use an over-the-counter product for vaginal yeast infections, such as Monistat, Gyne-Lotrimin, etc.

- Douche with a mild solution of 1 to 3 tablespoons of vinegar mixed in 1 quart of warm water. Repeat only once a day (up to 7 days) until the symptoms subside. Don't do this if you are pregnant or if you have a sexually transmitted disease.

- Limit sugar and foods with sugar.

### For Vaginal Dryness and Painful Intercourse:

- Don't use deodorant soaps or scented products in the vaginal area.

- Use a water soluble lubricant, such as K-Y Jelly, Replens, etc. Avoid oils or petroleum-based products.

- Use an estrogen cream for the vagina. Your doctor needs to prescribe this.

- Keep sexually active.

- Don't use antihistamines, unless truly needed.

### For Contact Dermatitis in the Vaginal Area:

- Avoid products that cause the problem (scented items, douches, etc.)

- Apply an over-the-counter hydrocortisone cream to the affected area. Use this infrequently, though. Hydrocortisone can, itself, lead to thinning of the vaginal tissue. Follow package directions.

- Put a cool compress on the affected area.

- Wash your underwear in a gentle detergent. Rinse it twice. Use only plain water for the second rinse. Don't use a fabric softener.

**18. Women's Health**

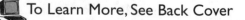

Sexual health is a part of overall health. Safe sex is good for both the body and the mind. Having sex on a regular basis helps maintain sexual function. Sexual health is more than having safe sex, though. It means feeling close or intimate with a partner. There are many ways to feel intimate. Sex is one of them. Hugging, kissing, and touching are others. Most older people want and are able to enjoy an active, satisfying sex life. This chapter covers changes in sexuality that come with aging. It gives tips for sexual health in later years. It also covers sexually transmitted diseases (STDs).

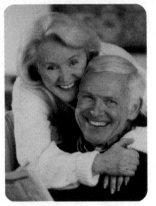

# 128. Sexual Changes with Aging

**Physical Changes For Men:**

- It may take longer to get an erection and to ejaculate.

- Erections may not be as hard or as large as in earlier years.

- The feeling that an ejaculation is about to happen may be shorter.

- After an ejaculation, more time needs to pass to get a second erection.

- Some males find they need more manual stimulation.

- The chances for impotence (see page 328) increase.

**Physical Changes For Women:**

- The vagina is drier. The walls of the vagina get thinner and less elastic. These things can make sex uncomfortable.

- It may take longer to feel aroused.

- Orgasms can be shorter or less intense than in years past.

**Changes from Health Conditions:**

For males and females, sexual health can be affected by a number of conditions. These include:

- Medicines. Antidepressants, tranquilizers, and certain high blood pressure medicines can slow you down and lower your sex drive. Ask your doctor if medicines you take affect your sexual response.

- Alcohol. Too much alcohol can reduce potency in men and delay orgasm in women. Limit alcohol to 1 drink per day, if any.

## *Sexual Changes with Aging, Continued*

- Heart attacks. Many people who have had a heart attack are afraid that having sex will cause another attack. The risk of this is very low. Follow your doctor's advice.

- Stroke. Sexual function is rarely damaged by a stroke and it is unlikely that an erection will cause another stroke. Using different positions or medical devices can help make up for any weakness or paralysis.

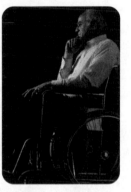

- Diabetes. Most men with diabetes do not have problems, but it is one of the few illnesses that can cause impotence (see page 328).

- Arthritis. Joint pain due to arthritis can limit sexual activity. In some cases, medicines can decrease sexual desire. Exercise, rest, warm baths, and changing the position or timing of sexual activity can be helpful.

- HIV and STDs. Anyone who is sexually active can be at risk for being infected with HIV and STDs. See "Prevention" in "HIV/AIDS" on page 294 and "Prevention" in "Basic Facts About STDs" on page 360.

- Cancer. Sexuality may suffer after cancer treatment. There are physical side effects of radiation therapy and chemotherapy on sexual desire and performance. Sexual expression may need to be put on hold during treatment, but touching and intimacy are still needed.

- Surgery. Surgery that involves the sex organs, such as hysterectomy, and prostatectomy can reduce the desire for sex. The good news is that most people do return to the kind of sex life they enjoyed before having surgery.

- Parkinson's disease or any condition in which symptoms or medicines' side effects affect sexual function. Ask your doctor for advice.

### Emotional Changes:

This country's emphasis on physical beauty and youth can interfere with feeling sexual. How people feel can affect what they are able to do.

- As persons age, they may feel more anxious about their appearance or ability to perform. This can interfere with the ability to enjoy sex.

- Not having a partner through choice, divorce, or death may make it difficult to deal with sexual feelings. Masturbation can bring sexual pleasure, but persons who have been taught that it is wrong are reluctant to do it.

19. Sexual Health

### *Sexual Changes with Aging, Continued*

- A lack of sexual desire can result in having sex less often. This may be due to lower hormone levels that come with aging, and to factors such as fatigue, stress, etc.

Some changes that come with aging can result in positive emotional changes:

- After menopause, both men and women may feel less anxious about having sex because they don't have to worry about a pregnancy. They may have sex more often if they chose not to have sex when the women menstruated.

- A woman may get more sexual pleasure due to having a drier, thinner, and smaller vagina which allows her to feel more friction and stimulation during sex.

- A couple may have more time and privacy for sex if their children are grown and spend less, if any, time at home.

### Self-Care:

**Tips for Sexual Health:**

- Have sex often. The more you do it, the more you will be able to.

- Express your needs. Let your partner express his or her needs, too. Talk about your fears, fantasies, etc.

- Spend more time on foreplay. Let your partner know where and how you want to be touched.

- Take the pressure off your partner. Tell him or her that you know sex can take longer. Express your need for intimacy, not just performance.

- Avoid or limit alcohol. A little alcohol can act as an aphrodisiac. Too much can interfere with sex and lead to unsafe sex.

- Ask your doctor or pharmacist if any medicines you take can affect your sex life. Find out if another medicine can be used without this side effect.

- Have sex when you are less tired, such as is in the morning.

- Stay as physically fit as you can. This allows more energy for sex.

- Plan time for sex, and being together. This promotes intimacy.
  - Make a point to spend at least 15 minutes of uninterrupted time with your partner each day.
  - Express your affection for each other every day.

*Continued on Next Page*

To Learn More, See Back Cover

**19. Sexual Health**

## Sexual Changes with Aging, Continued

### Self-Care, Continued

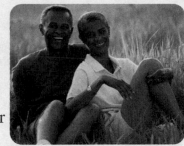

- Plan to spend part of a day alone together at least once a week. Make a date to take a walk in the park, go out for dinner, or share other activities you both enjoy.

- Schedule a weekend away together when you can.

- Go to bed at the same time.

■ Follow your doctor's advice for a chronic illness, if you have one, to help prevent possible problems with sexual satisfaction.

■ Practice safe sex to prevent sexually transmitted diseases. (See page 360.)

■ Give each other a massage or take a shower together.

■ Keep the T.V. out of the bedroom.

### Tips for Men:

■ See "Care" and "Prevention/Self-Care" for "Impotence" on pages 328 and 329.

■ Talk to your doctor about your concerns. Be open and honest.

### Tips for Women:

■ Discuss hormone replacement therapy (HRT) with your doctor. (See page 342.) Estrogen can help with vaginal dryness. It can help thicken the walls of the vagina.

■ Use a water-soluble lubricant, such as K-Y Jelly, Replens, etc. Don't use oil or petroleum-based products. These encourage infection.

■ Remain sexually active. Having sex often may lessen the chance of having the vagina constrict, helps keep natural lubrication, and maintains pelvic muscle tone. This includes reaching orgasm with a partner or alone.

■ Avoid using antihistamines unless truly necessary. They dry mucus membranes in the body.

■ Don't use deodorant soaps or scented products in the vaginal area.

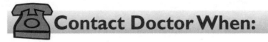

## Contact Doctor When:

■ You have pain or bleeding during sex.

■ You have signs and symptoms of an STD. (See "STDs Chart" on page 362.)

19. Sexual Health

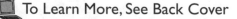

*Sexual Changes with Aging, Continued*

- You have sexual problems due to impotence (see on page 328).

- You have sexual problems due to an illness, surgery, or injury.

- You continue to have sexual problems after using self-care.

# 129. Basic Facts About STDs

Sexually transmitted diseases (STDs) are infections that pass from one person to another through sexual contact. Sexual contact includes vaginal, anal, and oral sex.

The most common STDs, in the U.S., in this order, are:

- Chlamydia
- Trichomoniasis
- Gonorrhea
- Genital Warts
- Genital Herpes
- Hepatitis B
- Syphilis
- HIV/AIDS

For information on Hepatitis B, see pages 291 and 292. For information on HIV/AIDS, see page 294. For information on the rest of the STDs listed above, see STDs Chart on page 362.

## Who Gets STDs?

Men and women of all ages who are sexually active, can get an STD. Every year, more than 12 million cases of STDs are reported in the U.S. One in 5 Americans carries an STD. Women are at greater risk for an STD from male/female intercourse than are men. More than 1 STD can be present at the same time. Gonorrhea and chlamydia, for example, can be picked up at the same time.

## Prevention

- There's only one way to guarantee you'll never get a sexually transmitted disease. Never have sex.

- Limiting your sexual activity to one person your entire life is a close second, provided your partner is also monogamous and neither of you have an STD.

- Avoid sexual contact with persons whose health status and practices are not known.

To Learn More, See Back Cover

19. Sexual Health

## Basic Facts About STDs, Continued

- Discuss a new partner's sexual history with him or her before beginning a sexual relationship. Be aware, though, that people are not always honest about their sexual history.

- Latex condoms for men and the female Reality condom can reduce the spread of STDs when used properly and carefully for every sex act. They do not eliminate the risk entirely.

- Plan ahead for safe sex. Practice what you'll say.

- Unless they are in a monogamous relationship in which neither partner has an STD, both women and men should carry latex condoms and insist that they be used every time they have sexual relations. Using spermicidal foams, jellies, or creams (especially those that contain Nonoxynol-9) and a diaphragm, can offer additional protection when used with a condom. Use water-based lubricants, such as K-Y Brand Jelly. Don't use oil-based or "petroleum" ones, such as Vaseline. They can damage latex condoms.

The female condom is shaped like the male condom, but is larger. It is made of polyurethane. This is thinner and stronger than latex. It is placed inside the vagina like a lining.

- Wash the genitals with soap and water before and after sexual intercourse.

- Ask your doctor to check for STDs every 6 months if you have multiple sex partners, even if you don't have any symptoms.

- Don't have sex while under the influence of drugs or alcohol (except in a monogamous relationship in which neither partner has an STD). These lower your inhibitions and can make you more prone to unsafe sex.

### Fast Response Counts

If you suspect you have an STD or know your partner is infected, see a doctor as soon as possible. Your sexual partner(s) should also be contacted and treated.

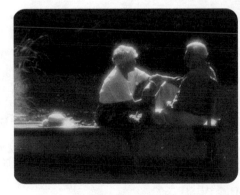

### Repeat Episodes

Once you've had an STD, you can get it again. You can't develop an immunity once you've been exposed.

# 130. STDs Chart

## Chlamydia

**Signs & Symptoms For Women:**

75% of women have few or no symptoms. When present, symptoms show up 2 to 4 weeks after infection and include:

- Slight yellowish-green vaginal discharge
- Vaginal irritation
- Need to urinate often and pain or burning feeling when urinating
- Abdominal pain

**Signs & Symptoms For Men:**

25% of men have few or no symptoms. When present, symptoms show up 2 to 4 weeks after infection and include:

- White discharge from the penis
- Burning or discomfort when urinating
- Pain in the scrotum

**Causes**

Specific bacterial infection

**Treatment**

- Oral antibiotics for the infected person and his or her partner(s).
- Avoiding sex until treatment is completed in the infected person and his or her partner(s).

## Genital Herpes

**Signs & Symptoms For Women and Men:**

- Sores with blisters on the genital area and anus and sometimes on the thighs and buttocks.
- Itching, irritation, and tingling in the genital area can occur 1 to 2 days before the outbreak of the blisters or sores. This is known as the prodrome.
- After a few days, the blisters break open and leave painful, shallow ulcers which can last from 5 days to 3 weeks.
- With the initial attacks, there may be flu-like symptoms (swollen glands, fever, body aches). Subsequent attacks are almost always milder and shorter.

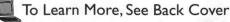 To Learn More, See Back Cover

19. Sexual Health

## STDs Chart, Continued

### Genital Herpes, Continued

- Attacks may be triggered by stress, fatigue, other illnesses, and vigorous sexual intercourse.

### Causes

- Herpes simplex virus type 1 or type 2. Either one can cause genital herpes, but type 2 is the common cause. Type 1 most often affects the oral area, showing up as fever blisters or cold sores. Oral sex can spread herpes to the mouth, lips, and throat.

- Genital herpes is contagious when blisters are present and up to 2 weeks after they are gone.

### Treatment

- There is no cure. Once infected, the virus remains with you forever. Symptoms occur, though, only during flare-ups.

- Antiviral medicine
- Self-care measures

### Self-Care

- Take a hot bath if you can tolerate it. This may help to inactivate the virus and promote healing.

- Bathe the affected genital area twice a day with mild soap and water. Gently pat dry with a towel or use a hair dryer set on warm. Using a colloidal oatmeal soap or bath may also be soothing.

- Use sitz baths to soak the affected area. You can get a sitz bath basin from medical supply or drug stores.

- Apply ice packs on the affected genital area for 5 to 10 minutes to relieve itching and swelling.

- Wear loose fitting pants or skirts. Don't wear pantyhose. Wear cotton, not nylon underwear.

- Squirt tepid water over the genital area while urinating to help with pain.

- Take a mild pain reliever. (See "Pain relievers" in "Your Home Pharmacy" on page 43.)

- Ask your doctor about using a local anesthetic ointment, such as Lidocaine during the most painful part of an attack.

- To avoid spreading the virus to your eyes, don't touch your eyes during an outbreak.

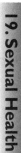

19. Sexual Health

*STDs Chart, Continued*

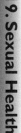

**19. Sexual Health**

## Genital Warts

### Signs & Symptoms

Often, there are no visible signs or symptoms. When present, warts:

- Can be soft or hard; pink, red, or yellow-gray in color

- Are inside the vagina, on the lips of the vagina or around the anus in women

- Are on the penis, inside the head of the penis, on the scrotum, or around the anus in men

- Appear 3 weeks to 6 months after being infected

### Causes

Human Papilloma Virus (HPV). There are about 25 types that can infect the genital area. Certain types increase the risk for cervical cancer in women.

### Treatment

- There is no cure.

- The warts can be removed medically by cryosurgery (freezing them); an acidic chemical that burns them; or laser surgery

- Women with a history of genital warts should get a Pap test every 6 months to check for cervical cancer.

## Gonorrhea

### Signs & Symptoms For Women:

Sixty to 80% have no symptoms. When present, they appear 2 to 10 days after infection and include:

- Mild vaginal itching and burning

- Thick, yellow-green vaginal discharge

- Burning when urinating

- Severe pain in lower abdomen

### Signs & Symptoms For Men:

- Pain at the tip of the penis

- Pain and burning during urination

- Thick, yellow, cloudy, penile discharge that gradually increases

 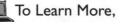

*STDs Chart, Continued*

| Gonorrhea, Continued | |
|---|---|
| **Causes** Specific bacterial infection. Can spread to joints, tendons, or the heart if not treated. In women, can cause pelvic inflammatory disease (PID). | **Treatment**<br>▪ Antibiotics<br>▪ Pain relievers<br>▪ Treating sexual partner(s) to avoid re-infection<br>▪ Follow-up cultures to determine if the treatment was effective |

## Syphilis

**Signs & Symptoms**

Three stages of progression:

▪ Primary stage. A large, painless, ulcer-like sore known as a chancre occurs 2 to 6 weeks after infection and generally appears around the area of sexual contact. The chancre disappears within a few weeks.

▪ Secondary stage. Within a month after the end of the primary stage, a widespread skin rash appears, on the palms of the hands, soles of the feet, and sometimes around the mouth and nose. The rash commonly has small, red, scaly bumps that do not itch. Other types of rashes, swollen lymph nodes, fever, and flu-like symptoms may also occur. Small patches of hair may fall out of the scalp, beard, eyelashes, and eyebrows.

▪ Latent stage. Once syphilis reaches this stage, it may go unnoticed for years, quietly damaging the heart, central nervous system, muscles, and various other organs and tissues. The resulting effects are often fatal.

**Causes**

Specific bacterial infection. Can lead to heart failure, blindness, dementia, or death, if not treated. {**Note:** An elderly person with signs of dementia should be evaluated for syphilis.}

19. Sexual Health

## STDs Chart, Continued

| Syphilis, Continued | |
|---|---|
| **Treatment**<br>■ Antibiotics (usually penicillin). If allergic to penicillin, another antibiotic can be taken. | ■ After treatment, a blood test is taken at 3, 6, and 12 months to be sure the disease is completely cured.<br>■ Once treatment is complete, you're no longer contagious. |

## Trichomoniasis

**Signs & Symptoms For Women:**

The parasite can be present in the vagina for years without causing symptoms. If they do occur, typical symptoms include:

■ Vaginal itching and burning

■ A yellow-green vaginal discharge

■ Burning or pain when urinating

■ Painful sexual intercourse

■ Pain during intercourse

■ Discomfort when urinating

**Signs & Symptoms For Men:**

Symptoms are not usually present. Men may infect their sexual partners and not know it. When present, symptoms include:

■ Discomfort when urinating

■ Pain during intercourse

■ Irritation and itching of the penis

**Causes**

A parasite

**Treatment**

■ The oral medication metronidazole (Flagyl). {**Note:** Don't drink alcohol for 24 hours before, during, and 24 hours after taking metronidazole. The combination causes vomiting, dizziness, and headaches.}

■ Treating sexual partners to prevent re-infection and spreading the infection further.

To Learn More, See Back Cover

19. Sexual Health

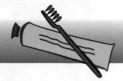

## 131. Teeth & Mouth Changes with Aging

As you age, changes occur with your teeth and mouth. Common changes are:

- Fewer taste buds on your tongue, especially for sugary and salty foods, but not for bitter tasting foods.

- Drier mouth. The tissues in your mouth get thinner and tend to hold less moisture. This makes your mouth more dry. Some medications can add to the problem. Examples are water pills, some antidepressants, and antihistamines. (See "Dry Mouth" on page 373.)

- Gum problems. Your gums may recede. This exposes the roots of your teeth and can promote cavities. (See "Periodontal Disease" on page 374.)

- Loss of natural teeth. Proper care of your teeth can prevent this. (See "Get Regular Dental Care" on page 19.) In persons over age 40, the number one cause of tooth loss is periodontal (gum) disease (see page 374).

More than half of persons over age 50 have at least one tooth replaced. A tooth or teeth can be replaced as crowns, bridges, partial or full dentures. Dental implants are another option.

## 132. Bad Breath

Bad breath (halitosis) is a social concern. It can also be a health issue.

### Prevention

- Practice good oral hygiene. (See "Get Regular Dental Care" on page 19.)

- If you wear dentures, clean and care for them as directed by your dentist.

- Don't smoke. Limit or avoid alcohol.

- Drink plenty of water and other liquids to prevent dry mouth.

### Signs & Symptoms

- A bad odor from the mouth. To detect this, wipe the back of your tongue with a piece of white, sterile gauze. After 5 minutes, smell the gauze for an odor.

- Unpleasant taste in the mouth

- You are told you have bad breath.

### Causes, Risk Factors & Care

Common causes of bad breath are:

- Bacteria on the back of the tongue

- Tooth and mouth problems, such as tooth decay or abscesses, infected gums, canker sores, etc.

20. Dental & Mouth Problems

## Bad Breath, *Continued*

- The strong odors of foods like garlic, onions, hot peppers, anchovies, deli meats, such as salami, and cheeses, such as blue cheese

- Smoking, alcohol, and mouthwashes with a high alcohol content.

- Poor oral hygiene or ill-fitting dentures

- Dry mouth (see page 373) or conditions that lead to it. "Morning breath" can be due to a dry mouth when you wake up.

Less often, bad breath is due to another condition such as an upper respiratory or sinus infection, or indigestion.

Most cases of bad breath can be treated with "Prevention" and "Self-Care", listed in this topic. If not, your dentist can prescribe special toothpastes, mouth rinses, brushes, tongue scrapers, and an antimicrobial solution.

### Self-Care:

Follow tips under "Prevention" and:

- Use a baking soda toothpaste. Brush your teeth and tongue. Carry a toothbrush and toothpaste with you to use after eating when you are not at home.

- If you can't brush after a meal, rinse your mouth with water.

- After eating, chew parsley, mint leaves, celery, or carrots.

- Try chlorophyll tablets.

- Don't rely on mouthwash or mints. They mask bad breath and contribute to it because they dry out the mouth.

- Eat at regular times. Eat nutritious foods. Limit sugary foods.

- Chew sugarless gum, suck on a sugarless mint, or suck on lemon or other citrus drops. These stimulate saliva secretion. Saliva helps deal with bacteria on the teeth and washes away food particles.

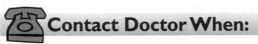

### Contact Doctor When:

- You have any of these problems with bad breath:
  - Bleeding, swelling, or pain in the mouth or throat
  - Indigestion, weight loss
  - Chronic cough
  - Digestion problems
  - Puffy, reddened gums

- You still have bad breath after using "Prevention" and "Self-Care" measures in this topic for 2 weeks.

**20. Dental & Mouth Problems**

# 133. Broken or Knocked Out Tooth

## Prevention

- Don't chew ice, pens, or pencils.
- Don't use your teeth to pry things open.
- If you smoke a pipe, don't bite down on the stem.
- If you grind your teeth at night, ask your dentist about a bite plate.
- If you play contact sports, wear a protective mouth guard.
- Wear a seat belt when riding in a car.
- Avoid sucking on lemons or chewing aspirin or vitamin C tablets. The acid wears away tooth enamel.

## Signs & Symptoms

- Loss of a tooth or part of a tooth
- Nicked or chipped tooth or teeth

## Causes & Care

A blow to the mouth or other injury or a strain on a tooth, such as from biting on a hard object can cause a tooth to be broken, knocked out, or chipped.

When a tooth gets knocked out, go to the dentist as soon as possible. Keep the tooth moist until you get to the dentist.

Your dentist may be able to reinsert the tooth if you get treatment within hours. Follow up treatment is also needed.

### Self-Care/First Aid:

**For a Broken Tooth:**

- To reduce swelling, apply a cold compress to the area.
- Save any broken tooth fragments and take them to the dentist.

**If Your Tooth has been Knocked Out:**

- Rinse the tooth with clear water.
- If possible, gently put it back in the socket or hold it under your tongue. Otherwise, put the tooth in a glass of milk or a wet cloth.
- If the gum is bleeding, hold a gauze pad, a clean handkerchief, or tissue tightly in place over the wound.

### Get Immediate Care When:

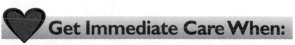

One or more teeth have been broken or knocked out. Try to get to a dentist within 30 minutes of the accident, if you can.

20. Dental & Mouth Problems

# Oral Cancer Warning Signs

The "Oral Cancer Warning Signs," listed below, can help detect oral cancer. See a doctor or dentist if you have any signs of oral cancer for 2 weeks. Any of these signs may be caused by oral cancer or by other, less serious problems. Don't wait for something to hurt. Pain is not usually an early symptom of oral cancer.

- A sore in the mouth that does not heal
- A lump or thickening in the cheek
- A white or red patch on the gums, tongue, or lining of the mouth
- Soreness or a feeling that something is caught in the throat
- A hard time chewing or swallowing
- A hard time moving the jaw or tongue
- Numbness of the tongue or other area of the mouth; swelling of the jaw that causes dentures to fit poorly or become uncomfortable

# 134. Canker Sores

Canker sores are small, round mouth sores in the lining of the mouth or on the tongue, gums, or lips. You can have 1 canker sore or a group of them.

## Prevention

- Avoid things that irritate the mouth, such as hot drinks and sharp objects.
- Use a toothbrush with soft bristles. Don't brush too hard.
- Use a toothpaste without sodium lauryl sulfate.
- Take a daily vitamin/mineral supplement as advised by your doctor.

## Signs & Symptoms

- A burning or tingling feeling before the sore appears
- Red-rimmed, shallow sores in the mouth
- Discomfort when you eat and talk

## Causes, Risk Factors & Care

Canker sores may be caused by any tear in the mouth's lining, from an uneven tooth, rough tooth brushing, dental work, a burn from a hot drink or food, etc. Vitamin/mineral deficiencies, emotional stress, and family traits may also trigger canker sores.

To Learn More, See Back Cover

## Canker Sores, Continued

Canker sores heal within 1 to 2 weeks. Self-care can help with symptoms and speed up healing. If needed, a mouthwash with tetracycline and/or an oral paste (amelxanox) can be prescribed.

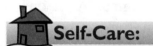

### Self-Care:

#### To Relieve Pain:

- Mix $\frac{1}{2}$ tsp. salt in 1 cup of warm water. Rinse the mouth with an ounce of this mixture 4 times a day. Don't swallow the water.

- Put ice on the canker sore or suck on a frozen popsicle.

- Avoid spicy foods and acidic drinks, like citrus juices.

- Use over-the-counter products, like Anbesol, Blistex, and aloe vera gel.

- Swish Mylanta or milk of magnesia around the mouth to coat the sore. Then spit the medicine out.

- Put the gel from a vitamin E capsule on the sore several times a day.

- Take an over-the-counter pain medicine. (See "Pain relievers" in "Your Home Pharmacy" on page 43.)

### Contact Doctor When:

- You have any of these problems with the canker sore:
  - Fever and/or swollen glands
  - Severe pain
  - A sore on the roof of the mouth or white spots in the mouth that do not heal in 1 to 2 weeks

- A canker sore disturbs your sleep or does not allow you to eat.

- A canker sore appears only after you start a new medicine.

- A canker sore has not healed after 3 weeks.

## 135. Cold Sores

Cold sores appear on or near the lips. They are painful and unpleasant. Nearly 1 in 3 people will have them. Cold sores are also called fever blisters.

### Prevention

To avoid getting or spreading cold sores:

- Don't share drinking glasses, towels, or cooking utensils.

- Don't touch cold sores with your fingers. If you do touch the cold sores, do not touch your eyes. This could cause a serious eye infection.

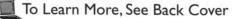 
**20. Dental & Mouth Problems**

## Cold Sores, *Continued*

- Wash your hands often.
- Avoid kissing or direct skin contact with the sores. This includes oral sex. The virus that causes cold sores can cause genital herpes, too.
- When in the sun, wear a hat and use a sunblock with a sun-protective factor (SPF) of 15 or more on the lips.
- Use a lip balm on cold or windy days.
- Ask your doctor about a prescribed antiviral medicine to take or apply when you feel a cold sore coming on.
- Try to figure out what triggers the sores. Once you identify a trigger, do what you can to avoid it.
- Get regular exercise.

## Signs & Symptoms

- Tingling feeling on or near the lips for 36 to 48 hours before the sore appears.
- Itching at the site (early sign)
- Small, red blisters with pus-filled centers
- Blisters form a yellow crust that lasts about 10 days
- One sore or a cluster of sores

## Causes, Risk Factors & Care

Cold sores are caused by the herpes simplex virus, either Type 1 (this is most often the cause) or Type 2 (the usual cause of genital herpes). A fever, cold, stress, cold or windy weather, and strong sun exposure are triggers for the virus.

Cold sores are very contagious. A person is at risk of catching them from another person or can re-infect themselves. You are able to spread the infection to others as soon as you begin to feel itching and/or tingling at the site and as long as the blisters are wet

At the first sign of cold sores use self-care. Prompt treatment may reduce the discomfort.

### Self-Care:

- Keep the sore clean and dry.
- Apply antiviral medication, if prescribed, to the affected area at the first sign of a cold sore or gently rub aloe vera on the sore.
- Apply ice to the sore or suck on frozen popsicles.
- Take an over-the-counter medicine for pain. (See "Pain relievers" in "Your Home Pharmacy" on page 43.)

*Continued on Next Page*

*Cold Sores, Continued*

*Self-Care, Continued*

- Try an over-the-counter treatment, such as Campho-Phenique, Blistex, or make a paste with cornstarch and water. Dab some on the sore with a cotton swab.

- Put witch hazel, alcohol, or petroleum jelly on the sore. Use a cotton swab.

- Learn to relax. Meditate, practice yoga, etc. Learn to deal with stress, too. (See "Manage Stress Checklist" on page 21.)

- Avoid foods that are sour, spicy, or acidic. These may irritate the sores.

- Take vitamin C and/or zinc supplements as directed by your doctor.

- Use cool compresses when the sores have crusted over.

- Try not to worry or be too self-conscious. This only makes the situation worse.

## Contact Doctor When:

- You have eye pain with the cold sore.
- Pain from the sore limits normal activity.
- The cold sore has lasted longer than 2 weeks.

- Cold sores appear 4 or more times a year.

- Cold sores appeared after you started a new medicine or are present while taking steroid medicines.

- Eczema (see page 125) occurs with cold sores.

## 136. Dry Mouth

Dry mouth is an abnormal dryness of the mucus membranes in the mouth. This happens when there isn't enough saliva or the composition of the saliva changes. Dry mouth is common in the elderly.

## Signs & Symptoms

- Dry, parched feeling in the mouth
- Lack of saliva
- Problems with talking and/or swallowing
- Lessened taste
- Bad breath
- Burning sensation in the mouth
- Dry mouth is worse after sleeping

## Causes, Risk Factors & Care

Dry mouth can be due to a side effect of many medications. These include antidepressants, antihistamines, water pills, and medicines for high blood pressure.

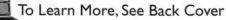 
20. Dental & Mouth Problems

## Dry Mouth, *Continued*

Dry mouth can also result from many health conditions. These include nasal congestion, gum disease, diabetes, stroke, and Sjögren's syndrome, an autoimmune disorder.

Treatment is aimed at relief and/or treating the underlying cause. If not treated, dry mouth may lead to severe tooth decay, infection, and poor nutrition.

### Self-Care:

- Try an over-the-counter artificial saliva, such as Xerolube.
- Avoid caffeine and alcohol.
- Have regular dental checkups.
- Drink at least 8 glasses of water each day. Avoid drinks with sugar.
- Avoid salty, spicy, or acidic foods.
- Don't use tobacco products.
- Chew sugarfree gum, suck on sugarfree candies and suckers.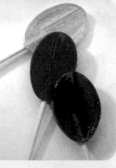
- Take a multivitamin that your doctor recommends.

- Use a humidifier in the bedroom.
- Keep your lips moist with lip balm.
- Breathe through your nose, not your mouth.
- Do not use mouthwashes with alcohol.
- Read about the side effects of medicines.

### Contact Doctor When:

- You have any of these problems with dry mouth:
  - Dry, burning eyes
  - Chewing or swallowing problems
  - Sore throat
  - Signs of an infection, such as fever and/or redness, or pus in the mouth
- The dry mouth is a chronic problem or there are marked changes on the tongue.

# 137. Periodontal (Gum) Disease

Periodontal disease refers to conditions that affect structures that surround the teeth. This includes the gums, the ligaments, and the bones.

To Learn More, See Back Cover

### Periodontal Disease, Continued

Sixty-five percent of persons over age 65 will lose one or more teeth due to periodontal disease. Aging itself is not the problem. Years of poor dental hygiene is.

## Signs & Symptoms

- Swollen, red gums that bleed easily. The gums may bleed during eating or teeth brushing.

- Teeth that are exposed at the gum line

- Loose teeth

- Bad breath; foul taste in the mouth

- Pus around the gums and teeth

## Causes, Risk Factors & Care

The cause is a buildup of bacterial plaque at the gumline. With **gingivitis**, the plaque along the gumline infects the tissue. If left untreated, it progresses to **periodontitis**. With this, the plaque builds up in deposits above and below the gumline. This creates pockets between the gums and the teeth. Pus collects in the pockets.

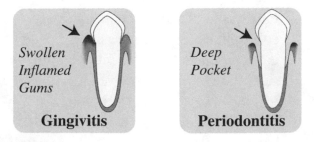

Swollen Inflamed Gums

**Gingivitis**

Deep Pocket

**Periodontitis**

When inflamed, these pockets expand and can hold more bacterial plaque. This breaks down the ligaments and bone that support the teeth.

Risk factors for periodontal disease include:

- Poor dental hygiene

- Smoking or chewing tobacco

- Crooked teeth or poorly-fitted dentures

- Vitamin C and folic acid deficiencies

- Family traits

- Diabetes

- Certain medicines, such as the anticonvulsant, Dilantin

Self-care and regular dental cleanings can prevent and treat many cases of periodontal disease. When these are not enough, your dentist may need to:

- Remove plaque. Deep cleaning is used to remove hardened plaque and infected tissue under the gum and to smooth the damaged root surfaces of the teeth.

- Prescribe medicine, such as Periostat, an antibiotic pill.

- Do periodontal surgery, if needed

- Anchor loose teeth to other teeth

- Pull teeth and replace them with dentures or dental implants

20. Dental & Mouth Problems

## Periodontal Disease, Continued

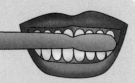

### Self-Care/Prevention:

- You can stop plaque buildup and prevent gum disease by brushing and flossing carefully every day.

  - Gently brush teeth twice a day with a soft nylon brush with rounded ends on the bristles.

  **Proper Brushing**

  - Use small circle motions and short back-and-forth motions.

  - Avoid hard back-and-forth scrubbing.

  - Gently brush your tongue which can trap germs.

  - Use a fluoride toothpaste to protect teeth from decay.

  - Use a piece of dental floss about 18 inches long.

  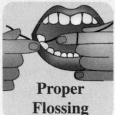

  **Proper Flossing**

  - Using a sawing motion, gently bring the floss through the tight spaces between the teeth.

  - Do not snap the floss against the gums.

  - Curve the floss around each tooth and gently scrape from below the gum to the top of the tooth several times.

  - Rinse your mouth after flossing.

- Check your work. Dental plaque is hard to see unless it is stained. Plaque can be stained by chewing red "disclosing tablets" sold at grocery stores and drug stores or by using a cotton swab to smear green food coloring on the teeth. The color left on the teeth shows where there is still plaque. Extra flossing and brushing will remove this plaque.

- Massage your gums as directed by your dentist. He or she may recommend an irrigating device, such as a Water Pik.

- Eat sugary foods infrequently. When you eat sweets, do so with meals, not in between meals.

- Finish a meal with cheese. This tends to neutralize acid formation.

- Include foods with good sources of vitamin A and vitamin C daily. Vitamin A is found in cantaloupe, broccoli, spinach, winter squash, liver, and dairy products fortified with vitamin A. Good vitamin C food sources include oranges, grapefruit, tomatoes, potatoes, green peppers, and broccoli.

 To Learn More, See Back Cover

## ☎ Contact Doctor When:

- You have signs and symptoms of peri-odontal disease listed on page 375.

- You need to schedule dental cleanings or other appointments as advised by your dentist.

# 138. Toothaches

## Prevention

- Get regular dental check-ups.
- Brush and floss your teeth daily.
- Eat nutritious foods.
- Use fluoridated water and toothpaste with fluoride
- Use a fluoride rinse and/or fluoride supplement (if prescribed)

## Signs & Symptoms

- Ache or pain in a tooth or in the area around the tooth
- Tooth pain after eating or drinking something hot or cold
- Bad breath

- Fever, earache, and/or swollen glands on the side of the face or in the neck. These occur with a tooth abscess, an inflammation and/or infection in the bone and/or tooth canal.

## Causes & Care

Causes for toothaches include:

- A cavity or tooth abscess
- Periodontal disease (see page 374)
- Temporary condition after having corrective dental work
- A food particle, such as a popcorn hull, stuck between the gum and a tooth
- Tooth grinding (bruxism). This can wear down your teeth and cause cracks in them.
- Sinus infection (see page 86)
- **Temporomandibular joint (TMJ) syndrome**. This is a medical condition that occurs when the muscles, joints, and ligaments of the jaw move out of alignment. Symptoms include earaches, headaches, pain in the jaw area that spreads to the face or the neck and shoulders, ringing in the ears, or pain when opening and closing the mouth.
- A symptom of angina (see page 192) or a heart attack (see page 202)

**20. Dental & Mouth Problems**

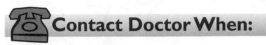

*Toothaches, Continued*

Treatment for a toothache depends on the cause. Self-care can help treat the pain until you see your dentist.

### 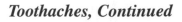 Self-Care:

- Take an over-the-counter pain reliever. (See "Pain relievers" in "Your Home Pharmacy" on page 43.)
- Hold an ice pack on the jaw.
- Never place a crushed aspirin on the tooth. Aspirin burns the gums and destroys tooth enamel.
- Don't drink very hot or cold liquids.
- Don't chew gum.
- Avoid sweets, soft drinks, and hot or spicy foods. These can irritate cavities and increase pain.
- Gargle with warm salt water every hour.
- For a cavity, pack it with a piece of sterile cotton soaked in oil of cloves (available at drug stores).

### Contact Doctor When:

- You have signs and symptoms of an abscessed tooth:
  - Persistent, throbbing, and severe pain
  - Earache, fever, general ill feeling
  - Bad breath and a foul taste in the mouth
  - Swollen glands on one side of the face
- You have any of these problems:
  - Tooth pain
  - Sensitivity to hot, cold, or sweet foods
  - Brown spots or little holes on a tooth
  - A change in your bite – the way your teeth fit together
  - Loose teeth
- You have a toothache only when eating or just after eating.

### Get Immediate Care When:

With the tooth pain, you have signs of a heart attack. (See "Heart Attack Warning Signs" on page 202.)

---

## For Information on Dental Health Contact:

American Dental Association
1-800-621-8099
www.ada.org

---

 To Learn More, See Back Cover

**20. Dental & Mouth Problems**

# SECTION III

## Emergencies

### Introduction

Would you know what to do in a medical crisis? Can you tell:

- If a problem needs emergency care?
- When you should see or call your doctor?
- If you can do first aid measures to take care of the problem?

This section can help you answer these questions.

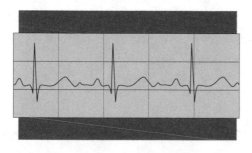

**Emergency Procedures**

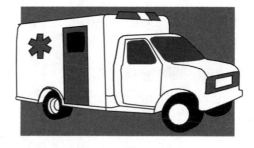

**Emergency Conditions**

## Recognizing Emergencies

Know which symptoms to watch for. According to the American College of Emergency Physicians, the following are warning signs of a medical emergency:

- Difficulty breathing, shortness of breath
- Chest or upper abdominal pain or pressure
- Fainting
- Sudden dizziness, weakness, or change in vision
- Change in mental status such as unusual behavior, confusion, difficulty rousing
- Sudden, severe pain anywhere in the body
- Bleeding that won't stop
- Severe or persistent vomiting
- Coughing up or vomiting blood
- Suicidal or homicidal feelings

Ask your doctor for signs and symptoms other than these that would require emergency care for you.

## Being Ready for Medical Emergencies

- Learn basic first aid skills. Take courses in CPR and first aid. These give hands-on practice in doing first aid the right way. Find out about them from your local:
  - Red Cross
  - American Heart Association
  - National Safety Council
  - Hospital
  - Police and/or fire department
  - Community education department
- Find out what services your health insurance company covers and what procedures you have to follow to get emergency care covered
- Carry the following information with you at all times:
  - Your name, address, phone number, and who to contact if you need emergency care
  - Your health insurance information
  - Important medical information. This could be on a medical alert tag, on a wallet card or on the back of your driver's license.
  - Emergency telephone numbers

## 139. First Aid Precautions

You can get organisms carried in blood that cause diseases, such as hepatitis B virus (HBV) and HIV, the virus that causes AIDS, from an infected victim's blood or other body fluids if they enter your body. These organisms can enter through cuts or breaks in your skin or through the lining of your mouth, nose, and eyes. When you give first aid, take these precautions especially if you don't know the person:

- Wear latex gloves that you can throw away whenever you touch a victim's body fluids, blood, or other

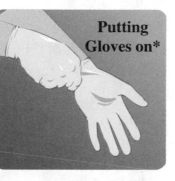

**Putting Gloves on\***

objects that may be soiled with his or her blood. If latex gloves are not available, put a waterproof material, such as a plastic bag, on top of the wound when you apply direct pressure. If possible, have the victim apply pressure to the wound with his or her own hand.

- Cover the victim's open wounds with dressings, extra gauze, or waterproof material.

- Use a mouth-to-mouth barrier device when you do rescue breathing. The victim could have blood in the mouth.

- Wash your hands with soap and water right away.

- Report every incident in which you are exposed to a victim's blood or other body fluids. Do this whether or not you use the precautions listed above.

- Before you give any medicine to a victim:

  • Find out if the victim has medicine prescribed for him or her to take, such as nitroglycerin for a heart condition. Ask where the victim keeps the medicine. Find out how much to give the victim. Ask the victim or read the directions on the medicine's label, if there is one.

  • Ask the victim for permission to give him or her the medicine.

  • Find out if the victim is allergic to any medicine.

## 140. CPR

{**Note:** The information given is not a substitute for formal training in CPR. CPR consists of rescue breathing and chest compressions. Follow Steps A, B, and C below, as needed.}

*CPR, Continued*

## A. Things to Check For

Tap or gently shake a collapsed person and ask, "Are you okay?" (A). If no re-

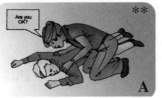

sponse, shout for help. Call 911! Check for breathing and a pulse.

### To Check for Breathing (all ages):

Put your ear very close to victim's mouth and nose. Listen for sounds of breathing for 5 seconds. Watch victim's chest to see if it rises and falls.

### To Check For Pulse:

- For adults and children age 1 and older: Press 2 fingers on the side of the neck in the groove

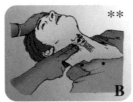

next to the voice box (B). Feel for pulse for 10 seconds.

- For infants under the age of 1: Press 2 fingers gently on the inside of the upper arm halfway between the elbow and the shoulder (C). Feel for a pulse for 3 to 4 seconds.

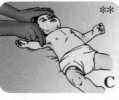

## Take Action

- If victim is breathing, check for other conditions in this book. Follow instructions.

- If victim is not breathing, but has a pulse, do "Rescue Breathing." (See below.)

- If victim is not breathing and has no pulse, do "CPR." (See page 384.)

## B. Rescue Breathing

For Victims Over 8 Years Old:

Do Rescue Breathing if victim has stopped breathing. Call 911! Shout for help.

1. If victim is not lying flat on his/her back, roll victim over, like a log, in one motion.

2. Open the victim's airway. With one hand, gently tilt the head back. Using 2 fingers (not the thumb) of the other hand, lift

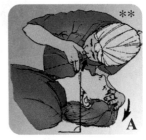

up the chin. If the airway remains blocked, tilt the head slowly and gently until the airway is open (A).

---

\*\* Illustrations are reproduced with permission from Basic Life Support Heartsaver Guide, 1993.
© Copyright American Heart Association

To Learn More, See Back Cover

## CPR, Continued

If you suspect a head, neck, or back injury, lift the chin without tilting the head back (B).

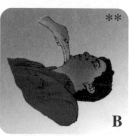

**B**

**3.** Once the airway is open, check for breathing. Check for 5 seconds. If victim is breathing, continue to hold airway open and keep checking until emergency help arrives.

If the victim is not breathing:

{**Note:** In step 4, a mouth-to-barrier device with a one way valve can protect you from diseases carried by blood (C).}

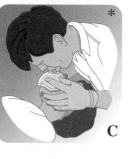

**C**

**4.** Pinch victim's nose shut. Place your mouth over victim's open mouth, forming a tight seal. Give two full breaths (D).

**D**

**5.** If victim's chest does not rise up, go to "Choking" (see page 385) and proceed.

**6.** If the chest rises, check for a pulse. If victim has a pulse, keep the airway open. Do rescue breathing until victim is breathing on his/her own or medical help arrives. If there is no pulse, do "CPR." (See page 381.)

**7.** To continue rescue breathing, give one full breath every 5 seconds for a minute. Check breathing and pulse for 5 to 10 seconds. Repeat cycle, if necessary.

### For Infants and Children Under 8 Years Old:

**1.** With infants, do not tilt head back too far to open the airway.

**2.** Do not pinch the nose of an infant to begin rescue breathing. Cover both the nose and mouth with your mouth and breathe slowly (1 to $1^1/_2$ seconds per breath) to make the chest rise.

**3.** With a small child, pinch the nose closed, cover the mouth with your mouth, and breathe at the same rate as for an infant (E).

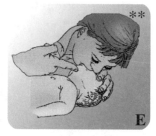

**E**

## CPR, Continued

# C. CPR

Do CPR only when victim is not breathing and has no pulse. Shout for help. Call 911! {**Note:** Use an automated external difribrillator (AED) device if available and you know how to use it.}

### For Victims Over 8 Years Old:

1. Do steps 1 to 6 of "Rescue Breathing" (See pages 382 and 383.)

2. If victim still has no pulse, begin chest compressions. Kneel at victim's side near the chest. Place the heel of one hand on the breast-

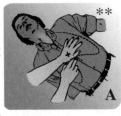

bone, $1^1/_2$ inch above the "V" where the ribs join the breastbone (A). Place the other hand on top of the one already in place and lock your fingers together.

3. Lean over victim and press straight down on the chest, using only the heels of the hands. Keep your arms straight.

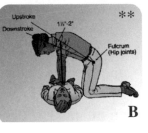

Depress the breastbone about 1 to 2 inches. Relax pressure completely, keeping your hands in place (B).

4. Do 15 compressions; pause and give 2 full breaths. Alternate compressions and breaths to do 80 to 100 compressions/minute.

5. After 1 minute, stop and check for a pulse.

6. Do CPR, as needed, until medical help arrives.

### For Infants Up to 1 Year Old:

1. Use the tips of the middle and ring fingers to compress the chest. Slip the other hand under the infant's back for support. Depress the breastbone to 1 inch at a rate of 100 times/minute.

2. Give 1 breath after every fifth chest compression.

3. Do CPR, as needed, until medical help arrives.

### For Children Ages 1 to 8:

1. Use the heel of one hand to compress the chest.

2. Depress the breastbone 1 to $1^1/_2$ inches at a rate of 80 to 100 times per minute.

3. Give 1 breath after every fifth compression.

4. Do CPR, as needed, until medical help arrives.

** Illustrations are reproduced with permission from Basic Life Support Heartsaver Guide, 1993.
© Copyright American Heart Association

# 141. First Aid for Choking (Heimlich Maneuver)

## For Victims Over 8 Years Old:

1. Ask, "Are you choking?" The victim may use the universal distress signal by clutching his throat with his hands (A). Do not interfere if the victim can speak, cough, or breathe.

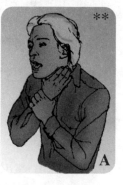

2. If the victim cannot speak, cough, or breathe, reach around the victim's waist from behind. Make a fist and place it above the victim's navel, but below the rib cage. Grasp your fist with your other hand. Press your fist into the victim's abdomen and give 6 to 10 quick, upward thrusts (B).

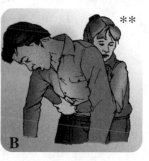

3. Check the victim. Repeat the procedure until the blockage is cleared or the victim becomes unconscious.

4. If the victim becomes unconscious, shout for help! Call 911! Then lay the victim on his back and check the airway. Place your finger in the back of victim's throat. Sweep from one side to the other to try to remove object. Do "Rescue Breathing." (See page 382.) If unsuccessful, sit straddling the victim's thighs. Place your hands, one on top of the other, above the navel, but below the breastbone. Press upward into the stomach and give 6 to 10 quick abdominal thrusts.

5. Repeat these steps: Finger sweep; rescue breathing; and abdominal thrusts until object is removed from airway. The victim should be seen by a doctor as soon as possible.

## For Infants Up to 1 Year Old:

1. Do not interfere if the infant is coughing or breathing.

2. If the infant is conscious, support the head and neck with one hand. Straddle the infant's face down over your forearm. Rest your arm on your knee for support. The infant's head should be lower than the rest of its body.

** Illustrations are reproduced with permission from Basic Life Support Heartsaver Guide, 1993.
© Copyright American Heart Association

To Learn More, See Back Cover

21. Emergencies Procedures

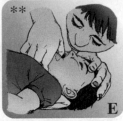

## Choking (Heimlich Maneuver), Continued

3. Use the heel of your hand and hit the infant's back between the shoulder blades 4 times. Use quick, forceful motions (C). If this does not work, go to step 4.

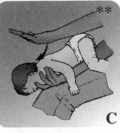

4. Turn the infant over on its back. Support its head with one hand, resting the infant on your forearm. Rest your arm on your legs for support. Place 2 fingers ¹/₂ inch below the nipple line and in between the nipples on the infant's chest. Give 4 quick downward thrusts.

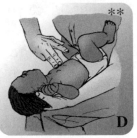

5. Repeat steps 3 and 4 until object is removed or the infant is unconscious. If the infant is unconscious go to step 6.

6. Shout for help. Call 911! Give back blows and chest thrusts as described for a conscious infant.

7. Perform tongue-jaw lift. With your thumb pressing down on the tongue and your fingers under the chin, lift the jaw upward. This pulls the tongue away from the back of the throat. If you see the object, remove it (E).

8. Attempt "Rescue Breathing." (See page 382.)

9. Give back blows and chest thrusts as described for a conscious infant.

10. Check for the object in the airway and remove it, if visible.

11. If the object is not visible, repeat steps 3 to 5. Don't give up!

12. If the object can be removed, check for breathing. (See "To Check For Breathing" on page 382.)

## For Children Ages 1 to 8:

1. If the child is conscious, give abdominal thrusts as for adults. Don't be too forceful.

2. If the child is unconscious, continue as for an adult, but do not perform blind finger sweep. Perform tongue-jaw lift instead, and remove object only if it is visible.

To Learn More, See Back Cover

## 142. Recovery Position

The recovery position may need to be used in many conditions that need first aid, such as unconsciousness. It should not be used when a person: Is not breathing; has a head, neck, or spine injury; or has a serious injury.

To put a person in the recovery position:

**1.** Kneel at his or her side.

**2.** Turn the victim's face toward you. Tilt the head back to open the airway. Check 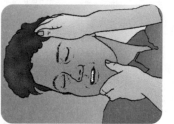 the mouth if the victim is unconscious and remove false teeth or any foreign matter.

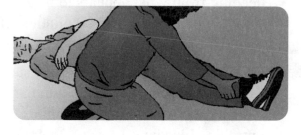

**3.** Place the victim's arm nearest you by his or her side and tuck it under the victim's buttock.

**4.** Lay the victim's other arm across his or her chest. Cross the victim's leg that is farthest from you over the one nearest you at the victim's ankles.

**5.** Support the victim's head with one hand and grasp his or her clothing at the hip farthest 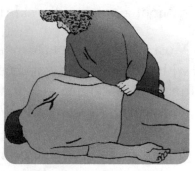 from you. Have him or her rest against your knees.

**6.** Bend the victim's upper arm and leg until each forms a right angle to the body. Pull the other arm out from under the victim's body. Ease it out toward the back from the shoulder down. Position it parallel to the victim's back.

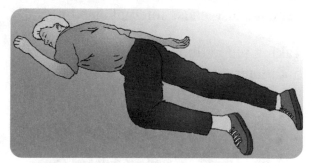

**7.** Make sure the head is tilted back to keep the airway open.

## 143. Bleeding

Bleeding can be external (visible or with a break in the skin) or internal (concealed without a break in the skin).

Most adults can donate a pint of blood without health consequences. Losing a quart of blood quickly, however, can lead to shock and even death. When bleeding occurs, the goal is to locate the source, stop or minimize the bleeding, and to help the body cope with the loss of blood.

## Signs, Symptoms & Causes

Bleeding can be external from cuts, scrapes, and punctures (see page 120), and from knife, gunshot, or other wounds.

Bleeding can also be internal from bruises (see page 114) and from blunt injuries that do not break the skin. A bleeding ulcer, an aneurysm, and bleeding disorders can also cause internal bleeding.

Taking blood thinning drugs can result in both internal and external bleeding.

## ♥ Get Immediate Care When:

- A body part has been amputated. (See "First Aid for Amputation" on page 390.)
- Shock occurs (see page 413).

- The bleeding is severe and/or blood spurts from the wound and is not controlled with direct pressure. (See "First Aid for Severe Bleeding" on page 389.)
- Bleeding comes from a deep wound (it appears to go down to the muscle or bone) and/or a bone is exposed.
- The skin on or around the wound site hangs open.
- With bleeding, there is a deformity at the site of the injury.
- The victim spits up true red blood.
- The victim has fractured ribs.
- Lethargy, fainting, dizziness, or mental status changes occur after a head trauma.
- Stools contain bright red blood or are maroon or black (not due to iron supplements).
- Bleeding from what appears to be a minor cut continues after 20 minutes of applied pressure.
- The victim has a bleeding disorder, such as hemophilia, or takes blood thinning medicine and is having a hard time controlling bleeding.

## ☎ Contact Doctor When:

- The victim has a bleeding disorder or is taking blood-thinning medicine and has a minor wound.

## Bleeding, Continued

- The cut or puncture that caused bleeding is from dirty or contaminated objects, such as rusty nails or objects in the soil or the puncture goes through a shoe, especially a rubber-soled one.

- A day or two after the injury, there are signs of infection (fever; redness, swelling, tenderness at the wound site; increased pain; general ill feeling; and/or swollen lymph nodes).

- The person has frequent nosebleeds; bruises easily; or has small red dots or clusters of small, pinpoint-sized red specks under the skin.

- In females, bleeding occurs after menopause.

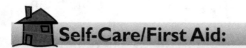
### Self-Care/First Aid:

### First Aid for Severe Bleeding:

Stay calm. Call 911 or take the victim to nearest hospital emergency department. In the meantime:

- Put on disposable latex rubber gloves, if available.

- Monitor for signs of shock: See "Shock" on page 413.

- Control bleeding.

- Apply direct pressure to the wound using a clean cloth or sterile bandage.

- Put pressure on the wound for at least 10 minutes. {**Note:** If the cut is large and the edges of it gape open, pinch the edge of the wound while applying pressure.}

- If bleeding continues before emergency help arrives, put extra cloths or bandages on top of existing ones and reapply pressure.

- Elevate the wounded area higher than heart level while applying pressure if there is no broken bone.

- Do not remove an object that is stuck in a wound. Pack it in place with padding and put tape around the padding so it doesn't move.

- If bleeding still continues after 15 to 20 minutes of direct pressure, apply pressure to a "pressure point." Use the pressure point closest to the bleeding site that is between the wound and the heart.

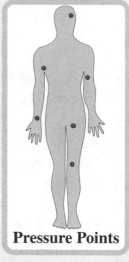

**Pressure Points**

*Continued on Next Page*

22. Emergency Conditions

## Bleeding, *Continued*

*Self-Care/First Aid, Continued*

- Continue to apply pressure to the bleeding site while you use flat fingers to put pressure on the pressure point. Do this until the bleeding stops. Do not apply a tourniquet except to save a life.

- Continue to monitor for signs of shock.

### First Aid for Amputation:

- Control bleeding. See "First Aid for Severe Bleeding" in this topic.

- Wrap the severed part in a clean, dry (not wet) cloth or sterile gauze. Place the wrapped part in a plastic bag or other waterproof container. Put these on a bed of ice. Do not submerge the severed part in cold water or ice.

### First Aid for Bleeding from the Scalp:

- Use a ring pad to apply pressure around the edges of the wound, not on the wound. Make a ring pad (shaped like a doughnut) with a bandage of narrow, long strips of cloth. Start with one end of the narrow bandage and wrap it around all four fingers on one hand until you form a loop. Leave a long strip of the bandage material to weave in and around the loop so it doesn't ravel.

- Don't wash the wound or apply an antiseptic or any other fluid to it.

- If blood or pink-colored fluid is coming from the ear, nose, or mouth, let it drain.

See also "Self-Care" for the cause(s) of bleeding: "Animal/Insect Bites," "Broken Bones," "Colon & Rectal Cancers," "Cuts, Scrapes, & Punctures," "Dislocations," "Head Injuries," "Hemorrhoids," "Neck/Spine Injuries," "Nosebleeds," "Rectal Problems," "Shock," and "Varicose Veins."

# 144. Choking

Choking happens when the airway is partly or completely blocked. When the airway is completely blocked, the brain doesn't get oxygen. Without oxygen, the brain can begin to die in 4 to 6 minutes.

## Prevention

- Chew all foods thoroughly before swallowing. Eat at a slow pace.

- Go easy on alcoholic beverages before you eat to lessen the chance of swallowing large pieces of food.

- Don't laugh and eat at the same time. This can draw food into the windpipe.

- If you wear dentures, make sure they fit.

To Learn More, See Back Cover

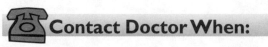

**Choking, Continued**

## Signs & Symptoms

When the airway is blocked completely, a choking victim can't talk, breathe, or cough. The victim may turn blue.

When the airway is partly blocked, a choking victim wheezes, coughs, and has fast and/or labored breathing and chest pain when breathing in.

## Causes

- Food goes down the windpipe or small objects get stuck in the throat and airway.

- Fluids, such as mucus or liquids swallowed the wrong way, block the airway.

- Snoring. Choking can occur when the tongue blocks the airway.

### Get Immediate Care When:

- The choking victim is unconscious or unable to breathe. Do "First Aid for Choking (Heimlich Maneuver)" on page 385.

- The choking victim has fast and/or labored breathing

### Contact Doctor When:

- A choking victim has received "First Aid for Choking (Heimlich Maneuver)".

- Wheezing, a cough that doesn't go away, or symptoms of pneumonia (see page 104) occur after a choking incident.

### Self-Care/First Aid:

- If you or someone else cannot breathe, cough, or speak, give "First Aid for Choking (Heimlich Maneuver)" on page 385.

- If you or someone else is choking, but able to breathe and speak:
  - Cough to clear the airway.
  - Take a slow, deep breath to get a lot of air into the lungs.
  - Give a deep, forceful cough. Try to breathe in deeply enough to be able to cough out 2 or 3 times in a row before taking a second breath.

## 145. Dehydration

Dehydration is when the body loses too much water and needed minerals (electrolytes). This can result from:

- Not getting enough water or other fluids

- Losing too much water or other body fluids

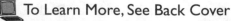
22. Emergency Conditions

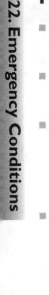

*Dehydration, Continued*

- Loss of electrolytes, such as sodium and potassium

## Prevention

- Drink plenty of fluids when you sweat, exercise, or are in a hot climate.

- Avoid drinks with alcohol and/or caffeine.

- If vomiting, follow "Self-Care" in "Vomiting & Nausea" on page 189. If you have diarrhea, follow "Self-Care" in "Diarrhea" on page 157.

- If you take water pills, weigh yourself daily. Let your doctor know if you lose more than 3 pounds in 1 day or more than 5 pounds in 1 week.

## Signs & Symptoms

Signs and Symptoms of severe dehydration are:

- Severe thirst (sometimes)

- Sunken and dry or tearless eyes

- Dry mouth, tongue, and lips

- No urine or a low amount of urine that is dark yellow

- Headache; lightheadedness, especially when getting up quickly

- Dry skin that doesn't spring back after being pinched

- Dizziness, confusion, weakness

- Increase in breathing and heart rate

## Causes & Care

Causes of dehydration include:

- Diarrhea (see page 156), vomiting (see page 189), and/or fever (see page 283)

- Heavy sweating

- Overuse of water pills

- Heat exhaustion or heat stroke (see page 405)

- Uncontrolled diabetes

- Severe injury that results in loss of blood or body fluids

- Fever

Fluids and electrolytes must be replaced. See "Self-Care/First Aid for Dehydration" in this topic. If this can't be done by mouth, IV fluids need to be given.

## ♥ Get Immediate Care When:

- Signs of severe dehydration, listed above, are present

- After being in hot conditions, 2 or more signs of heat exhaustion are present. (See "Signs and Symptoms" in "Heat Exhaustion & Heat Stroke" on page 406.)

*Dehydration, Continued*

- You have Type 2 diabetes with signs of dehydration, listed on page 392. {**Note:** You may have high blood sugar without ketones in your urine. This is a serious condition that often comes after an illness, such as the flu, that has caused dehydration.}

## Contact Doctor When:

Vomiting or severe diarrhea lasts longer than 2 days.

## Self-Care/First Aid:

**First Aid to Replace Water and Mineral Salts:**

Drink about 2 cups of fluid per hour (if vomiting isn't present). Fluids include:

- Mixture of 4 teaspoons of sugar, $\frac{1}{2}$ teaspoon of salt and 4 cups of water.

- Mixture of $\frac{1}{2}$ teaspoon salt, 1 teaspoon of baking soda, 8 teaspoons of sugar, and 8 ounces of orange juice with enough water to make 1 liter (8 cups) of liquid

- Sports drinks, such as Gatorade, PowerAde, and All Sport

- Broths

- Flat cola, ginger ale, 7-Up, or other clear sodas

- Popsicles

- Weak tea with sugar

- Gelatin (solid or liquid)

{**Note:** If you have high blood pressure, heart disease, diabetes, or a history of stroke, find out what fluids your doctor prefers you take.}

See also "First Aid for Heat Exhaustion" on page 407; "Self-Care in "Diarrhea" on page 157, "Self-Care" in "Fever" on page 285, and "Self-Care in "Vomiting & Nausea" on page 189.

# 146. Electric Shock

## Prevention

- Don't use an electrical appliance near water. Use hair dryers and curling irons that have built-in shock protectors.

- Install ground-fault circuit-interrupters (GFCIs) in wall outlets in bathrooms, kitchens, basements, garages, and outdoor boxes. With GFCIs, when an electrical appliance falls into water, the current is instantly cut off.

*22. Emergency Conditions*

### Electric Shock, Continued

- Don't turn electrical switches on or off or touch an electric appliance while your hands are wet, while standing in water, or when sitting in a bathtub.

- Replace worn cords and wiring.

- Cover all electric sockets with plastic safety caps.

- Remove the appropriate fuse or switch off the circuit breaker before doing electrical repairs. Turning off the appliance or light switch is not enough.

- To avoid being harmed by lightning:

  - Heed weather warnings.

  - Take shelter in a building, if you can. Stay away from windows, appliances, water pipes, and telephones with cords.

  - Stay in your car (if it is not a convertible) rather than out in the open.

  - If you are caught outside, avoid tall trees, open water, and high ground. Crawl in a ravine or other low-lying place. If you are out in the open, curl up on the ground, head to knees with your head touching the ground. Don't touch items that contain metal.

## Signs & Symptoms

- Slight shocking sensations

- Muscle spasms or muscle and tissue damage under the skin's surface

- Seizures

- Interrupted breathing

- Third-degree burns (where the electricity enters and exits the body)

- Irregular heartbeats or cardiac arrest

- Unconsciousness

- Death

## Causes

- Touching a low-voltage current source, such as an electric socket or worn cord

- Touching high-tension wires that fall during a storm or touching someone who is still touching a live current

- Mixing water and electricity

- Being struck by lightning

## ♥ Get Immediate Care When:

- The person received a shock from a high voltage wire or was struck by lighting. Call 911!

- The person received a shock from a low-voltage current and his heart keeps skipping beats.

---

To Learn More, See Back Cover

### Electric Shock, Continued

## ☎ Contact Doctor When:

After being treated for an electric shock, the person has a fever or coughs up sputum.

## 🏠 Self-Care/First Aid:

- Do not touch the victim until power is shut off. If the source is a high voltage wire, call 911! If the source is a low voltage current, do these things until emergency care arrives:

  - Switch off the current, if possible, by removing the fuse or switching off the circuit breaker.

  - Do not touch the person who is in contact with electricity.

  - If you can't turn off the current source, use a board, wooden stick, rope, or other non-conducting device to pull the victim away from the source of the electric current. Make sure your hands and feet are dry and you are standing on a dry surface.

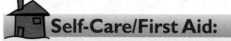

- If it is safe for you to touch the victim:

  - Check for heartbeat and breathing. Feel for a pulse along the neck, under the earlobe, on the chest, or on the wrist. Watch the rise and fall of the chest to see if the person is breathing. If you find no heartbeat and no breathing, do CPR. (See "CPR" on page 381.)

  - If there is a heartbeat but no breathing, do rescue breathing. (See "Rescue Breathing" on page 382.)

  - Check for burns and treat as third-degree burns. (See "Burns" on page 115.)

# 147. Fainting & Unconsciousness

## Signs & Symptoms

An unconscious person is hard to rouse, can't be made aware of his or her surroundings, and is unable to move on his own. Unconsciousness requires medical care. Fainting is a brief loss of consciousness. It can last from seconds to minutes. One episode of fainting that lasts only a few seconds may not be a serious problem. Let your doctor know if you faint, especially if you faint more than once.

*Fainting & Unconsciousness, Continued*

## Causes & Risk Factors

Things that can lead to feeling faint or fainting include:

- Irregular, too fast or too slow heartbeat
- A sudden change in body position, like standing up too quickly (postural hypotension)
- Extreme pain; sudden emotional stress, fright, or anxiety
- Standing a long time in one place or being in hot, humid weather
- Taking some prescribed medicines, such as some that lower high blood pressure; tranquilizers; and antidepressants.
- Excessive amounts of alcohol or some over-the-counter medicines

Causes of unconsciousness include:

- Very low or extremely high blood sugar
- Anemia or any condition in which there is a rapid loss of blood; shock
- Heart and circulatory problems, such as abnormal heart rhythm, stroke, etc.
- Heat stroke, heat exhaustion, or hypothermia
- Head or spinal injury; epilepsy
- Drug overdose, poisoning, or a severe allergic reaction

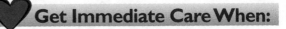

## Get Immediate Care When:

- The person is not breathing and does not have a pulse. Call 911! (See "CPR" on page 381.)
- The person has signs of a heart attack (see "Heart Attack Warning Signs" on page 202) or a stroke (see "Stroke Warning Signs" on page 229). Call 911!
- The person who fainted had sudden, severe back pain.
- With unconsciousness, the person is more than 50 years old and this is the first episode; the person has a known heart problem, or fainting or unconsciousness occurred for no apparent reason.
- The person had signs of a low or high blood sugar before unconsciousness. (See "Signs & Symptoms for Low Blood Sugar (Hypoglycemia) and High Blood Sugar (Hyperglycemia)" on page 280.)

## Contact Doctor When:

- Fainting occurred with pelvic or abdominal pain or with black stools.
- Fainting occurred in a person taking medicine, such as for high blood pressure, or the fainting occurred after starting a new medicine or increasing the dose of a medicine.

To Learn More, See Back Cover

22. Emergency Conditions

*Fainting & Unconsciousness, Continued*

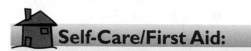
## Self-Care/First Aid:

### For Unconsciousness:

- Check for breathing and a pulse. If no pulse, call 911! Do CPR (see page 381). If the victim has a pulse but is not breathing, call 911! Do "Rescue breathing" (see page 382).

- Check for a medical alert or information. Call the emergency number if there is one. Follow instructions.

- Don't give the person anything to eat or drink, not even water.

### To Reduce the Risk of Fainting:

- Follow your doctor's advice to treat any medical condition which may lead to fainting. Take medicines as prescribed, but let your doctor know about any side effects.

- Get up slowly from bed or from a sitting position.

- Avoid turning your head suddenly.

- Don't wear tight-fitting clothing around your neck.

- Avoid excessive exercise in hot, humid conditions. Drink a lot of liquids when you do exercise.

- Avoid stuffy rooms and hot, humid places. When you can't, use a fan.

- Drink alcoholic beverages in moderation, if at all.

### For Fainting:

- Catch the person before he falls.

- Have the person lie down with the head below the level of the heart. Raise the legs 8 to 12 inches. This promotes blood flow to the brain. If a victim who is about to faint can lie down right away, he may not lose consciousness. If the person can't lie down, have the victim sit down, bend forward, and put his head between his knees.

- Turn the victim's head to the side so the tongue doesn't fall back into the throat.

- Loosen any tight clothing.

- Apply moist towels to the person's face and neck, but keep the victim warm, if the surroundings are chilly.

- Don't slap or shake anyone who's just fainted or give him anything to eat or drink.

- Don't allow the person who fainted to get up until the weakness passes.

*Continued on Next Page*

22. Emergency Conditions

*Fainting & Unconsciousness, Continued*

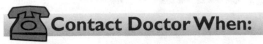

## Get Immediate Care When:

A fishhook is stuck in an eye.

*Self-Care/First Aid, Continued*

**For a Low Blood Sugar Reaction:**

- Have a sugar source, such as: $1/2$ cup of fruit juice or regular (not diet) soda; 6 to 7 regular (not sugar free) hard candies; 3 glucose tablets; or 6 to 8 ounces of milk.

- If you don't feel better after 15 minutes, take the same amount of sugar source again. If you don't feel better after the second dose, call your doctor.

## Contact Doctor When:

- You can't remove the fishhook.

- Twenty-four to 48 hours after the accident, signs of an infection occur at the wound site (increased redness, pain, and/or swelling; red streaks that extend from the area; pus, and/or fever).

- You have not had a tetanus shot in the last 5 years.

## 148. Fishhook Accidents

Parts of a fishhook are the shank and the barb. The upper end of the shank connects the fishing line. The barb is the curved and sharp end that hooks the fish. Because it is sharp, the barb can cut or penetrate the skin.

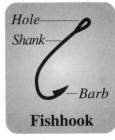

*Hole* — *Shank* — — *Barb* **Fishhook**

## Self-Care/First Aid:

**For Knicks or Surface Cuts to the Skin:**

Treat for a cut. (See "First Aid for Minor Cuts and Scrapes" on page 121.)

**For a Fishhook Stuck Near the Surface of the Skin:**

- Put ice or cold water on the wound area. This temporarily numbs it.

*Continued on Next Page*

## Signs, Symptoms & Care

A fishhook can knick or cut the skin; get stuck in the skin near its surface; or become embedded in the skin.

First aid treats most fishhook accidents.

To Learn More, See Back Cover

22. Emergency Conditions

## Fishhook Accidents, Continued

### Self-Care/First Aid, Continued

- Take a piece of fishing line. Loop one end and tie it to the hook near the surface of the skin.

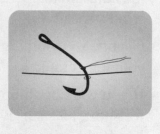

- Grasp the shaft end of the hook with one hand and press down about $1/8$th inch to disengage the barb.

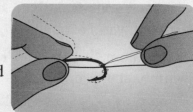

- Keep pressing the hook down and jerk the fishing line in a motion parallel to the skin's surface to make the shaft of the hook lead the barb out of the skin.

- Wash the wound area well with soap and water. Treat for a puncture wound. (See "First Aid for Punctures That Cause Minor Bleeding" on page 122.)

## For a Fishhook Deeply Embedded:

- Put ice or cold water on the wound area. This temporarily numbs it.

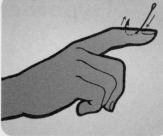

Push on the shaft of the hook until the barb protrudes.

- With wire cutters, snip the hook at either the shank or the barb.

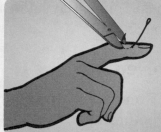

- Pull the hook out.

- Wash the wound area well with soap and water. Treat for a puncture wound. (See "First Aid for Punctures That Cause Minor Bleeding" on page 122.)

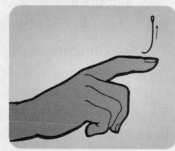

22. Emergency Conditions

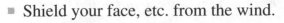

# 149. Frostbite & Hypothermia

Frostbite freezes the skin. It can damage tissue below the skin, too. Most often, frostbite affects the toes, fingers, ear-lobes, chin, and tip of the nose.

Hypothermia is when body temperature drops below 96°F. The body loses more heat than it can make. This is usually brought on by staying in a cold place for a long time.

## Prevention

### To Prevent Frostbite and Outdoor Hypothermia:

- Stay indoors as much as possible when it is very cold and windy.

- Wear clothing made of wool or polypropylene. These fabrics stay warm even when wet. Layer your clothing. Wear 2 or 3 pairs of socks instead of 1 heavy pair and wear roomy shoes. Do not wear items that constrict the hands, wrists, or feet. Wear outerwear that is wind and waterproof.

- Wear something to keep your head and ears warm. The major source of heat loss is through the head.

- Don't drink alcohol or smoke ciga-rettes.

- Shield your face, etc. from the wind.

- Be aware of the "Wind-Chill Factor." Listen to weather reports which give the adjusted temperature with the wind's speed.

- Change wet clothing when exposed to cold temperatures.

- If you walk or climb in cold weather for sport, take survival bags that are lined with space blankets.

### To Prevent Indoor Hypothermia:

- Keep your indoor thermostat set at 65°F or higher. Also keep a supply of warm clothing, blankets, etc. on hand in the event of a power outage. If you are elderly or live alone, have someone check on you regularly to see that you are kept warm enough.

- If your home is below 65°F, dress warmly and wear a hat.

## Signs & Symptoms

### For Frostbite:

- Cold, numb skin that swells and feels hard and solid

- Loss of function and absence of pain

- Skin color changing from white to red to purple; blisters

- Slurred speech; confusion

To Learn More, See Back Cover

*Frostbite & Hypothermia, Continued*

**Frostnip** is a less serious problem. The skin turns white or pale and feels cold, but the skin does not feel hard and solid.

### For Hypothermia:

With mild hypothermia, symptoms include: Shivering, slurred speech; memory lapses; and the abdomen and back feel cold.

With moderate hypothermia, shivering stops but the skin feels ice cold and looks blue. The person may act confused, drowsy, irritable, and/or stuporous. Muscles may be rigid and stiff and pulse rate and breathing slow down.

With severe hypothermia, the person has dilated pupils, no response to pain, and loss of consciousness. The person appears to be dead. Death occurs in half or more of persons with severe hypothermia.

## Causes & Risk Factors

### For Frostbite and Frostnip:

Frostbite and frostnip can occur when temperatures drop below freezing. Both can set in very slowly or very quickly. This will depend on how long the skin is exposed to the cold and how cold and windy it is.

### For Hypothermia:

- Exposure to cold temperatures (wet or dry). Many factors increase the risk. Examples are: Wet clothing or lying on a cold surface; circulation problems, diabetes, and stroke; and old age. The elderly are more prone to hypothermia if they live in a poorly heated home and are not clothed warmly enough.

- Immersion. This can be from 6 hours or less of exposure to cold water immersion. It can also be from water immersion, or exposure on land to cold, wet weather near freezing, for up to 24 hours.

- Shock (see page 413)

### ♥ Get Immediate Care When:

- Any of these problems are present:
  - No breathing and/or no pulse. Call 911! (See CPR on page 381.)
  - Pale or blue colored skin, lips, and/or nailbeds
  - Decreased level or loss of consciousness; fainting
  - Body temperature less than 95°F
  - Rigid and stiff muscles
  - Mental confusion, drowsiness
  - Slow pulse rate and breathing or a hard time breathing
  - Stumbling, lack of coordination

**22. Emergency Conditions**

### Frostbite & Hypothermia, Continued

- Signs and symptoms of frostbite (see page 400)
- With a low body temperature, the person had a recent infection and now has signs of sepsis (lethargy, chills, vomiting, looks sick, and delirium).

### ☎ Contact Doctor When:

- Any of these persons have had prolonged exposure to the cold:
  - Elderly persons
  - Persons with a history of alcoholism or drug abuse
  - Persons whose immune systems are depressed due to disease and/or medication, such as chemotherapy
- The person has continued and persistent shivering after being warmed or his body temperature is not rising to normal after 4 hours of warming.

{**Note:** Reassess symptoms. The damage from exposure to the cold may not be completely noted for 72 hours.}

- After being exposed to the cold, symptoms (shivering, cold skin, and body temperature) have not improved after first aid.

### Self-Care/First Aid:

**First Aid For Frostbite Before Emergency Care:**

- Get the victim out of the cold and into a warm place.
- Loosen or remove wet and/or tight clothing. Remove jewelry.
- Don't rub the area with snow or soak it in cold water.
- Warm the affected area by soaking it in a tub of warm water (101°F to 104°F).
- Stop when the affected area becomes red, not when sensation returns. (This should take about 45 minutes. If done too fast, thawing can be painful and blisters may develop.)
- If warm water is not available, cover the victim with blankets, coats, sweaters, etc. or place the frostbitten body part in a warm body area, such as the armpit or on the abdomen.
- Keep the exposed area elevated, but protected.
- Don't massage a frostbitten area.
- Protect the exposed area from the cold. It is more sensitive to reinjury.
- Don't break blisters.

*Continued on Next Page*

To Learn More, See Back Cover

*Frostbite & Hypothermia, Continued*

*Self-Care/First Aid, Continued*

**First Aid for Frostnip:**

- Warm the affected area. Put the affected area in warm water (101°F to 104°F).

{**Note:** After warming the area, the skin may be red and tingling. If not treated, frostnip can lead to frostbite.}

- Protect the exposed area from the cold. It is more sensitive to reinjury.

**For Moderate to Severe Hypothermia:**

Call 911!

**First Aid Before Emergency Care:**

- Handle the victim gently.
- Get the victim out of the cold and into a warm place, if possible.
- Remove wet and/or cold clothing. Remove jewelry.
- Change to warm and dry garments.
- Place the victim on dry blankets and cover him with blankets, coats, sweaters, etc. Place covers, etc. around the victim, too, and cover the top of the victim's head.

- Keep the victim in a flat position.
- If available, place hot packs on the victim's body areas of high heat loss such as the groin, armpits, and neck.

**For Mild Hypothermia:**

- Move the victim from a cold to a warm place, if possible. If indoors, raise the temperature in the room.
- Change to warm and dry garments.
- Give warm, non-alcoholic, drinks.
- Place the victim in a tub of hot water (106°F or less), but leave the arms and legs out and keep them elevated.
- Take and recheck temperature to see if first aid measures are raising body temperature back to normal.

# 150. Head Injuries

Any blow to the head can result in a head injury. Head injuries can cause damage to the scalp, the skull, or the brain itself.

## Prevention

Prevent falls and injuries. (See "Home Safety Checklist" on page 23 and "Personal Safety Checklist" on page 24.)

*Head Injuries, Continued*

## Signs & Symptoms

- Bruise, cut, dent, or blood on the scalp
- Severe headache
- Stiff neck
- Vomiting
- Blood or fluid that comes from the mouth, nose, or ear
- Loss of vision, blurred or double vision, pupils of unequal size
- Confusion, drowsiness, or personality change
- Inability to move any part of the body or weakness in an arm or leg
- Convulsions
- Loss of consciousness

Watch for signs and symptoms of a serious head injury during the first 24 hours. Symptoms may not occur, though, for as long as several weeks.

### ♥ Get Immediate Care When:

- The victim with a head injury has no pulse and/or is not breathing. Call 911! See "CPR" on page 381. Do not tilt the head back or move the head or neck when you do "Rescue Breathing."

Instead, pull the lower jaw (chin) forward to open the airway. Place your thumb(s) or fingers on the jawbone, just in front of and below the earlobes to do this.

- The victim of head injury has bleeding from the scalp, mouth, nose, or ears, or is unconscious longer than 5 minutes. Call 911!
- Any of these problems occurred after a head injury:
  - Convulsions
  - Drowsiness or it is hard to awaken the victim
  - Headache that lasts longer than 1 or 2 days or gets worse with time
  - Inability to move arms or legs, weakness in limbs
  - Blurred or double vision or pupils of unequal size
  - Slurred speech
  - Nausea, vomiting, dry heaves
  - Memory loss, confusion, dizziness, disorientation, personality change

### ☎ Contact Doctor When:

The head injury victim sees stars or feels unusual in any way.

🖥 To Learn More, See Back Cover

*22. Emergency Conditions*

*Head Injuries, Continued*

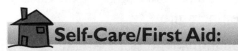

## Self-Care/First Aid:

### For a Serious Head Injury:

- Call 911! In the meantime, keep the head, neck, and back perfectly still until emergency care arrives. Do not move someone with a suspected head, neck, or spine injury unless the person must be moved because his or her life is in danger. Any movement of the head, neck, or back could result in paralysis or death. Hold the head, neck, and shoulders perfectly still. Use both hands, one on each side of the head.

- If the victim is bleeding from the scalp, see "First Aid for Bleeding from the Scalp" on page 390.

### First Aid for Minor Head Injuries:

- Apply an ice pack to the injured area to reduce swelling or bruising. Change it every 15 to 20 minutes for 1 to 2 hours. Do not put ice directly on the skin. To make an ice pack, put ice cubes into a plastic bag with a little cold water and seal it. Wrap it in a clean towel and apply to the bump or bruise. Or, cover a bag of frozen vegetables with a towel and place on the injured area.

- Cover an open, small cut with gauze and first aid tape or a bandage.

- Resume normal activities once you know there is no serious head injury.

- Take an over-the-counter medicine for pain. (See "Pain relievers" in "Your Home Pharmacy" on page 43.)

# 151. Heat Exhaustion & Heat Stroke

Heat exhaustion is a warning that the body is getting too hot. Heat stroke is a medical emergency. Many people die of heat stroke each year; most are over 50 years of age.

## Prevention

- Drink lots of liquids, especially if your urine is a dark yellow. Drink water, sport drinks, such as Gatorade, etc.

- Do not stay in or leave anyone in closed, parked cars during hot weather.

- Avoid drinks with alcohol or caffeine.

- Use caution when you must be in the sun. At the first signs of heat exhaustion, get out of the sun. If possible, avoid the midday heat. Do not do vigorous activity during the hottest part of the day (noon to 4 p.m.).

22. Emergency Conditions

*Heat Exhaustion & Heat Stroke, Continued*

- Wear light, loose-fitting clothing, such as cotton, so sweat can evaporate. Wear a wide-brimmed hat with vents. Use an umbrella for shade.

- If you feel very hot, try to cool off. Open a window. Use a fan. If possible, use an air conditioner.

- Check with your doctor about sun exposure if you take water pills, mood-altering or antispasmodic medicines, and some antibiotics, such as tetracycline.

- Limit your stay in hot tubs or heated whirlpools to 15 minutes. Don't use them when you are alone.

## Signs & Symptoms

### For a Heat Stroke:

- Very high temperature (104°F or higher)

- Hot, dry, red skin; no sweating

- Deep breathing and fast pulse, then shallow breathing and weak pulse

- Dilated pupils

- Confusion, delirium, hallucinations

- Convulsions; loss of consciousness

These signs and symptoms can occur suddenly, with little warning.

### For Heat Exhaustion:

- Normal, low, or only slightly elevated body temperature

- Cool, clammy, pale skin; sweating

- Dry mouth, thirst

- Fatigue, weakness; dizziness

- Headache

- Nausea, sometimes vomiting

- Muscle cramps

- Weak or rapid pulse

## Causes & Risk Factors

In hot weather, or during vigorous activity, the body perspires. As sweat evaporates from the skin, the body is cooled. If this personal cooling system fails, especially with long periods of intense heat, heat exhaustion or a heat stroke can occur. Factors that increase the risk include:

- Changes in the skin caused by the normal aging process

- Poor circulation, heart, lung, and kidney diseases

- The inability to perspire due to medicines, such as water pills

- Any illness that causes weakness, fever, vomiting, or diarrhea

- Being in places without fans or air conditioners during hot, humid weather

To Learn More, See Back Cover

*Heat Exhaustion & Heat Stroke, Continued*

- Not being able to get to public air conditioned places and/or waiting for buses and other types of public transportation in hot, humid weather.
- Overdressing

## Get Immediate Care When:

- Signs and symptoms of a heat stroke (see page 406) are present. Call 911! See "First Aid Before Emergency Care" in the next column.
- The person is too dizzy or weak to stand; has nonstop vomiting; or has pale, cool, and clammy skin.

## Contact Doctor When:

Two or more of these signs of heat exhaustion are present:

- Dry mouth
- Fatigue, weakness; dizziness
- Headache
- Nausea, sometimes vomiting
- Weak and rapid pulse
- Muscle cramps
- Feeling lightheaded or faint

## Self-Care/First Aid:

**First Aid Before Emergency Care:**

- Lower the body temperature.
  - Move the person to a cool place indoors or under a shady tree. Place the feet higher than the head.
  - Remove the person's clothing. Wrap the person in a cold, wet sheet, sponge the person with towels or sheets that are soaked in cold water, or spray the person with cool water. Fan the person. If using an electric fan, use caution. Keep the person with wet items far enough away from the fan so as not to cause electric shock.
  - Put ice packs or cold compresses on the neck, under the armpits, and on the groin area.
- Place the person in the recovery position (see page 387) once his or her temperature reaches 101°F. Do not lower the temperature further.

**First Aid for Heat Exhaustion:**

- Move the person to a cool place indoors or in the shade.
- Loosen clothing.

*Continued on Next Page*

22. Emergency Conditions

*Heat Exhaustion & Heat Stroke, Continued*

*Self-Care/First Aid, Continued*

- Give fluids, such as cool or cold water. If available, add $\frac{1}{2}$ teaspoon of salt to 1 quart of water and sip it or drink sport drinks, such as Gatorade.
- Have salty foods, such as saltine crackers, if tolerated.
- Lie down in a cool, breezy place.

# 152. Neck/Spine Injuries

Anything that puts too much pressure or force on the neck or back can result in a neck and/or spinal injury. Suspect a neck injury, too, if a head injury has occurred.

## Prevention

- Prevent falls and accidents. See "Home Safety Checklist" on page 23 and "Personal Safety Checklist" on page 24.
- Use padded head rests in your car to prevent whiplash.
- Check the water's depth before diving into it. Do not dive into water that is less than 9 feet deep. Never dive in an above-ground pool.

## Signs & Symptoms

### For a Whiplash Injury:

- Neck pain and stiffness
- Having a hard time raising the head off of a pillow

### For a Serious Injury:

- Severe pain in the back and/or neck or immediate neck pain
- Inability to open and close the fingers or move the toes
- New feelings of numbness in the legs, arms, shoulders, or any other part of the body
- Appearance that the head, neck, or back is in an odd position
- New loss of bladder or bowel control
- Blood or other discharge from the nose or ears following the injury
- Paralysis
- Unconsciousness

## Causes

Neck and spinal injuries are usually due to falls, accidents, and hard blows.

To Learn More, See Back Cover

## Neck/Spine Injuries, *Continued*

### ♥ Get Immediate Care When:

- The injured person does not have a pulse and/or is not breathing. Call 911! Do "CPR" (see page 381). {**Note:** When doing rescue breathing, do not tilt the head back or move the head or neck. Instead, pull the lower jaw (chin) forward to open the airway. Place your thumb(s) or fingers on the jawbones, just in front of and below the earlobes, to do this.} You must keep the neck and/or back perfectly still until emergency help arrives. Do not move someone with a suspected neck or spine injury unless the person must be moved because his life is in danger. Any movement of the head, neck, or back could result in paralysis or death. Hold the head, neck, and shoulders perfectly still. Use both of your hands, one on each side of the head. (See "To Immobilize the Neck and/or Spine" in the next column.)

- The injured person has one or more signs and symptoms of a serious injury (see page 408). See "To Immobilize the Neck and/or Spine" in the next column.

- Any of these problems occur after a recent injury to the neck and/or spine that did not get treated with emergency care at the time of the injury:

- Severe pain
- Numbness, tingling, or weakness in the face, arms, or legs
- Loss of bladder control

### ☎ Contact Doctor When:

A whiplash injury is suspected or pain from any injury to the neck or back lasted longer than 1 week.

### 🏠 Self-Care/First Aid:

Follow the measures below before emergency care arrives.

**To Immobilize the Neck and/or Spine:**

- Tell the victim to lie still and not move his or her head, neck, back, etc.

- Place rolled towels, articles of clothing, etc., on both sides of the neck and/or body. Tie and wrap in place, but don't interfere with the victim's breath- 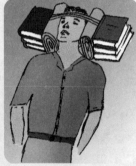 ing. If necessary, use both of your hands, one on each side of the victim's head, to keep the head from moving.

*Continued on Next Page*

## Neck/Spine Injuries, Continued

### Self-Care/First Aid, Continued

**To Move Someone With a Suspected Neck or Spinal Injury:**

Immobilize the neck and spine and:

- Find a door or other rigid board.

- Several people should carefully lift and move the person onto the board, being very careful to keep the head and neck in a straight line with the spine. The head should not rotate from side to side or forward to backward.

- Make sure one person uses both of his or her hands, one on each side of the victim's head, to keep the head from moving. If you can, immobilize the neck and/or spine by placing rolled towels, articles of clothing, etc. on both sides of the neck and/or body. Tie and wrap in place, but don't interfere with the victim's breathing.

**To Move Someone With a Suspected Neck Injury from a Diving or Other Water Accident:**

Before emergency care arrives:

- Protect the neck and/or spine from bending or twisting. Place your hands on both sides of the neck and keep in place until help arrives.

- If the person is still in the water, help the person float until a rigid board can be slipped under the head and body, at least as far down as the buttocks.

- If no board is available, several people should take the person out of the water. Support the head and body as one unit. Make sure the head does not bend in any direction.

### For Non-Emergency Injuries:

If You Suspect a Whiplash Injury:

- See your doctor as soon as you can so the extent of injury can be assessed.

- For the first 24 hours, apply ice packs to the injured area for up to 10 minutes every $1/2$ hour.

- After 24 hours, use ice packs or heat, whichever works best, to relieve the pain. Ways to apply heat:

  - Take a hot shower for 20 minutes a few times a day.

  - Use a hot-water bottle, heating pad (set on low), or heat lamp directed to the neck for 10 minutes several times a day. (Use caution not to burn the skin.)

- Use a cervical pillow or a small rolled towel placed behind your neck.

*Continued on Next Page*

To Learn More, See Back Cover

### Neck/Spine Injuries, Continued

#### Self-Care/First Aid, Continued

- Wrap a folded towel around the neck to help hold the head in one position during the night.

- If your arm or hand is numb, ask your doctor about a cervical-traction device.

- Take an over-the-counter medicine for pain. {**Note:** See "Pain relievers" in "Your Home Pharmacy" on page 43.}

# 153. Poisoning

Poisoning can result from harmful substances that are swallowed, inhaled, or that come in contact with the skin.

## Prevention

- Follow your doctor's advice on taking medicines, vitamins, minerals, and herbal remedies. If you have a hard time remembering if you took your medicines, use containers with sections that specify doses and times.

- Wear protective clothing, masks, etc. when using chemicals that could cause harm if inhaled or absorbed by the skin.

- Use volatile substances, such as gasoline and wood stain, only in areas that are well ventilated, such as outdoors.

- Store hazardous materials and medicines in their original containers.

- Keep all harmful substances locked up and out of the reach of children and grandchildren. Teach them not to touch items with a skull-and-crossbones on it.

- Store all medicines and vitamins in containers with child-resistant tops. Don't call medicines or vitamins "candy" in front of children. Vitamins with iron can be deadly to a small child.

- Flush unused medicines down the toilet. Rinse the containers before throwing them away.

- Buy a bottle of syrup of ipecac and replace it yearly. This is used to induce vomiting after certain poisons have been swallowed. Buy activated charcoal, too. This may be needed when certain chemicals are swallowed. Call Poison control Center [(1-800-POISON1 (764-7661)] before giving either of these.

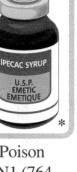

- Install carbon monoxide detectors in your home and garage. Have your furnace, chimney, and flue checked by a qualified person every year. Don't run cars and lawn mowers in the garage. Don't use gas ranges for heat. Use portable heating devices, coal burning stoves, etc., as directed.

*Poisoning, Continued*

## Signs & Symptoms

Signs and symptoms depend on the poisonous substance. They range from a skin rash to an upset stomach to unconsciousness. Some poisons can cause death.

## Causes

- Medicines, such as aspirin, tranquilizers, and sleeping pills

- Household cleaners, such as bleach, drain cleaners, ammonia, and lye

- Insecticides and rat poison

- Vitamins and minerals, if taken in toxic amounts

- Alcohol and drugs

- Rubbing alcohol, iodine, hair dye, mouthwash, and mothballs

- Some indoor plants and outdoor plants and berries

- Gasoline, antifreeze, oil, and other chemicals for the car

- Lighter fluid and paint thinner

- Carbon monoxide. This has no color, odor, or taste.

- Airplane glue and formaldehyde

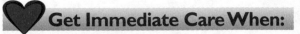 Get Immediate Care When:

- The person does not have a pulse and/ or is not breathing. Call 911! (See "CPR" on page 381.)

- The person is unconscious or having convulsions. Call 911!

- A substance has been swallowed, inhaled, or absorbed by the skin that:

  - Has a "Harmful or fatal if swallowed" warning on the label or a skull-and-crossbones sign

  - You suspect is poisonous

  {**Note:** Before getting immediate care, call the Poison Control Center at 1-800-POISON1 (764-7661).}

- After being in a closed space with a heater or furnace on, are signs of carbon monoxide poisoning present? Call 911!

  - Unconsciousness

  - Lethargy, confusion, or agitation

  - Sudden shortness of breath

  - Severe headache

  - Seizure

  - Signs of shock (see page 414)

  - Chest pain or irregular heartbeat

*Poisoning, Continued*

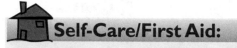
### Self-Care/First Aid:

Follow measures in the "Prevention" section of this topic. In addition:

**For Swallowed Poisons:**

- If the victim is unconscious, shout for help. Call 911! Do "CPR" as needed.
- Once conscious, place the victim in recovery position (see page 387).
- Call the Poison Control Center. Follow instructions. Do this step first if the first 2 steps do not apply.

If and when you need to call the Poison Control Center, your doctor, or local hospital, be ready to give this information:

- The name of the substance taken
- The amount taken
- When it was taken
- A list of ingredients on the product label
- Age, gender, and weight of the person who took the poison; how the person is feeling and reacting; and any medical problems the person has

- Lay the victim on his left side to keep the windpipe clear, especially if the victim has vomited.
- Keep a sample of the vomit and the poison container.

**For Inhaled Poisons:**

- Move the victim to fresh air (outdoors if possible) right away. Try not to breathe the fumes yourself.
- Follow the first 3 steps above for "Swallowed Poisons," as needed.
- Get medical attention.

**For Chemical Poisons on the Skin:**

- Flood the skin with water for 10 to 15 or more minutes and remove contaminated clothing.
- Gently wash the skin with soap and water. Rinse well.
- Get medical attention.

## 154. Shock

Shock occurs when the circulation system fails to send blood to all parts of the body. With shock, areas of the body are deprived of oxygen because blood flow or blood volume is too low to meet the body's needs. The result is damage to the limbs, lungs, heart, and brain.

*Shock, Continued*

## Signs & Symptoms

- Weakness, trembling
- Restlessness, confusion
- Pale or blue-colored lips, skin, and/or fingernails
- Cool and moist skin
- Weak, but fast pulse
- Rapid, shallow breathing
- Nausea, vomiting
- Enlarged pupils
- Extreme thirst
- Loss of consciousness

## Causes & Care

Causes include a heart attack; severe or sudden blood loss from an injury or serious illness; and large drop in body fluids, such as following a severe burn or severe vomiting and/or diarrhea.

Shock requires emergency medical care.

## Get Immediate Care When:

Signs and symptoms of shock (see above) occur. Call 911!

## Self-Care/First Aid:

**First Aid for Shock Until Emergency Care Arrives:**

- Check for breathing and a pulse.
- Lay victim flat, face-up, but do not move if you suspect a head, back, or neck injury.
- Do rescue breathing or CPR, as needed. (See "CPR" on page 381.)
- If victim vomits or has trouble breathing, raise to a half-sitting position (if no head, back, or neck injury).
- Raise victim's feet about 12 inches. Use a box, etc. Do not raise the feet or move the legs if hip or leg bones are broken. Keep the victim lying flat.
- Loosen tight clothing. Keep victim warm using a coat, etc. Place insulation between the person and the ground.
- Monitor for breathing and pulse every so often.
- Do not give any food or liquids. If the person wants water, moisten the lips.
- Reassure the person. Make him or her as comfortable as you can.
- If the person vomits, roll him or her on the side so the vomit does not back up into the windpipe and lungs.

22. Emergency Conditions

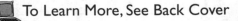 To Learn More, See Back Cover

# Index

# B

## I

Impotence 328–29; and peripheral vascular disease 206; physical causes 328; psychological causes 328–29

Impotence Center 329

Incisional hernia 170

Incontinence 183–86. *See also* Urinary incontinence.

Infections: with burns 117; with calluses or corns 120; cervix 352; with diabetes 280; with dry skin 124; ear 74, 79; with eczema 126; foot 247, 251; with ingrown nails 130; kidney 186; leg 255; lymph nodes 265; respiratory 94; signs of 284; sinus 86–87, 91, 94; skin 42, 43; throat 88–89; urinary tract 186–89; uterus 352; vagina 352

Inflammation, reducing 44

Influenza. *See* Flu.

Influenza vaccine 36

Informed consent 32

Ingrown toenails 129–30

Inguinal hernia 170, 171

Injured toe 251–52

Insect bites 107–10: to the eye 63

Insect in ear, treatment 77

Insect stings 130–32

Insomnia 297–99

Insurance 47–50: checklist 48; and doctors 25–26

Intercourse (*see also* Sexual activity): anal 180, 182, 295; painful 152, 345, 350, 355

Internal injury, signs of 351

Intestinal obstruction 160, 180, 189, 223

Ipecac, syrup of, uses 44

Iron sources 269

Irregular heartbeat 223

Irritable bowel syndrome (IBS) 156, 173–75

Itching: rectum 179–82; skin 43

IvyBlock 132

## J

Jaundice 152, 161, 290

Jock itch 330

Joints, inflammation 231–34

## K

Kaopectate 42

Kegel exercises 185

Ketoprofen 44

Kidney disease 44, 123, 197, 328

Kidneys 43, 186: dialysis 33

Kidney stones 175–77, 183, 188, 253

Knee joint replacement 263

K-Y Jelly 187

## L

Labyrinthitis 89, 189, 223

Lactaid 161

Lactose intolerance 151, 156, 160, 161

Laryngitis 83–84

Laxatives, uses/warnings 43

Leg and Ankle Pain Chart 254–57

Leg cramps 89, 257, 258, 259

Leg pain 254–59: chart of symptoms 254–57

# M

## S